P9-EEM-249

Realities
of
Contemporary
Nursing

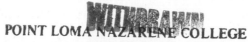
POINT LOMA NAZARENE COLLEGE
Ryan Library
3900 Lomaland Drive, San Diego, CA 92106-2899

610.73
H219r

Realities
of
Contemporary
Nursing

Second Edition

Persis Mary Hamilton, RN, MS, EdD

Associate Professor
College of Nursing and Health Sciences
University of Guam

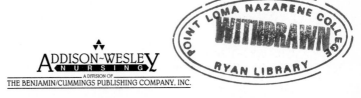

POINT LOMA NAZARENE COLLEGE
WITHDRAWN
RYAN LIBRARY

ADDISON-WESLEY
NURSING
A DIVISION OF
THE BENJAMIN/CUMMINGS PUBLISHING COMPANY, INC.

Menlo Park, California • Reading, Massachusetts • New York • Don Mills, Ontario
Wokingham, UK • Amsterdam • Bonn • Paris • Milan • Madrid
Sydney • Singapore • Tokyo • Seoul • Taipei • Mexico City • San Juan, Puerto Rico

Executive Editor: Patricia L. Cleary
Acquisitions Editor: Erin Mulligan
Managing Editor: Wendy Earl
Production Coordinator: Bradley Burch
Administrative Assistant: Dorothy Zinky
Text and Cover Designer: Brad Greene
Copy Editor: Antonio Padial
Proofreader: Kristin Barendsen
Indexer: Karen Hollister
Composition and Film Coordinator: Vivian McDougal
Compositor: Greene Design
Manufacturing Supervisor: Merry Free Osborn
Printer and Binder: R.R. Donnelley and Sons
Cover Printer: New England Book Company

The quilt pictured on the cover, "Kyoto," was designed by Miriam Nathan-Roberts. Photography credits may be found on page 451.

Copyright © 1996 by Addison-Wesley Publishing Company, Inc.

All rights reserved. No part of this publication may be reproduced, stored in a retrieval system, or transmitted, in any form or by any means, electronic, mechanical, photocopying, recording, or any other media or embodiments now known or hereafter to become known, without the prior written permission of the publisher. Manufactured in the United States of America. Published simultaneously in Canada.

Care has been taken to confirm the accuracy of the information in this book. The authors, editors, and publisher, however, cannot accept any responsibility for errors or omissions or for consequences from the application of the information in this book and make no warranty, express or implied, with respect to its contents.

Library of Congress Cataloging-in-Publication Data
Hamilton, Persis Mary.
    Realities of contemporary nursing / Persis Mary Hamilton. — 2nd ed.
      p.   cm.
    Includes bibliographical references and index.
    ISBN 0-8053-2020-2
    1. Nursing—Vocational guidance. 2. Nursing—Practice. I. Title.
    [DNLM: 1. Nursing. 2. Philosophy, Nursing. WY 16 H219r 1996]
  RT82.H35 1996
  610.73—dc20
  DNLM/DLC
  for Library of Congress   95-8827
                                               CIP
ISBN 0-8053-2020-2
 2 3 4 5 6 7 8 9 10—DOC—99 98 97 96

Addison-Wesley Nursing
A Division of The Benjamin/Cummings Publishing Company, Inc.
2725 Sand Hill Road
Menlo Park, California 94025

Dedicated to
the memory of my beloved sister
Patricia Alice Tangemann Dahlin

◇ Preface

The first edition of *Realities of Contemporary Nursing* was written to help new graduates cope with the "reality shock"* they so often experience when they first begin to practice nursing. The need for such a text has not ended, nor has the purpose of this text. However, since the first edition was published, nursing has undergone many changes. This new edition addresses those changes, and continues to meet the need for a realistic text about nursing for new members of the profession.

Philosophical Viewpoint

Realities of Contemporary Nursing is about *being* a professional nurse in contrast to *doing* clinical nursing. The text presents nursing as an authentic, emerging profession, encompassing all the characteristics of a true profession, with its own history, credentials, organizations, ethical codes, and educational system. While its essence is caring, nursing is based on science, and functions within legal constraints and theoretical frameworks. Nurses think critically, exhibit cultural competence, lead and manage others, use personal and professional power, and to an increasing extent, practice autonomously. The text encourages nurses to acknowledge and assume their professional identity.

This text begins with the history, education, credentials, organization, essential functions (thinking, being, caring), and place of nursing in the health-care system. It then explores nursing ethics, legal issues, change, power, politics, and managing nursing care. Finally, *Realities of Contemporary Nursing* addresses the needs of practicing nurses in relation to stress management, collective bargaining, and career management. The appendices include a list of members of the National Council of State Boards of Nursing and a directory of nursing and health-related organizations.

* Kramer M. *Reality Shock, Why Nurses Leave Nursing.* CV Mosby, 1974.

Features to Enhance Learning

Several features enhance the effectiveness of the book as a teaching-learning tool. Each chapter opens with a photograph that emphasizes the essence of the chapter. Then, a vignette of a real-life situation points to the practical value of the content. The writing style and reading level contribute to understanding. Unique terms are defined in vocabulary lists within the text. Numerous tables and figures illustrate concepts. Exercises and samples personalize the content, such as inventories and sample resumés. Chapter 1 includes a full color timeline to illustrate the progression of nursing through the ages. Each chapter provides learning objectives, a summary of the content, ciritcal thinking questions, learning activities, annotated readings, and a reference list.

The *Instructor's Manual* is available to instructors on adoption of the book. Chapters in the manual correspond to those of the text, and include a summary, learning objectives, lecture outline, critical thinking questions, learning activities, instructional aides, and a test-bank of multiple choice questions keyed to the learning objectives. The test key includes rationales for distractors.

Acknowledgments

Many people contributed to the success of this second edition, which was complicated by my move to Guam, about 7,000 miles from the editorial offices of Addison-Wesley Nursing. Therefore, I am particularly grateful for the contributions of the following people:

Patti Cleary, executive editor, for initiating this edition and providing leadership, counsel, wisdom, and sensitivity throughout the process.

Erin Mulligan, acquisitions editor, for quickly and skillfully assuming responsibility for the project in midstream.

Dorothy Zinky, administrative assistant, for serving as communicator, rapid-response specialist, coordinator par excellence, encourager, and good friend.

Wendy Earl, managing editor, and Bradley Burch, production coordinator, for their creativity and professionalism.

David F. Singletary, my husband, for his support, patience, acceptance, and computer wizardry.

Margaret Craig, contributor of Chapter 5, respected nurse educator, colleague, and fellow adventurer in the Western Pacific.

Roberta O'Grady, contributor of Chapter 6, Stanford University classmate, leader in maternal-child health and the public health community, and friend.

Faculty members and students at the College of Nursing and Health Sciences, University of Guam, for the enrichment they provide.

To many reviewers, for their expertise and thoughtful suggestions for change. I am deeply indebted to each of you.

Countless clients, students, colleagues, mentors, instructors, family members, and friends who have influenced my life. Those human experiences, melded with many years of learning and teaching, created the examples and conclusions of this text.

Persis Mary Hamilton

◇ Reviewers

Fay L. Bower, RN, MSN, DNSc, PhD, FAAN, Clarkson College

Jeanne Clement, RN, CS, MS, EdD, Ohio State University

Kathleen Hartnett, RN, MS, Queensborough Community College

Ann Hill, RN, MSEd, IVY Tech, Central Indiana

Marilyn Hopkins, MSN, DNSc, California State University, Sacramento

Barbara Hughes, RN, MSN, Temple University

Trish Hughes, RN, EdD, Pacific Lutheran University

Mary Kuhl, RN, MSN, PhD, Kaskaskia College

Virgil Parsons, RN, DNSc, San Jose State University

Nancy E. Rooker, RN, MS, Elgin Community College

Carolyn Schultz, RN, EdD, Pacific Lutheran University

Sharon Vincent, RN, MSN, Augusta College

Joy Wachs, RN, PhD, Eastern Tennessee State University

Loretta Wetmore, RN, MSEd, MSN, Broward Community College

Betty L. Whigham, RN, MEd, ARNP, Hillsborough Community College

Judith Wilkinson, RN, MSN, Johnson County Community College

Mary Woodside, RN, BSN, Consultant, Labor Relations,
    Sacramento, California

◈ Contents

Chapter 1   Nursing Throughout History 1

Chapter 2   Education of Nurses 31

Chapter 3   Credentialing: Licensure and Certification 63

Chapter 4   Nursing Organizations 89

Chapter 5   Critical Thinking, Cultural Competence, and Caring . . 117
             with Margaret M. Craig, RN, MSN
             Director of Nursing Program
             Greenfield Community College
             Greenfield, Massachusetts

Chapter 6   Health Care Systems 141
             with Roberta S. O'Grady, RN, MA, MPH, DrPH
             School of Public Health
             University of California, Berkeley, California

Chapter 7   Ethical Concerns 187

Chapter 8   Legal Issues 225

Chapter 9   Change, Power, and Politics 263

Chapter 10   Managing Nursing Care 293

Chapter 11   Effective Stress Management 337

Chapter 12   Collective Bargaining 367

Chapter 13   Career Management 395

Appendix A   Members of the National Council
             of State Boards of Nursing 441

Appendix B   Directory of Selected Nursing
             and Health-Related Organizations 445

Photography Credits 451

Index 453

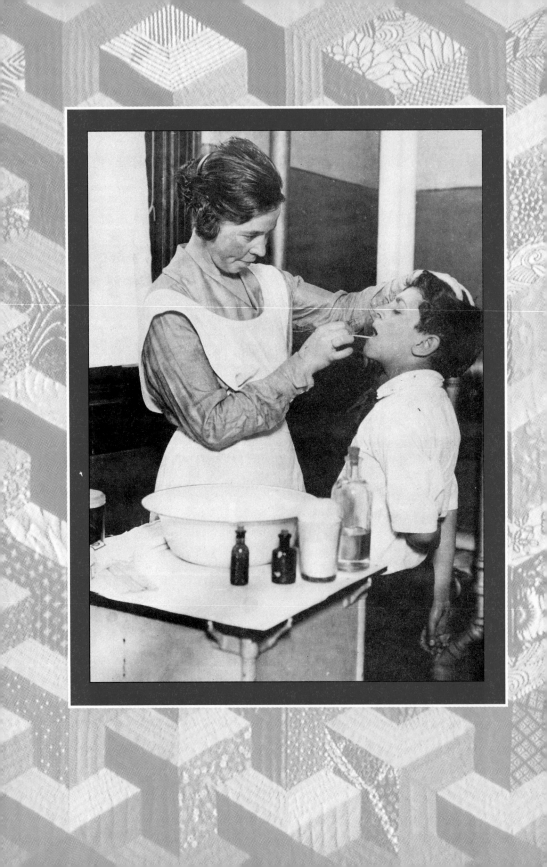

Nursing Throughout History

◆ Learning Objectives

- Explain how religion and culture, politics and war, and technology and medicine influenced nursing throughout history.

- Give a rationale for the emergence of feudalism, monasticism, and guilds in medieval Europe.

- Discuss the effects of the Renaissance and Reformation on health care today.

- Explain the meaning and origin of the term "dark ages of nursing."

- Identify some social reforms spurred by conditions of the Industrial Revolution.

- Explain the importance of Florence Nightingale to modern nursing.

- Describe the influences on nursing of the politics, technology, and medicine of colonial America.

- Describe some influences on nursing of the Civil War, World War I, World War II, the Korean War, and the Vietnam War.

- Discuss the criteria of a true profession as they relate to nursing.

- Identify some of the challenges nursing faces in the twenty-first century.

Anna bent to hear the whispered words of her client. "Thank you, thank you for listening." Anna reached for her client's hand. She could feel the tendons and vessels through the thin, smooth skin. Anna had just begun her first clinical course in nursing at the skilled nursing facility. Mrs. Selby was her only patient. Anna learned from the nursing history that Mrs. Selby had been a nurse for over 50 years. As she bathed her, Anna asked about her years of nursing. Mrs. Selby began slowly, but as she spoke, the pace quickened.

She had entered nursing school when nurses stood in the presence of physicians and marriage was grounds for dismissal. She had mixed and given penicillin when it was the only injectable antibiotic, boiled syringes, sharpened needles, and washed out intravenous tubing for reuse. She had cared for polio victims in iron lungs, wrapped agitated psychiatric patients in wet sheets, and applied Kenny packs to polio victims. She had consoled desperate women, septic from back-alley abortions, and youths dying from kidney failure before dialysis machines were invented. She had set up oxygen tents, given IPPB treatments, and marveled at the first cardiac monitors. She had met planeloads of military casualties from Korea and civilian refugees from Vietnam. During her long life she had seen the influence of technology, culture, and war upon nursing practice. Her pride and satisfaction were evident.

Mrs. Selby was tired now, but Anna continued to hold her hand. She looked deeply into Mrs. Selby's eyes as if to see for herself the things this remarkable woman had experienced and felt a bond she didn't want to break. Anna knew now why she was in nursing school. She wanted to learn more of the history and future of nursing, her chosen profession.

The history of nursing is rooted in the distant past. Even the word *nursing* comes from the language of ancient Rome. In Latin *nutrire* means to nourish, nurture, or suckle a child. Because the need for nurturance and care is as old as humankind, Donahue called nursing the oldest of arts and the youngest of professions (1985). Even though its essential function—to care for those who cannot care for themselves—has not changed, the practice of nursing has changed, influenced by religion and culture, politics and war, and technology and medicine. Understanding how those influences affected nursing gives direction and hope for the future.

◆ Nursing in Prehistoric Times

Although there are no written records of early societies, it is speculated that the culture of isolated tribes living today reveal something of prehistoric societies. In these tribes, women assume major responsibility for nourishing, nurturing, and caring for children and sick family members. Those who exhibit special healing skill often become healers or *shaman*. One function of the shaman is to exorcise the evil spirits believed to cause illness by using incantations, charms, massage, hypnosis, and herbal mixtures. Ancient healers sometimes drilled holes in the skull (trephining), perhaps to provide a means of escape for the evil spirits that caused disease (Haggard 1980).

◆ Nursing in Ancient Civilizations

Mesopotamia, the Cradle of Civilization

Ancient records indicate that by 5000 BC a complex civilization had developed in Mesopotamia, a portion of the region called the Fertile Crescent. Its culture blossomed in the warm climate and fertile soil of the valleys of the Tigris and Euphrates Rivers, and separate city-states grew up. By 2100 BC, these states united to become the Babylonian Empire (Roberts 1993). The Babylonians were students of astronomy, mathematics, and numerology. They developed horoscopes to predict the future, and gave numbers such as 3, 7, and 13 magical significance. They believed that displeasing the gods caused illness, and they used diet, rest, massage, purging, and vile-tasting formulas to banish those spirits. Their records describe midwifery and care of people with heart disorders, tuberculosis, jaundice, tumors, and the plague. Physicians and nurses were held accountable for their actions by the strict Code of Hammurabi, which prescribed severe penalties for malpractice, such as amputation of the hand of a surgeon who bungled an operation (Rhodes 1985).

Egypt

The Egyptian civilization was developed by people who settled along the Nile River before 4000 BC. Health care was an important part of the culture and religion. A record of these people, dating back to 1500 BC, describes over 250 diseases, many surgical and dental procedures, and more than 700 medicines. It tells of schools of medicine and midwifery and describes the first known physician, Imhotep, a surgeon, priest, and architect. Advanced concepts of sanitation and hygiene were practiced, and community planning helped maintain public health by protecting the water from pollution. Strict laws regulated diet, exercise, bodily cleanliness, and sexual relations. Dying persons were isolated in "houses of death." Because of beliefs about life after death, embalming became a highly developed skill. Slavery was accepted, providing the nation with a labor force. Women enjoyed freedom and dignity, managed the household, and nursed the young and the sick (Roberts 1993).

Israel and Judaism

The Hebrew people descended from Abraham (Israel), a shepherd from Ur of Chaldea. By the time of King Hammurabi, about 1950 BC, the Hebrews were well established in the Jordan River Valley. They built towns, raised sheep and cattle, and cultivated the land. The country flourished, and Jerusalem became a religious and political center. About 1700 BC, famine drove the people of Jerusalem (Jews) to Egypt. At first they prospered, then they were enslaved for 400 years. Under the leadership of Moses, an adopted son of the pharaoh, they escaped and returned to Palestine to reestablish the nation of Israel. Moses was educated in the learning of Egypt and was likely taught the history of his people by his mother (Exodus 2). He instituted a theocentric (god-centered) form of government and the Mosaic Code, which contained many Egyptian hygienic rules. In time, invading powers conquered, enslaved, and scattered the people.

Yet they maintained their Jewish identity, religion, and culture, suffering relentless persecution wherever they went. In 1948, they again established the nation of Israel in Palestine.

The ancient Hebrews wrote historical narratives and detailed codes of conduct found in the Old Testament and Talmud. These codes regulated every aspect of personal, family, and national life. They affirmed one omnipotent god who punished disobedience with sickness and death. Blood had symbolic cleansing power, and animal sacrifice was a regular priestly duty. Rules governed women during menstruation, pregnancy, and childbirth. The Hebrews required circumcision of male infants at eight days of age, isolation of people with communicable diseases, and care of widows, orphans, strangers, and the poor. Dietary laws forbade eating blood, scavengers, or diseased animals, and the Sabbath was set aside for rest (Deuteronomy 12). Women nursed the sick, cared for the young, and held a place of honor in the home.

India, Hinduism, and Buddhism

Until 3000 BC, when Aryan people migrated to India from the West, the Himalayan mountains isolated India from the rest of the world. The Aryans found a warm climate, rich vegetation, and a race of dark-skinned people. By 2500 BC, an advanced culture developed geometry, trigonometry, the decimal system, and a written script. From 1600 to 500 BC, the Vedic language and the Brahman (Hindu) religion prevailed. It divided the people into four castes or social levels, affirmed *pantheism* (everything is a part of god), *nihilism* (nothingness is desirable), *transmigration*, and *reincarnation* (rebirth of the soul into human or animal forms). Believers worshiped ancestors, revered animals such as monkeys and cows, and forbade killing or eating them. Priests directed the worship of numerous deities, interpreting and enforcing a code of conduct. The code was written in the *Vedas*, sacred books that served as historical documents. These writings promoted hygienic practice, offered magical cures for disease and infertility, and revealed a team approach to health care and a high level of surgical and medical knowledge. Women cared for children and sick family members (Wells 1956).

About 530 BC, Siddhartha Gautama, a prince of the warrior class who had become an ascetic, announced himself Buddha, the Enlightened. He taught that perfection consists of attaining nothingness by means of severe penance. His philosophy rejected the caste system and made inner peace available to everyone (Roberts 1993).

China, Taoism, and Confucianism

About 3000 BC, Mongolian people from central Asia migrated to China, settling first in the lush Yellow River Valley, then in the Yangtze River Valley and beyond. Over time, three religions took root: Taoism, Confucianism, and Buddhism, each affecting health care.

Taoism, the oldest, was based on Tao, the Way, an intermingling of heaven and earth, a balance between yin and yang found everywhere. Disease and demons were combated by such means as noisy firecrackers and tea made of ashes of paper on which magic symbols had been written. Huang Ti, the Yellow Emperor, is credited with writing the great medical compendium, *Nei Ching* (Veith 1966). It tells how to promote health and prevent, assess, and treat disease. Assessment involved looking, listening, asking, and feeling, especially the pulse, the primary diagnostic gauge. Treatment included herbal medicine, nourishment, acupuncture, and moxibustion. *Acupuncture* is the insertion and twisting of needles along 12 meridians of the body. *Moxibustion* is the burning of mounds of plant fiber on the meridians until blisters form. Smallpox vaccination and medicinal herbs are described. Surgery was limited to repairing wounds and castrating males for court service. There is no record of hospitals, probably because the family took care of its own. Women were valued for their ability to produce sons and to manage and care for family members (Unschuld 1985).

About 500 BC, Confucius became prominent as a political reformer, basing his reforms on moral principles. He taught a negative version of the Golden Rule: What you do not wish done to you do not do to others; he viewed women as inferior to men. *Confucianism* stressed the value of knowledge and etiquette, family cohesion, and reverence for ancestors. His teachings failed to produce change and by 200 BC, *Buddhism* gained widespread acceptance (Wells 1956).

The Americas

It is likely that the American continents were settled before 10,000 BC by people from Central Asia who crossed the Bering Strait into North America. These people left traces of their cultures on both the Atlantic and Pacific coasts. Aztec, Mayan, Incan, and Toltec civilizations flourished, then died. They all believed that sickness was caused by displeasing the gods and that health was a result of balancing the body, nature, and the supernatural. Warriors wore protective charms and purified their bodies with sweats and mineral baths. Shamans and priests performed healing rituals. Aztec medicine, surgery, and midwifery was highly developed. The Aztecs treated illness with minerals and herbs, massage, bloodletting, trephining, suturing wounds, extracting teeth, and amputating limbs. Women were respected, assisted with childbirth, and nursed the sick and elderly (Wells 1956). Sand painting, a unique therapy, developed in what is now the southwestern United States. To effect cures, the shaman created intricate designs of colored sand (Smith 1991).

Greece and Greek Polytheism

In about 1400 BC, Aryan tribes from Northern Europe invaded and conquered the city-states they found on the Aegean peninsula. There they built a civilization that was to influence human affairs for centuries. A common language, religion, and literature, along with the quadrennial Olympic Games, united the people. The Greeks told mythical tales of gods with human attributes. Apollo was the god of health and medicine. Asklepios, son of Apollo and a human mother, was the chief healer. He was pictured holding the wand of Mercury, a wayfarer's staff entwined by sacred serpents of wisdom, the original caduceus. Nurses cared for the sick and injured in *iatrion* (clinics for ambulatory patients) and *xenodochia* (shelters for strangers). Slavery was an accepted social institution (Roberts 1993).

In time, a branch of priests became itinerant physicians. Their records were compiled into a medical text, credited to a priest named *Hippocrates* (450–377 BC), the "father of medicine." The text taught that disease was not the work of spirits, demons, or deities but the result of natural laws. It named four humors of the body: blood, phlegm, yellow bile, and black bile and attributed health to balance between them and illness to an excess or deficiency of humors. Case histories described signs, symptoms, and environmental influences on health. The *Hippocratic method* came to mean intellectual honesty, careful observation, study of the patient rather than the disease, assisting nature to effect a cure, and ethical practice as defined by the *Hippocratic oath*. Other literature described nursing procedures, such as poultice application, bathing, diet therapy, and comfort measures. Because women were not admitted to the "mysteries" of an art, men probably provided nursing care outside the home. The unique culture of the Greeks lead to the "birth of reason" and produced Socrates, Plato, and Aristotle, men who sought truth by observation and reason rather than by intuition and revelation (Wells 1956).

Italy and Roman Polytheism

Ancient Italy was settled by people from surrounding lands. The city of Rome was founded about 753 BC. In time, its army became a dominant force, conquering and absorbing other city-states. By 290 BC, Rome was the chief city of central Italy. By 31 BC, under a succession of aggressive leaders, Rome had become an empire that included most of the lands around the Mediterranean Sea. Yet, by 476 AD, the empire had crumbled, as waves of Huns, Goths, and Vandals plundered it (Roberts 1993).

The brutal culture of the Roman Empire condoned slavery, crucifixion, gladiator contests, human sacrifice, and authorized immense differences between citizen and noncitizen, bond and free. Caesars ruled the empire, appointing governors and armies to occupy conquered lands. Their religion named a god or goddess for almost every physiologic function or disease, such as Scabies to cure scabies and Febris to reduce fevers. Other gods included Jupiter, Juno, Janus, Mars, and the Greek gods Hygeia and Asklepios. Pleasing the gods brought health and prosperity. Displeasing them brought sickness and death (Wells 1956).

The Romans adopted the achievements of those they conquered. From Greece they took art, money, textiles, sailing ships, and religion and adapted the Greek alphabet to the Latin language. They sent enslaved Greek physicians throughout the empire to care for their soldiers. Using the Hippocratic method of observation, Aretaeus described diphtheria, pneumonia, emphysema, epilepsy, tetanus, and diabetes. Pedanius wrote *De Materia Medica*, a compendium of over 600 preparations of medicinal herbs. Celsus described the four cardinal signs of infection: heat, pain, redness, and swelling. Pliny reported on occupational diseases such as mercury poisoning and asbestosis. Galen, a Greek assigned to care for gladiators and athletes, described numerous surgical procedures, including tracheostomies and caesarean births. Women nursed sick family members, served as midwives, and enjoyed more freedom and power than in other cultures of the day (Rhodes 1985).

Roman culture was known for its laws, monetary system, and military strategy, but its greatest attainments were in engineering, many of which affected public health. The Romans drained marshes and built aqueducts, good roads, central heating systems, and cemeteries (Wells 1956). Roman interest in military power led to improved medical care for soldiers, first aid on the battlefield, ambulance services, *nosocomi* (trained orderlies) to provide nursing care, and *valetudinaria* (military hospitals) to house the sick and wounded (Donahue 1985).

Christianity

At the height of Roman imperial power, Jesus of Nazareth was born in Palestine. The religion he began was destined to influence nursing for centuries to come. When he was about 30 years old, Jesus gathered 12 disciples and began to proclaim the fatherhood of God and a kingdom of heaven available to all by a life of inner purity and service to others. He taught in parables and gave a positive version of the Golden Rule: Whatsoever ye would that men do to you, do ye even so to them (Matthew 7:12). Many believed he performed miracles and healed the sick. When the crowds hailed him "the Messiah," both Jewish and Roman officials decided Jesus had become too dangerous. They arrested, tried, and crucified him. His disciples reported his resurrection and began preaching his message throughout the Roman Empire.

People of many walks of life became converts: physicians like Luke, leaders like Paul, and notable women like Phoebe. In 312 AD, Emperor Constantine espoused Christianity and established himself as absolute ruler. "By 400 AD, it was probably as dangerous *not to be* a Christian as it had been *to be* one in 100 AD" (Donahue 1985 p. 93). At first, Christianity was a simple faith, but with time its doctrine, rituals, and organization proliferated. As the Roman empire waned, the power of the church increased, and a rigid male hierarchy took control. The bishop of Rome, the Pope, became the supreme ruler of the Holy Roman Empire. In 330, Emperor Constantine split from Rome, moved to Istanbul, and established the Eastern branch of the church (Wells 1956).

As Christianity spread, many women of wealth and learning heeded its teachings to care for the poor and sick. Marcella made her home into a convent for women. In 385 Paula assisted Jerome with a Latin translation of early church writings known as the *Vulgate*, and in 390 Fabiola founded the first Christian hospital of Rome in her villa (Donahue 1985).

Islam

In 570 AD, the founder of Islam was born in Mecca, the commercial and religious center of Arabia. Muhammad, an uneducated shepherd, joined the service of a rich widow, married her, and gained community status. Mecca was the site of the black stone of Kaaba, chief god of Arabia, to which Arabs made annual pilgrimages. Muhammad rejected Kaaba and taught there was but one true god, Allah. He declared that physical and spiritual death awaits unbelievers, there is one brotherhood of men with direct access to god without priests, women have identity only as adjuncts of men, and alcohol and pork are forbidden. These and other doctrines are found in the sacred book of Muslims, the Koran, dictated by Muhammad to his disciples (Roberts 1993). After Muhammad's death in 632, a power struggle among his followers led to schism and the formation of the Shiite and Sunite branches. In spite of this schism, the faithful set out to spread their religion. Armed with the "sword of Islam," they conquered Turkey, Persia, Arabia, Egypt, Palestine, North Africa, and Spain, creating the Byzantine Empire (Wells 1956).

Nestorians in Arabia

Nestorians were an early group of Christians who founded hospitals and medical schools in Greece. By a twist of fate they influenced health care for many centuries. When the Roman Pope declared them heretics in 450, the Nestorians went to Persia, taking with them Greek and Roman literature. There they built medical schools where Greek, Indian, Chinese, and Arabian teachings were respected. In these schools Arabs, Christians, and Jews studied together. Although the study of anatomy was limited by Islamic rules, the schools excelled in clinical medicine, chemistry, drug therapy, and humane treatment of lepers and the mentally ill. Patients were separated by diagnosis and attended by male nurses, because Muslim law restricted women to the home. Avicenna authored the *Canon of Medicine*, a text used for the next 600 years. Rhazes, the "father of pediatrics," studied childhood communicable diseases. Thus, for more than 1000 years, Eastern medicine preserved ancient Greek medicine while Western medicine slowly decayed (Rhodes 1985).

◆ Nursing in Medieval Europe

The years between the fall of Rome in 476 and the fall of Constantinople in 1453 divide ancient and modern times. The interval between is called the *Middle Ages* or medieval period. The first 500 years is termed the *Dark Ages* because conditions were so chaotic. War, exorbitant taxation, abysmal poverty, ignorance, superstition, sickness, and misery prevailed. Communicable diseases ravaged the populace. At intervals, for 300 years, the bubonic plague (black death) swept across Europe. In the pandemic of 1348, one-third to one-half of the population died. To forestall the spread of the plague, maritime cities adopted a *quaranta*, a 40-day detention period for vessels entering their ports. Thus, isolation for a set period became known as *quarantine* (Wells 1956).

The Parabolani brothers of Rome were known for their nursing care of plague victims. The Augustinian sisters established the Hôtel Dieu in Lyons in 542, the Hôtel Dieu in Paris in 650, and the Santo Spirito Hospital in Rome in 717. A famous medical school was established in 848 at Salerno. In Northern Europe, two secular nursing orders, the Alexian Brothers and Bequines of Belgium, cared for the sick and the poor (Donahue 1985).

During the chaotic Middle Ages people had no personal safety. As a result, three social systems developed by which people exchanged autonomy for safety: feudalism, guilds, and monasticism (Wells 1956). *Feudalism* was based on a lord-vassal relationship. The lord owned the land and assumed responsibility for protecting his vassals (serfs) from harm. The serfs worked the land, paid fees to the lord, and fought in his militia. *Guilds* were unique social organizations that emerged about 750 in England and 1050 on the continent. At first they were voluntary associations of artisans formed to give mutual aid to families of guild members. Youths contracted to work for master craftsmen in exchange for bed and board and an opportunity to learn a trade. From 1350 to the rise of the factory system about 1700, guilds held a near-monopoly on all trades. They became the model for health care societies of modern Germany and the apprenticeship system of early nursing education. *Monasticism* reflected a widespread belief that salvation required self-denial and withdrawal from the world. Monastic orders for both men and women grew up around strong leaders. Members lived together in walled monasteries. Each order had its own rules of conduct and dress. Novitiates, new members, entered as probationers and, when proven, took the vows of the order. To signify humility and obedience, women shaved their heads and covered them with a veil. Each order developed a unique habit (uniform) and crucifix which hung from the rosary (prayer beads). The cap, uniform, and pin of early nursing schools were modifications of the veil, habit, and crucifix of these orders (Donahue 1985).

◆ Nursing During the Crusades

From 700 to 1000, the Holy Roman and Byzantine empires coexisted. In 1094, when the Turks mounted an especially threatening force against Greece, Emperor Comnenus of Constantinople appealed to Pope Urban II for help. The Pope seized the chance to engage Christians in a holy war against Islam to recapture the site of the holy sepulcher in Jerusalem from the "infidel Seljuk Turks." He organized the first crusade in 1097, during which knights looted and captured city after city until they reached Jerusalem, taking it in 1099. He ordered the second crusade to consolidate initial gains, but this provoked the Muslims to mount a counterattack, ending in 1187, with recapture of Jerusalem by the Muslims. The loss provoked a third, fourth, and fifth crusade. The sixth and final crusade ended in 1244, with Jerusalem, the battered prize, in Muslim hands. There it remained until 1918, when British and French forces captured the city and gave it to Muslim Jordan (Wells 1956).

Nursing orders such as the Knights Hospitallers of St. John cared for the sick and wounded along the crusade routes. A Maltese cross adorned their habits. Years later, the Nightingale School of Nursing adopted that cross as its symbol. The Knights continued for centuries, becoming so expert in disaster relief that they were consulted when the International Red Cross was formed in 1864 (Donahue 1985).

◆ Nursing During the Renaissance and Reformation

During the years between 1350 and 1600, two great social movements revolutionized Europe: the Renaissance and the Reformation. Scholars began to question traditional beliefs, and the scientific method became the basis of knowledge. The *Renaissance* began in Italy and spread to Western Europe. Copernicus, Descartes, Galileo, and Newton made revolutionary discoveries that lead to inventions such as the telescope, microscope, barometer, thermometer, and pendulum clock. Using the microscope, Leeuwenhoek described protozoa, bacteria, and human spermatozoa. Vesalius, a Flemish anatomist, published the first authoritative text of human anatomy. Pare, a French surgeon, used ligatures to tie off bleeding vessels. Harvey initiated experimental physiology by using animals to demonstrate the circulation of blood. Artists changed their focus from religion to living people. Leonardo da Vinci, Michelangelo, and Raphael depicted anatomically correct figures, as did the Dutch master, Rembrandt, whose "Lesson in Anatomy" became a classic (Donahue 1985).

The *Reformation* began as a result of theological debate and widespread abuses within the Roman Catholic church. The spread of ideas quickened because of two innovations: the manufacture of paper from China and printing with movable type from Korea. By the time the Church initiated reform, Martin Luther (1483–1546), a mendicant monk, led a rebellion. His followers, called Lutherans, and other Protestants declared independence from the Pope and asserted the right of nations to choose religious affiliation. The Western world was divided into Catholic and non-Catholic countries. Many Protestant groups arose: Lutheran, Presbyterian, Anabaptist, Anglican, Quaker, and Puritan. Though they all called themselves Christian, each interpreted scripture differently. The Thirty Years' War (1618–1648) ensued, and many groups migrated to the New World to practice their faith as they saw fit (Roberts 1993).

◆ The Dark Ages of Nursing

The Reformation had no direct effect on hospitals in Catholic countries, but in Protestant ones, the government closed or took control of hospitals operated by Catholic orders. In England in 1525, Henry VIII confiscated the property of some 600 charitable endowments. Monks and nuns of nursing orders were expelled, and no one was prepared to take their places (Donahue 1985). Administrators recruited women of the lowest social strata to fill nursing positions. The work was hard, the hours long, the pay poor, and corruption rampant. Thus, the period from 1550 to 1860 is called the *dark ages of nursing*. The age coincided with the rise of the factory system. In his 1844 novel, *Martin Chuzzlewit*, Charles Dickens describes the sad state of nursing through the persons of Sairey Gamp, a home nurse, and Betsy Prig, a hospital nurse:

> She was a fat old woman, this Mrs. Gamp, with a husky voice and a moist eye.... She wore a very rusty black gown, rather the worst for snuff, and a shawl and bonnet to correspond.... The face of Mrs. Gamp—the nose in particular—was somewhat red and swollen, and it was difficult to enjoy her society without becoming conscious of a smell of spirits.... Mrs. Prig was of the Gamp build, but not so fat; and her voice was deeper and more like a man's. She had also a beard.

◆ Nursing During the Industrial Revolution

During the period called the Industrial Revolution, poverty, famine, and plague devastated Europe. Life was cheap and ignorance widespread. Factories paid starvation wages for long days of dangerous work. Child labor, widespread disease and alcoholism, and squalor cried out for social reform. Many groups sought to minister to the sick and poor, including the Sisters of Charity of St. Vincent de Paul and the Brothers of St. John of God. The Sisters developed a nurse training program for women with a two-month probation, followed by a five-year apprenticeship, and in 1640 established the Hospital for Foundlings in Paris. Many others responded to the terrible social conditions. One of the best known was John Howard (1727–1789), an Englishman who spent his life and fortune exposing conditions in the prisons, hospitals, and asylums. His vivid portrayals shocked the public conscience and helped bring reform. Elizabeth Guerney Fry, a deeply religious Quaker, was especially concerned for women prisoners and their children. She established the Institute of Nursing Sisters, the first organized district nurses (Donahue 1985).

Kaiserswerth

Inspired by prison reforms in England and Holland, Pastor Theodor Fliedner and his wife Frederike established the Deaconess Institute at

Kaiserswerth, Germany, in 1836. Originally a refuge for released prisoners, it expanded to become a hospital and training school for deaconesses. The three-month program included pharmacology, home care, and hospital care. Graduate deaconesses earned no wages and took no vows but had lifetime care in an arrangement known as the *motherhouse system*. Kaiserswerth's reputation spread, and emissaries from abroad came to learn how to set up similar programs. One such motherhouse was founded in 1849 in Pennsylvania (Donahue 1985).

Florence Nightingale, the Founder of Modern Nursing

Florence Nightingale was born May 12, 1820, the second daughter of prominent English parents. She enjoyed wealth and social position and was probably better educated than most men of her day (Donahue 1985). At an early age, Nightingale expressed interest in becoming a nurse, but her parents disapproved, expecting her to marry and take her place in society. Instead, she began a systematic study of public health, hospitals, and nursing care. She traveled widely. In Rome, she met Sir Sidney Herbert and his wife, respected Britishers interested in hospital reform. In 1847, Nightingale took the three-month Kaiserswerth course of study, later calling it her "spiritual home." In 1853, she took additional training with the Sisters of Charity in Paris. On returning to London, she began working with the committee supervising the Establishment for Gentlewomen During Illness, a hospital for women. She became its superintendent and transformed its operation within one year (Dolan et al 1983).

Reports from the Crimean War of appalling conditions in field hospitals inspired public outrage and demand for change. In 1854, Sir Sidney Herbert, then Secretary of War, recruited Nightingale to go to Crimea and institute reform. With energetic commitment and 37 select nurses from various nursing orders, Nightingale accepted the challenge. Within six months, the death rate in one hospital of 3500 patients dropped from 42.7% to 2.2%. Obstacles of every kind created huge demands of time and energy. Nightingale contracted Crimean fever, nearly died, and remained a semi-invalid the rest of her life. In 1856, she returned to London, a national heroine. Public contributions created the Nightingale Fund, and Longfellow wrote "The Lady with a Lamp" in her honor.

In the years that followed, Nightingale was appointed to many commissions and wrote extensively on health, statistics, sanitation, hospitals, and nursing education. Her two best-known books are *Notes on Hospitals* (1858) and *Notes on Nursing: What It Is and What It Is Not* (1860). She insisted that nurses should spend their time caring for patients, instead of doing menial jobs, be educated, use their knowledge to improve patient care, have social standing, and continue to learn throughout life. She declared that nursing schools should be run by nurses, independent of hospitals and physicians. Nightingale opposed state licensure for nurses, arguing that individual merit would be "leveled down." She insisted on cleanliness and order but never accepted the germ theory, believing to her death in the spontaneity of disease (Dock & Stewart 1938, Dolan et al 1983, Donahue 1985).

In 1860, the Nightingale Training School for Nurses opened as an independent educational institution financed by the Nightingale Fund. It was strongly opposed by physicians who wrote, "nurses are in much the same position as housemaids and require little teaching beyond that of poultice-making." Nonetheless, the school prospered, serving as a model for nursing education, with graduates in demand around the world. This remarkable woman died in 1910, having raised the status of nursing from degradation to honor (Donahue 1985).

International Red Cross

The International Red Cross was established in 1864, through the efforts of J. Henri Durant, a Swiss banker. He credited Nightingale's work in Crimea as the inspiration for his idea of a humanitarian agency to provide care for war casualties, regardless of their allegiance. Twelve nations signed the original Treaty of Geneva, agreeing to honor Red Cross nurses as noncombatants, respect their hospitals, and permit humanitarian services for either side in a war. The treaty recognized a common flag, a red cross on a white background. Muslim nations use a red crescent; Israel, a red star. In 1882, at the urging of Clara Barton, the United States ratified the treaty (Dock & Stewart 1938).

◆ Nursing in Colonial America

Exploration and colonization of the New World came in the wake of the Renaissance and Reformation. Nations sought power, trade, and wealth in the New World. Colonists sought religious freedom and economic opportunity. Beginning in 1519, Spain founded colonies around the globe and established the first hospital in Mexico City in 1524. France established colonies in Nova Scotia, Canada, and New Orleans. Ursuline sisters opened the first training school for nurses in 1640, and in 1642 Jeanne Mance founded Hôtel Dieu of Montreal. A century later, the sisters in the Order of Grey Nuns became Canada's first district nurses.

Beginning in 1607, England laid claim to the Atlantic coast, exchanging colony charters for taxes. Slaves began arriving from Africa in 1619. In 1620, Pilgrims and Puritans settled the Massachusetts Bay Colony. The Dutch East India Company established New Amsterdam on Manhattan Island, English Catholics settled in Maryland, dissident members of the Massachusetts Colony founded Connecticut and Rhode Island, and William Penn founded a Quaker colony in Pennsylvania.

Although colonists came to America for similar reasons and endured common hardships, they remained isolated and antagonistic toward one another for over 150 years. Indian massacres, starvation, nutritional disorders, infectious diseases, and complications of pregnancy took a high toll. Nursing and medical care consisted of folk remedies. Quacks abounded. Any educated man could declare himself a physician. Prior to the American revolution, there were but five hospitals. In truth, they were almshouses with infirmaries for the homeless and poor, where residents nursed each other. One of these was Bellevue on Manhattan Island, founded in 1658 by the Dutch East India Company to care for sick sailors and African slaves arriving on company ships. Donahue (1985) describes Bellevue as a "house of horrors" with a death rate of more than 50%. Care did not improve until 1884, when the city hired Alice Fisher, a Nightingale nurse from England to initiate reform (Robinson 1946).

In the United States the first hospital dedicated solely to the treatment of the sick was Pennsylvania Hospital, founded in 1751 at the urging of Benjamin Franklin. There, patients were segregated according to diagnosis, and insanity was considered an illness rather than a moral defect. In that day the insane often were shackled in filthy dungeonlike rooms. For a fee the public could visit, stare, and laugh. In *Inquiries and Observations upon Disease of the Mind*, published in 1812, Dr. Benjamin Rush advocated the humane treatment of mentally ill persons, but reform was slow to come.

In 1786 the Quakers founded the Philadelphia Dispensary to provide outpatient care for the poor, offering free obstetric, medical, and surgical services. In 1791 New York Hospital opened. It gained notice because its attendants received lectures on anatomy, physiology, maternity nursing, and child care. During the 1800s many religious nursing orders came to America, including the Irish Sisters of Mercy, the Episcopal Sisterhood of the Holy Communion, the Lutheran deaconesses from Kaiserswerth, and the Sisters of Charity, begun by Mother Seton in Emmitsburg, Maryland (Dock & Stewart 1938).

◇ Nursing During the Revolutionary War

In 1776, the colonies declared independence from England. Their hastily mobilized army had no medical or nurse corps. Volunteers nursed the wounded in private homes and public buildings. Smallpox, dysentery, and scarlet fever ravaged the camps. Food was scarce, clothing was meager, ether was unknown, and amputation was the most common surgery. In spite of all these obstacles, the beleaguered army prevailed, and the United States became a separate nation.

The practice of medicine in colonial America differed little from its practice in medieval times. As the discoveries of Pasteur, Lister, Koch, and others became known across the Atlantic, treatment and hygienic practice began to change. Tincture of opium, coca, ipecac, and digitalis were introduced. In 1796 Jenner demonstrated that cowpox was the source of a safe and effective smallpox vaccine. Although some physicians were schooled in Europe, most were self-taught or learned as apprentices from established physicians. In 1800, there were only four medical schools in the United States. Then, for-profit schools began to appear, many granting degrees in but one year of lecture-only study. Soon there were more than 400 such schools. Formation of the American Medical Association (AMA) in 1847 led to reform. The Flexner Report of 1910 gave a damning indictment of medical education, grading each school. In time, the worst schools closed for lack of foundation grants.

During this period, men took control of medicine, excluding even midwives from practice. A Boston physician gloated, "one of the first and happiest fruits of improved medical education in America [is] that females are excluded from practice" (Robinson 1946). A notable exception was Elizabeth Blackwell (1821–1910), the first woman physician in the United States. After she was denied admission to 29 medical schools, Geneva College in New York accepted her "as a lark." Although ridiculed, she graduated first in her class, only to find that no hospital would admit her patients. In 1857, she founded New York Infirmary, a 40-bed hospital staffed solely by women. It later became the first medical school for women in the United States (Sigerist 1934).

◆ Nursing During the War Between the North and South

As the United States grew, adding territories that became states, a profound difference developed between the South, with a landed gentry supported by slave labor, and the North, with a citizenry of free individuals. When the South seized federal forts in 1861 and seceded from the Union, the Civil War began. Neither side had field hospitals, a medical corps, a nurse corps, or ambulance service. Although ether and chloroform were introduced as general anesthetics in the 1840s, they were scarce on the battlefield. The need for nurses was critical. Sisters of various religious orders worked beside hundreds of volunteers. Catholic Sisters of Mercy staffed the Red Rover, the first hospital ship. Dorothea Dix, a schoolteacher, became superintendent of the first army nurse corps. Mother Mary Ann Bickerdyke challenged corrupt medical officers, and Jan Stuart Woolsey and her sisters worked for standards of selection and training of army nurses. Harriet Tubman and Susie Taylor, African-American nurses, served the Union army with distinction. In the end, more than 618,000 men died from injury or disease (Donahue 1985). Although the Union was preserved and slavery abolished, the South was ravaged, and legal segregation of the races continued for another century.

◆ Nursing During the Nineteenth Century

Between 1800 and 1900, 30 million immigrants arrived in America from all parts of the world. The population of coastal cities exploded,

Job Description of Hospital Staff Nurses in 1887*

In addition to caring for your 50 patients, each nurse will follow these regulations:

1. Daily sweep and mop the floors of your ward. Dust the patient's furniture and window sills.
2. Maintain an even temperature in your ward by bringing in a scuttle of coal for the day's business.
3. Light is important to observe the patient's condition. Therefore, each day fill kerosene lamps, clean chimneys, and trim wicks. Wash windows once a week.
4. The nurses' notes are important in aiding the physician's work. You may whittle nibs [pencil points] to your individual taste. Keep pencil handy.
5. Each nurse on duty will report every day at 7:00 AM and leave at 8:00 PM except on the Sabbath, on which day you will be off from 12:00 noon to 2:00 PM.
6. Graduate nurses in good standing with the director of nurses will be given an evening off each week for courting purposes, or two evenings a week if you go to church regularly.
7. Each nurse should lay aside from each payday a goodly sum of her earnings for her benefit during her declining years so she will not become a burden. For example, if you earn $30 a month, you should set aside $15.
8. Any nurse who smokes, uses liquor in any form, gets her hair done at a beauty shop, or frequents dance halls will give the director good reason to suspect her worth, intentions, and integrity.
9. The nurse who performs her labors and serves her patients and doctors faithfully and without fault for a period of five years will be given an increases of five cents a day by the hospital and administrator, provided there are no outstanding hospital debts.

*Source: An advertisement in a Western newspaper, 1887.
Reproduced from Collins J: California Nurses Association Bulletin, Sept–Oct, 1962.

and the economy industrialized. A network of railroads spread from coast to coast, and multitudes migrated to the West in search of gold and land. A series of inventions significantly changed life, including a process to manufacture steel, refrigeration, linotype, electric light, the typewriter, telephone, phonograph, and automobile. Discovery of the alkaloid of morphine in 1815 led to research using quinine, strychnine, atropine, and codeine. Graduate nurses worked 72 to 90 hours a week, often living in dormitories controlled by hospitals. They had no job security or retirement plan other than their own savings. (See

the accompanying box.) In 1893 Lillian Wald began the famous Henry Street Settlement in New York and helped found the National Organization for Public Health Nursing. In 1888 and 1895 the first occupational health nurses, Betty Moulder and Ada Stewart, began their work. In 1898, while serving in Cuba during the Spanish-American War, Clara Maas became a yellow fever research subject. Her death, ten days after the bite of an infected mosquito, led to the identification of the cause of the disease (Donahue 1985).

◇ Nursing During the Twentieth Century

As the century began, World War I and a devastating influenza epidemic demoralized the world, but the creation of the League of Nations rekindled optimism. Against great opposition, the women's movement sought personal and political power for women. In 1916, Margaret Sanger was imprisoned for opening the first clinic in America offering information on birth control. In 1920 the 19th Amendment to the Constitution gave women the right to vote. In 1925, Mary Breckinridge founded the Frontier Nursing Service, providing the first organized midwifery service in the Appalachian Mountains of Kentucky. The depression and drought of the 1930s brought social and economic havoc to the nation, temporarily halting the women's movement. Thousands migrated to western states. Although nursing services were needed, jobs were scarce, wages were low, and nurses were unwilling to join the strident labor movement of the day. The government, under Franklin Roosevelt's New Deal, began many social programs, notably Social Security.

World War II and Its Aftermath

The 1930s saw changes that would culminate in war: antisemitism and nationalism in Germany and Italy, and expansionism in Japan. World War II changed every aspect of life, particularly nursing. In 1941 the United States entered the war, and in 1945 dropped the first atomic bombs. As in other wars, qualified nurses were in demand, and Congress created the US Cadet Nurse Corps. It consisted of a 30-month basic program paid for by the government and offered by existing schools of nursing. Participating schools had to meet National

League of Nursing Education standards and were required to admit all qualified students, regardless of race or religion. Graduates, when registered, were commissioned as military officers. As the war progressed, casualties mounted, but the prognosis of the wounded was vastly improved by penicillin and sulfonamide, prepackaged intravenous plasma and blood, physical therapy, and group psychotherapy. As in other wars, nurses distinguished themselves and gained stature in the public eye.

At war's end in 1945, the United Nations and the World Health Organization were formed. But peace did not come. Communist nations, led by the United Soviet Socialist Republic, and noncommunist ones, led by the United States, began a "cold war" that lasted until 1990. In 1949, Congress created the US Air Force Nurse Corps. In 1950, the Korean War brought renewed bloodshed. Nurse-physician teams initiated emergency care units called Mobile Army Surgical Hospitals (MASH). The success of these units confirmed the contribution nurses could make in demanding situations and led to the development of intensive care units and emergency medical treatment teams.

A soaring birth rate following World War II, the "baby boom," ended with the advent of the contraceptive "pill" in the late 1950s. A poliomyelitis epidemic paralyzed and killed thousands before vaccines developed by Salk in 1955 and Sabin in 1961 halted its spread. Because the disease paralyzes the muscles of respiration, the first respirators (iron lungs) were invented. Sister Kenny, an Australian nurse, antagonized physicians by introducing a system of hot wet packs to relieve the agonizing muscle spasms. Eventually the medical establishment endorsed her treatment, but nursing leaders frowned on her autonomous intervention and Sister Kenny remained a maverick to her death.

In 1956, Russia launched Sputnik, and, to catch up, the United States initiated an ambitious space exploration program, landing men on the moon in 1970. Huge federal expenditures spurred research, advancing technology in computers, food preservation, communication, and lightweight materials. All these technologies influenced nursing.

Vietnam, Civil Rights, and Feminism

During the 1960s, US involvement in the Vietnam War and a civil rights movement tore the nation apart. Assassins killed President John Kennedy, civil rights leader Martin Luther King, and presidential candidate Robert Kennedy. Countless youths dropped out of work and school and "tuned in" to street drugs. In 1973, the troops left Vietnam, but thousands suffered post-traumatic stress disorder, drug addiction, and damage from substance abuse.

During this same period, hospitals installed intensive care units and recovery rooms. Nurses learned to start intravenous infusions, monitor electrocardiograms, and use complex equipment. Disposable supplies replaced reusable ones, hospitals bought sophisticated diagnostic and therapeutic machines, and health costs soared. Research brought advances in genetics, organ transplantation, pharmacology, and immunology. It also created ethical dilemmas never before encountered.

A growing workforce of educated women, awakened by the publication in 1963 of *The Feminine Mystique* by Betty Friedan, led to a revival of feminism. In 1964, Congress passed Title VII of the Civil Rights Act prohibiting discrimination in employment on the basis of sex, religion, race, and national origin. A 1964 report by President Kennedy's Commission on the Status of Women uncovered widespread disregard of the law. This led to formation of the National Organization for Women and an effort to pass an Equal Rights Amendment to the US Constitution. Although conservatives blocked its passage, the push for equal opportunity for women continued on many fronts.

Nurses gained positions of power in the health care industry and greater autonomy in their practice. In 1973, the American Nurses Association initiated the certification program in specialty practice. Master's programs in clinical specialties opened in major universities, as did doctoral degrees in nursing. By 1990, certified nurse practitioners and clinical nurse specialists worked individually and in joint practice with physicians. Economic pressure to reform the health care system promised to increase the stature and opportunity for nurses in advanced practice roles.

◆ Nursing in the Twenty-First Century

As nursing moves into the twenty-first century, it faces enormous challenges. An ongoing epidemic of blood-borne disease, civil war in many lands, substance abuse, homelessness, violence, and poverty threaten public health and personal safety. Immigrants with diverse cultures swell the population. Health care is inadequate or unavailable to many. These challenges present opportunities for nursing as never before. While holding on to its commitment to care, nursing can meet these challenges by applying the intellectual energy, technical skill, organizational ability, cultural competence, and ethical standards that typify the profession.

◆ The Mark of a Profession

With the challenge of the twenty-first century before us, nurses may wonder if nursing has at last achieved the status of a true profession. Margretta Styles suggests that "professionalism is something that comes from within the individual, a self-image which nurses have of themselves, a way of life, a commitment to the ideals of the profession" (1982). Ever since Abraham Flexner compared social work to law, medicine, and theology, scholars have debated the issue of professional status. A profession, he said, is: (1) basically intellectual, carrying with it great responsibility; (2) learned in nature, because it is based on a body of knowledge; (3) practical, rather than theoretical; (4) internally well-organized; (5) motivated by altruism; and (6) teachable through educational discipline (Flexner 1915).

Since Flexner's time, many writers have proposed other criteria that characterize professions. Moloney (1992) compared 14 such lists and found 12 criteria they all included. Using Moloney's list, we can evaluate nursing to see if it is a profession:

1. *Knowledge-based.* Scientific research is the most reliable means of gaining knowledge. Nursing has developed a large body of knowledge through research. In addition, nursing uses knowledge from chemistry, mathematics, biology, and the behavioral, physical, and social sciences. Indeed, nursing is knowledge-based.

2. *Theory-based.* The development of nursing theory requires broad scholarship in the sciences, recognition of phenomena, creation of new connections, and the design and control of research studies. Nurse theorists continue to develop a body of theory on which nursing practice is based. Yes, nursing is theory-based.

3. *Altruistic.* Throughout history, unselfish caring has been the hallmark of nursing. In fact, if altruism were the sole criterion, nursing would have qualified as a profession from the beginning. Yet,

altruism is not enough. Modern nursing uses both "heart" and "head." It employs knowledge and theory, together with other-directed caring to assist clients and families adapt effectively to attain maximum wellness. Indeed, nursing is altruistic.

4. *Codes of ethics.* The International Council of Nurses and member organizations throughout the world each have codes of ethics. While the words may differ, the standards and principles these codes affirm are the same. Yes, nursing has a code of ethics.

5. *Autonomy.* Autonomy is the freedom to make decisions that are consistent with a scope of practice. Autonomy requires nurses to be responsible and accountable for their clinical decisions. Of all the criteria of a profession, autonomy has been most difficult for nursing to achieve. As Sister Kenny discovered, nurses have not always supported autonomy, perhaps because they had not yet defined their role. Today, however, the role of nursing is defined and independent nursing practice well-established. Indeed, nursing is becoming increasingly autonomous.

6. *Service.* The essence of nursing is service, caring for people who cannot care for themselves. Service does not mean martyrdom. It means assisting clients to attain maximum physical and emotional wellness. Yes, nursing is service.

7. *Competence.* Nurses value clinical competence because it is essential for safe practice. Because it is achieved and maintained through education and experience, nurses and their professional organizations support accreditation of nursing programs, licensure of individuals, and continuing education. Indeed, nursing values competence.

8. *Commitment.* Commitment means dedication to a calling rather than merely doing a job. Nursing, the art and science of human caring, demands wholehearted commitment. In return, it gives practitioners untold satisfaction and joy. Yes, nursing requires commitment.

9. *Professional association.* For more than a century, nurses in America have supported their own professional organizations (see Chapter 4). These organizations provide structure and leadership for nursing. Indeed, nursing has its own professional organizations.

10. *Prestige.* Prestige is the perception that someone has influence, success, and rank. Nursing has gained that status because its

members demonstrate leadership in health care, practice in autonomous roles, earn respectable salaries, maintain ethical standards, and exhibit caring behaviors. Indeed, nursing is a prestigious profession.

11. *Authority*. Nurse practice acts give nurses authority to practice nursing. Neither physicians nor physician's assistants are licensed to practice nursing. Only nurses have that authority. Because nurse practice acts differ from state to state, nurses must know what their license authorizes them to do. Diers (1989) put it well when she said, "Physicians are authorized to practice medicine, which is to diagnose, treat, prescribe, and operate on disease, not people. Everything else is nursing." Indeed, nursing has authority.

12. *Trustworthiness*. Trustworthiness means being accountable for one's acts. Nurses are legally and ethically responsible for their practice. As licensed professionals, nurses must meet standards of practice; failure to do so leads to charges of malpractice. As ethically responsible professionals, nurses faithfully fulfill their commitments to employers and clients. Yes, nurses are trustworthy.

Indeed, nursing meets all 12 criteria of a profession. It is a proud and extraordinarily satisfying profession with a rich history and a challenging future.

◇ Summary

Nursing is the art and science of caring for others. Throughout history it has been influenced by the religion and culture, politics and war, technology and medicine of each age. The influences of past centuries have left their mark on nursing. The impact of each of these factors in the twenty-first century are enormous. They remind us that although nursing is the oldest of arts, it is the youngest of professions, and meets all twelve criteria of a profession.

Critical Thinking Questions

1. Throughout history, women have nursed the sick and injured. Traditional wisdom explains this behavior as an extension of the mothering role. Using your insightful thinking (refer to the box "Questions That Stimulate Effective Thinking" in Chapter 5), consider other factors that might account for this behavior.

2. An assumption is an idea or concept we take for granted (for instance, people never questioned the assumption that the world was flat). Assumptions may be correct or incorrect. What assumptions did the Nightingale School of Nursing probably make in choosing the Maltese Cross as its symbol? That is, what things can you logically conclude that they were taking for granted?

3. The author argues that nursing is a true profession. Practice your rational thinking (refer to the box "Questions That Stimulate Effective Thinking" in Chapter 5) by tracing the main points of the author's argument. What evidence, if any, does the author give for the conflicting side of this argument?

Learning Activities

1. Select ten events of history you believe had the greatest influence on nursing. Were they from religion, culture, politics, war, medicine, or technology?

2. In a group discussion, compare the teachings of Jesus, Muhammad, and Gautama relative to care of the sick.

3. Visit three hospitals: military, secular, and affiliated with a religious group. Compare the philosophy, services, and staff morale of each.

4. Read *Martin Chuzzlewit* by Charles Dickens.

5. In a group, discuss the question, "If Florence Nightingale could visit a nursing school today, what would surprise, please, or displease her most?"

6. Peruse issues of the *American Journal of Nursing* published before 1920. Identify ten issues that concerned nursing in those years. Which are still concerns today?

7. Debate the proposition: "Nursing has achieved the status of a profession."

Annotated Reading List

Nightingale F. *Notes on Nursing: What It Is, and What It Is Not.* Lippincott, 1992.

In this valuable reprint, Florence Nightingale speaks on such subjects as ventilation, noise, light, cleanliness, and observations of the sick. She reminds us that "this knowledge is distinct from medical knowledge, which only a profession can have." In the first half of the book, twelve nurse-theorists and thinkers reflect on the person, message, and impact of Nightingale on modern nursing. Nurses cannot help but be enlightened and inspired as they read the words of this powerful woman.

Moloney MM. *Professionalization of Nursing: Current Issues and Trends,* 2nd ed. Lippincott, 1992.

The author addresses the degree to which nursing has become a profession. She offers various definitions of professions, describes nursing's progress toward professional status, and develops strategies for attaining the goals of full professional status. The author presents this still-debated issue in five parts: an introduction to professionalization of nursing, perspectives on professionalization of nursing, control of nursing education, control of nursing practice, and strategies to advance the professionalization process.

References

Dock LL, Stewart IM. *A Short History of Nursing,* 4th ed. Putnam's Sons, 1938.

Dolan JA, Fitzpatrick ML, Hermann H. *Nursing in Society: A Historical Perspective,* 15th ed. Saunders, 1983.

Donahue HP. *Nursing: The Oldest Art, an Illustrated History.* Mosby, 1985.

Flexner A. Is social work a profession? *School Society.* 1:26 1915.

Haggard HW. *Devils, Drugs, and Doctors: The Story of the Science of Healing from Medicine-Man to Doctor.* Lippincott, 1980.

Moloney MM. *Professionalization of Nursing, Current Issues and Trends.* Lippincott, 1992.

Nightingale F. *Notes on Hospitals*. Appleton & Co., 1860.

Nightingale F. *Notes on Nursing*. Appleton & Co., 1858.

Rhodes P. *An Outline History of Medicine*. Butterworth-Heinemann, 1985.

Robinson V. *White Caps: The Story of Nursing*. Lippincott, 1946.

Roberts JM. *History of the World*. Oxford University Press, 1993.

Rush B. *Medical Inquiries and Observations upon the Diseases of the Mind*. Kimber and Richardson, 1812.

Sigerist HE. *American Medicine*. Norton, 1934.

Smith JZ. Healing cults. In *The Encyclopedia Britannica*, 15th ed. 1991.

Styles M. *On Nursing: Towards a New Endowment*. Mosby, 1982.

Unschuld PU. *Medicine in China: A History of Ideas*. Norton, 1985.

Veith I. *Huang Ti Nei Ching Su Wen, The Yellow Emperor's Classic of Internal Medicine*, New Edition. University of California Press, Berkeley, 1966.

Wells HG. *The Outline of History*, 5th ed., vols 1 & 2. Doubleday, 1956.

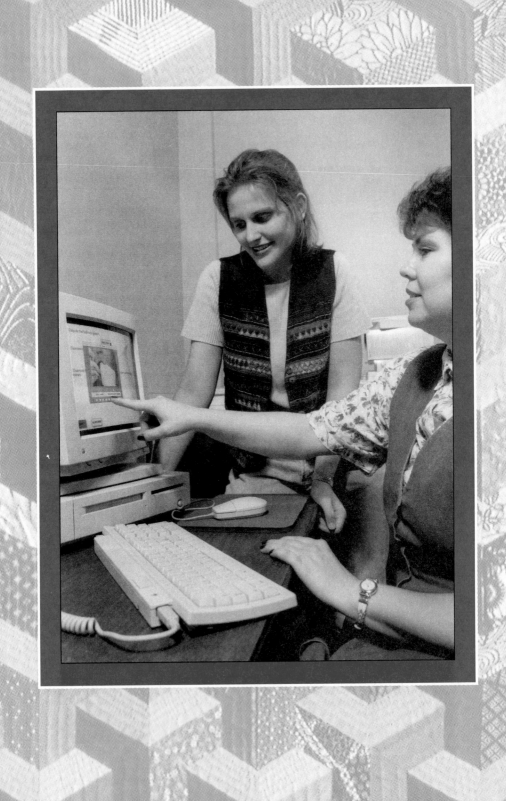

Education of Nurses

◆ Learning Objectives

- Compare the educational preparation and scope of practice of licensed practical nurses with that of certified nursing assistants.

- Compare the history, administration, and length of diploma, associate degree, and bachelor's degree nursing programs.

- Discuss articulation between practical nurse, associate degree, and bachelor's degree programs.

- Discuss factors that motivate ADN and diploma graduates to enroll in bachelor's degree programs.

- Discuss the value to nurses and hospitals of preceptorship and internship programs.

- Discuss grandfathering, interstate endorsement, scope of practice, titling, and competency expectations as they relate to the issue of entry into practice.

- Discuss mandatory versus voluntary continuing education requirements for licensure.

- Describe types of nursing literature and ways to select it.

- Discuss nursing research: its process, written report, ethical considerations, and evaluation of nursing research.

- Discuss three conceptual models of nursing practice, comparing their central themes, definitions of nursing, and concepts of the nursing process.

Eden's large family had gathered for the annual spring dinner at Gramma's home. Three generations were there, soon to be four. They had stuffed themselves on delicious foods and sat back to visit. Aunt Jona turned to Eden and said, "Won't you be graduating from nursing school pretty soon?"

Eden replied proudly, "I certainly will, in six weeks, two days, and about two hours! You'll all be invited to the ceremony." Eden's cousin, Tony, leaned forward and said, "I know someone who went to nursing school for only one year; why have you been going for so long?" Before Eden could reply, someone else said, "I thought nursing schools were in hospitals, how come you go to a community college?" Eden's pregnant cousin brightened, "I see a nurse practitioner at the prenatal clinic almost every visit. Is that what you're going to be when you graduate?" Eden explained that she was going to be a registered nurse, not a practical nurse. Registered nurses study for two or more years while practical nurses study for 12 to 18 months. She added, "I do go to hospitals for clinical experience, just my classes are at the college. No, I won't be a nurse practitioner, that takes much more education."

As Eden attempted to enlighten her family she realized how little she knew about nursing education. She was relieved when the conversation shifted to other topics. However, the questions people asked left her wondering. Why are there so many kinds of nurses? What are the differences between them?

◆

Unlike medicine that focuses on disease and injury, nursing focuses on human responses to health problems. Consequently, nursing provides a broad range of health care services, from the most basic to the most complex. To deliver these services, nursing needs a wide spectrum of caregivers. These caregivers include orderlies, nursing assistants, practical-vocational nurses, registered nurses, and advanced practice nurses. Historically, caregivers fell into two groups: practical nurses and trained (educated) nurses. The term *trained* reflected the early notion that nurses, like animals, respond to stimuli in fixed patterns. At first, practical nurses learned their skills in apprenticeships, with little or no formal instruction, while educated nurses learned in more structured programs. Although two divisions of nursing remain to this day, both have changed significantly.

◆ Practical Nursing

Certified Nursing Assistants

The first practical nurses in the United States worked in the homes of people in the community, giving nursing care to new mothers, babies, and sick family members. They were self-taught or learned from other caregivers. In time, hospitals hired them as nursing assistants and orderlies, but their knowledge and skills varied widely. To meet the need for better prepared workers, hospitals and schools began offering basic nursing classes. Nowadays, most states regulate nursing assistant programs. Typical state-accredited programs are 120 to 150 hours long and include instruction in basic nursing skills such as personal hygiene, bathing, and food preparation. They are offered by vocational schools and hospitals, and graduates receive certificates such as Certified Nursing Assistant (CNA) and Home Health Aide (HHA). The scope of practice for these caregivers consists of assisting clients with activities of daily living under the supervision of a licensed health care practitioner.

Licensed Practical Nurses

The first formal preparation for practical nurses in the US began in 1890 at the YWCA in Brooklyn, New York. It was known as the Ballard School after Miss Lucinda Ballard, who provided the operating funds. In the three-month course of study, students learned to care for invalids, the aged, and children in home settings. Other early practical nursing programs included the School of Practical Nursing in Brooklyn, New York, founded in 1893; the Thompson School for Practical Nurses in Brattleboro, Vermont, begun in 1907; and the Household Nursing Association in Boston, now called Shepard-Gill School of Practical Nursing (Johnston 1966). In 1908, the American Red Cross began teaching classes in home nursing. In 1918, the Surgeon General of the US Army asked the Red Cross to begin training nurse's aides for military hospitals. The number and reputation of practical nursing schools grew, and before long, civilian hospitals began to hire graduates.

In the mid-1930s the American Nurses Association (ANA) became concerned about the increasing number of "subsidiary" workers. As a result, representatives of the ANA, National League of Nursing Education, and National Organization for Public Health Nursing formed a Joint Committee to Outline Principles and Policies for the Control of Subsidiary Workers in the Care of the Sick. The committee recommended that "workers of this type should be subject to control under compulsory licensure to provide satisfactory control of their use." In 1938, New York enacted the first mandatory practical nurse practice act. By 1949, 28 states, Hawaii, and Puerto Rico had passed licensing laws. By 1959, all 50 US states and territories and Canada had licensed practical nurses (LPN) or licensed vocational nurses (LVN), as they are called in Texas and California (Johnston 1966).

In 1941, educators in various practical nursing schools founded the Association of Practical Nurse Schools. A year later they opened membership to individuals, and the name was changed to the National Association of Practical Nurse Education (NAPNE). NAPNE developed the first nationally endorsed curriculum for practical nurses. In 1949, practical nurse leaders organized the National Federation of Licensed Practical Nurses. The National League for Nursing (NLN) established a Council on Practical Nursing, and in 1966 the Chicago Public School Program became the first NLN-accredited practical nurse program in the US.

Today, practical nurse education varies from state to state and school to school. Programs are accredited by state licensing boards and offered in high schools, hospitals, adult education departments, trade-technical schools, community colleges, and universities. Programs last 12 to 18 months, and students gain clinical experience in structured settings such as hospitals and extended care facilities. The scope of practice of practical nurses consists of meeting the health needs of clients in stable condition in hospitals, homes, and long-term care facilities, under the supervision of a registered nurse or physician. Graduates of state-accredited programs take the National Council Licensure Examination for Practical Nurses (NCLEX-PN) and work under provisions of their state nurse practice act.

In recent years nurse educators have designed career ladders to help LPN-LVNs become RNs. These ladders seek to avoid duplication by giving credit for past experience. In some colleges, articulation (joining together) of practical-vocational and registered nurse education is built into the curriculum plan, with all nursing students taking a one-year basic nursing course. At the end of the year they can "stop out" and seek licensure as a LPN-LVN or continue, completing RN licensure requirements. In other schools, LPN-LVNs are credited with the first year of a nursing program. When they have completed prerequisite courses, they enroll in the second year of the nursing curriculum. In California, by regulation, "the additional education required of licensed vocational nurse applicants [to take NCLEX-RN] shall not exceed a maximum of 30 semester or 45 quarter units" (Board of Registered Nursing 1994).

◆ Registered Nurse Education

Early Schools of Nursing

The first European nursing schools began in hospitals of religious and secular orders. After completing study, student novices took vows and became full members of the order. Students of early hospital-based schools received diplomas when they graduated. When colleges and universities began to offer nursing education, students who completed the nursing curriculum received academic degrees. Thus, hospital-based nursing education became known as *diploma programs,* and college-based education became known as *degree programs.*

The United States was nearly 100 years old when the Civil War (1861–1865) created a dire need for prepared nurses. In 1869, a committee of the American Medical Association said "it is just as necessary to have well-instructed nurses as to have intelligent and skillful physicians" (Culpepper & Adams 1988). They recommended that county medical societies supervise nursing education. Nightingale would have agreed that nurses need quality instruction, but she would have insisted that nursing schools operate independently of both hospitals and physicians. In 1872, the New England Hospital for Women and Children (NEHWC) established the first nursing school in the United States. When Linda Richards graduated from the 12-month program, she became the first educated nurse in America. In 1873, hospitals such as Bellevue initiated programs designed after the Nightingale school, except that they were not autonomous. In 1874, Canada founded its first "Nightingale" school at General and Marine Hospital in St. Catherine's. Others schools began at Toronto General, Children's Hospital at Toronto, and Winnipeg General. In 1879, Mary Eliza Mahoney became the first "trained" African-American nurse when she completed the NEHWC program. In 1888, Mills School, a nursing school for men, was organized at Bellevue Hospital (Dolan 1983).

Because students provided nursing service at minimal cost to hospitals, there was a massive proliferation of schools. By 1909, there were 1105 hospital-based, two-year, and three-year diploma schools in the US and 70 in Canada. These schools ignored the Nightingale principle that student experience was for learning, not service. There was no school accreditation process and no standard curriculum. Hospitals developed programs to meet their service needs rather than the educational needs of students. Curricula differed widely from school to school. Often the hospital director of nurses served as the school superintendent and graduates served as instructors. Few were educated beyond basic nursing, yet they taught most of the courses, including the sciences. Sometimes the hospital dietitian taught nutrition, and medical staff members gave lectures about diseases. Typically, the curriculum was laid out in blocks of study paralleling medical specialties, with rotations through the diet kitchen and operating room. Courses in anatomy, physiology, nutrition, pharmacology, history of nursing, and professional adjustment rounded out the curriculum. If the host hospital could not provide a specialty such as psychiatry, the school might omit it from the curriculum, or the students might be sent to another hospital for the experience (Dock & Stewart 1938).

Students worked split shifts on hospital units during the early and late hours of the day, with classes in between. Most days were 12 to 15 hours long with one day off per week. Many students contracted tuberculosis and other communicable diseases, but they had no sick leave and had to make up all lost time before they could graduate. Juniors and seniors worked evening and night shifts but were expected to attend classes that met during the day. In those early schools most students were young single women who entered soon after completing high school. They lived in dormitories near hospitals under strict rules that controlled their lives. Marriage was grounds for dismissal.

By 1912, most programs were three calendar years long. For the first four to six months, students were on probation, and instructors evaluated the aptitude and ability of these probationers (probies). When students completed this period, they were "capped" and recited a nursing pledge at a symbolic ceremony resembling the taking of religious vows. After this ceremony students became freshmen. As they progressed through the program, they became juniors and finally seniors. Status was designated by uniform changes such as adding ribbons to the cap or wearing white instead of black stockings. On completion, graduates received a diploma and a school pin. Because hospitals were not degree-granting institutions, they could not award an academic degree or give academic credit. Most schools were segregated by race and sex.

Studies Bring Change

As the nation matured and scientific knowledge grew, nursing leaders recognized that nursing education needed to change. In 1912, M. Adelaide Nutting led a study for the American Society of Superintendents of Training Schools entitled *The Educational Status of Nursing*. Her study revealed appalling working and living conditions of students and poor teaching. The lack of well-educated nurses in World War I led to three studies of the National League of Nursing Education, conducted by Isabel M. Stewart. In 1917, the first study, *Standard Curriculum for Schools of Nursing*, contained an instructional plan and detailed course outlines. In 1927, the second study, *Curriculum for Schools of Nursing*, used job analysis to define the qualifications and functions of nurses. In 1937, the third study, *A Curriculum Guide for Schools of Nursing*, involved nurse educators across the nation in curriculum development (Stewart 1943). In 1923, the Winslow-Goldmark Report, *Nursing and Nursing Education in the United States*, concluded that public health nurses, supervisors, and instructors needed additional study beyond basic nursing. It recommended endowment for university schools of nursing (Committee for the Study of Nursing Education 1923). In 1923, under the leadership of Annie W. Goodrich, Yale University founded a School of Nursing, followed by Western Reserve University, Vanderbilt University, University of Toronto, and many others. In 1932, these schools established the Association of Collegiate Schools of Nursing to promote university-level nursing education and encourage research.

In 1925, the Committee on the Grading of Nursing Schools began an eight-year study of nursing education. In 1928, the committee concluded that the "need of a hospital for cheap labor should not be considered a legitimate argument for maintaining a...school. The decision...to conduct [a school of nursing] should be based solely upon the kinds and amounts of educational experience...[a] hospital is prepared to offer" (Stewart 1943). In 1934, in its final report, the committee suggested that a collegiate level of education should be instituted "dominated neither by hospital, nor treasury, nor nursing traditions" (Stewart 1943). In 1932, Dr. George Weir led a study of nursing education in Canada for the Canadian Nurses Association and Canadian Medical Association. His report urged higher standards and better qualified instructors (Gibbon & Mathewson 1947).

In 1948, Esther L. Brown studied society's need for nursing and published her findings in *Nursing for the Future*. She said the proper place for basic schools of nursing was in colleges and universities, not hospitals, and recommended that nursing recruit members of minority groups and men. That same year, in a study of nursing shortages, the Ginzberg Report recommended that nursing teams consist of four-year and two-year registered nurses and one-year practical nurses. In 1958, the American Nurses Association (ANA) and American Nurses Foundation published *Twenty Thousand Nurses Tell Their Story*. Part of a five-year sequence of studies of nursing functions, these studies formed the basis for the ANA nursing functions, standards, and qualifications (ANA 1958). In 1967 the ANA and National League for Nursing (NLN) set up the National Commission for Study of Nursing and Nursing Education to probe the supply and demand for nurses, their roles, functions, and education. Its final report, *An Abstract for Action*, called for greater government funding for nursing research and for state master-planning committees for nursing education (National Commission 1970).

In 1984, the National Commission of Nursing Implementation Project began its efforts to seek consensus about suitable education and credentialing for basic nursing practice, effective models for care, and ways to develop and test nursing knowledge. Their 1989 report described many innovative strategies. In 1991, the Department of Health and Human Services sponsored a study by the Secretary's Commission on the National Nursing Shortage to implement a 1989 report calling for increased financial support for nursing education.

Space in this chapter does not allow a description of the many other studies, but this sampling exemplifies their nature and importance.

Diploma Programs

Diploma programs of today differ greatly from the service-oriented programs of yesteryear. They meet NLN accreditation criteria and associate with colleges and universities. Because each school has unique historic roots, it is difficult to generalize, but diploma programs typically

- are administered, controlled, and housed in or near a sponsoring hospital

- charge tuition

- offer courses in nursing, arts, and sciences, some of which may be taken in a nearby college

- take three academic or calendar years to complete

- meet accreditation standards of state licensing boards and usually are NLN accredited

- employ faculty with bachelor's and master's degrees in nursing who meet state licensing board qualifications and often have dual assignments in both the school and the hospital

- use the sponsoring hospital, affiliated hospitals, and community agencies for clinical experience

- use nationally published nursing textbooks

- have a clearly stated philosophy, conceptual framework, learning objectives, and evaluation criteria

- accord students the rights and responsibilities identified by the school of nursing

- prepare graduates to manage, teach, and provide direct care for individuals, families, and groups in structured settings, using the nursing process

- prepare graduates to take the National Council Licensure Examination for Registered Nurses (NCLEX-RN)

- on completion of the program, award a diploma

Diploma education provides a unique learning experience. Because of the hours spent in direct client care, students become skilled in basic nursing functions. They learn to work within the bureaucratic structure of a hospital and to function in the role of a staff nurse in a process called *professional socialization*. As a result, graduates of diploma schools make the transition from student to practicing nurse with relative ease, rapidly becoming productive members of the health care team. The list of competencies of diploma graduates, compiled by the National League for Nursing Council of Diploma Programs, is available from the National League for Nursing, 350 Hudson Street, New York, NY 10014.

Associate Degree in Nursing Programs

The Associate Degree Nursing (ADN) program is a relative newcomer to nursing education and is the first educational program established on the basis of research. In 1951 Mildred L. Montag suggested the ADN in her doctoral dissertation as a solution to the shortage of nurses after World War II. In her proposal, ADN programs were to be theory-based, situated in community colleges, two years in length, and designed to prepare graduates to take the licensing examination for registered nurses. Employing hospitals were to provide supervision while the new graduates refined their clinical skills. Such supervision, similar to that provided in diploma schools, was to be given by experienced nurses.

In 1952, a pilot project called the Cooperative Research Project in Junior and Community College Education for Nursing was begun by Teachers College, Columbia University. The five-year project included seven colleges and one hospital school located in six regions of the US. The results of the project showed that programs could be established in community colleges, use clinical facilities in the community, attract quality students, and be cost effective. Graduates met learning objectives and passed the registered nurse licensing examination.

ADN programs have been so successful that today most of the RNs in the US are ADN graduates. Students are attracted to this type of education because of its short duration, relatively low cost, location near their homes, and accredited status (Williams 1989). Although most ADN programs are in community colleges, some are in four-year institutions that also offer a bachelor of science in nursing (BSN) degree. The University of the State of New York offers an ADN through the Regents External Degree Program. It is described later in this chapter.

ADN students differ from the young, single white women who once typified nursing students. The average age of ADN students is 30 years; most work part or full time; half have children; many are single parents and have other interests, abilities, and degrees; and more are men and racial minorities than in other programs (Williams 1989). Many ADN programs grant credit to LPN-LVNs for first-year nursing courses, permitting them to enter as second-year students if they have met science and general education prerequisites. Curricula are built on high school chemistry, mathematics, and English. Typically, ADN programs

- are administered, controlled, and situated in departments of colleges and universities

- charge tuition (less in public colleges, more in private ones)

- include academic courses in nursing, arts, and sciences

- take two or more academic years to complete within the lower division

- meet accreditation standards of the state licensing boards and regional higher education accrediting agencies, and may or may not be NLN-accredited

- employ faculty with master's and doctoral degrees who meet both college and licensing board qualifications

- use community hospitals and agencies for clinical experience

- use nationally published nursing textbooks

- have a philosophy, conceptual framework, learning objectives, and evaluation criteria

- accord students the same rights and responsibilities as other college students

- prepare graduates to manage, teach, and provide direct care for individuals, families, and groups in structured settings, using the nursing process

- prepare graduates to take the NCLEX-RN

- fulfill college requirements for an associate degree

The list of competencies of ADN graduates, complied by the NLN Council of Associate Degree Programs, is available from the National League for Nursing, 350 Hudson Street, New York, NY 10014.

Bachelor of Science Degree in Nursing Programs

Near the end of the nineteenth century, the increasing complexity of nursing led to preparatory courses of theoretical instruction. One of the earliest was taught at St. Mungo's College in Glasgow, Scotland in 1883. In 1887 the University of Texas assumed responsibility for the John Sealy Hospital in Galveston and its nursing school. Although the superintendent occupied a place on the university committee, students were not enrolled in the university. In 1901, a true prenursing course was developed by M. Adelaide Nutting at Johns Hopkins School of Nursing in Baltimore, Maryland. This six-month course offered basic sciences and nursing principles with related clinical practice. Within ten years, 86 schools of nursing in the United States and Canada required similar preparatory courses.

Between 1907 and 1910, many university hospitals took over schools of nursing or established their own. Frequently the universities placed these schools under the auspices of medical schools. Nursing students were admitted and registered as regular students, but the school was not an independent unit within the university, and some did not offer college degrees. By 1917, several universities granted graduates of nursing programs nonnursing degrees. By 1919, eight universities offered BSN degrees. These consisted of two academic years of liberal studies followed by a typical three-year diploma program. In 1923, Yale University School of Nursing became the first independent school of nursing within a university. Considering that women did not have the right to vote until 1920, these early baccalaureate programs were exceptional. Many people of the day believed that higher education was wasted on women. Others viewed nursing as an unacceptable vocation for women of good social standing and moral character. In spite of these attitudes, the number of BSN programs grew. By now, there are about 460 BSN programs in United States.

Generic Baccalaureate Programs

Following World War II, curricula of BSN programs began to resemble majors of other four-year professional degrees. Today these programs typically

- are administered, controlled, and situated in departments, schools, and colleges within universities and colleges

- charge tuition (less in public colleges, more in private ones)

- include academic courses in nursing, arts, sciences, and humanities

- take four academic years to complete, with concentration in the upper division

- meet accreditation standards of state licensing boards, regional higher education accrediting agencies, and the NLN

- employ faculty with master's and doctoral degrees who meet both college and licensing board qualifications

- use community hospitals and various agencies for clinical experience

- use nationally published nursing textbooks

- have a clearly stated philosophy, conceptual framework, learning objectives, and evaluation criteria

- accord students the same rights and responsibilities as other college students

- prepare graduates to manage, lead, teach, and provide care to individuals, families, groups, and communities—directly, or through delegation—in structured and unstructured settings, using the nursing process with emphasis on assessment, analysis, planning, implementation, and evaluation

- prepare graduates to take the NCLEX-RN

- fulfill college or university requirements for a baccalaureate degree

Baccalaureate Programs for Registered Nurses

Programs that offer a bachelor's degree for RNs with diplomas or associate degrees are the fastest growing branch of nursing education. Many factors account for this rise: (1) the 1965 ANA position paper stating that a BSN should become the minimum entry level for professional nursing practice; (2) upward mobility of nurses in administration, education, community health, and advanced clincial practices; (3) societal approval of lifelong learning; (4) mandated continuing education for licensure and certification; and (5) self-actualization. Called by such names as Capstone, Two plus Two, and Second Step, the programs vary greatly. In some, RNs enter as lower division students and take all prerequisite and major course requirements. In others, students receive credit for selected academic and nursing courses. Still others admit only ADNs, and the BSN major is entirely in upper division. Courses include pathophysiology, nursing theory, pharmacology, advanced nursing practice, statistics, research, leadership-management, and community health.

Alternative Programs

Many universities offer innovative programs to meet the needs of working adults who seek nursing degrees. One such program, the New York Regents External Degree program, offers both an ADN and BSN degree. The program is designed to allow students to earn a degree by using college courses, proficiency examinations, and/or special assessments. Fees are charged for enrollment, examinations, and record keeping. The ADN curriculum is equivalent to a generic two-year nursing program, and the BSN is equivalent to a generic four-year nursing program. Both programs are accredited by the NLN. There are no prerequisites, although nursing experience is an advantage. Clear learning objectives for each unit of study are measured by written tests and performance examinations at testing centers throughout the US (New York Regents External Degree 1994).

The California Statewide Nursing Program offers baccalaureate and master's degrees for nurses in a distant education plan. The curricula are standardized, and courses are taught on a rotating basis, year-round, at sites throughout the state by qualified faculty who live in the area. Courses are designed for adult learners in one-unit modules with in-class learning activities and out-of-class assignments. California State University at Dominguez Hills awards a BSN degree or MSN degree to students who complete the programs (Degree and Certificate Programs for RNs 1994).

Master's Degree Programs

Master's degree programs prepare nurses for careers in education, administration, consultation, and advanced clinical practice. Although all programs include advanced theory and practice in nursing, they vary enormously. Some include study of both a clinical specialty, such as community health, and a functional role, such as educator. Some emphasize clinical practice, preparing students for advanced practice in a clinical area such as gerontology. Typically, master's degree programs build on a BSN and require 24 to 48 semester units (30 to 60 quarter units) of graduate study. Entrance requirements usually include a BSN from an NLN-accredited program with a 3.0 grade point average, an RN license, at least one year of work experience, completion of a prerequisite course in statistics, and a Graduate Record Examination or Miller Analogy test score. The goals of the applicant must match the resources of the school. To accommodate students who work while pursuing graduate education, many programs offer classes at off-campus sites, in the evening, on weekends, and by telecommunication systems. Generic master's degree programs teach basic nursing theory and skills at the master's level. Prerequisites vary, but often they build on a bachelors degree in a nonnursing field. After the two to three-year program, graduates earn a master's degree in nursing and are eligible to take the NCLEX-RN.

Doctoral Degree Programs

Doctoral degrees in nursing are relative newcomers to graduate education. Prior to their appearance, nurses who wished to pursue doctoral study earned degrees in related fields such as sociology, education, psychology, and physiology. Many nurses still do. For this reason, a variety of degrees are found among nursing leaders, including doctor of education (EdD), doctor of philosophy (PhD), doctor of public health (DPH), doctor of nursing science (DNSc), and doctor of science in nursing (DSN). Regardless of the name, the core of doctoral study is in-depth inquiry, scientific research into a specific field of learning. The doctoral dissertation reports research findings in a formalized pattern. Generic doctoral programs in nursing admit students with bachelor's or master's degrees in a non-nursing field. They include basic nursing theory and skills and a research project in nursing. Graduates earn a doctor of nursing degree (ND), a professional degree equivalent to a bachelor's, and are eligible to take the NCLEX-RN.

◆ Entry into Practice

For years nurses have debated minimum educational preparation for entry into professional practice. Unfortunately, they did not begin by identifying outcomes of education: specific knowledges, skills, and attitudes of a professional nurse. Instead they focused on the degree earned and number of years of formal education. In 1923, the Winslow-Goldmark Report said that schools of nursing need to be "recognized and supported as separate educational components with, not just training in nursing, but also a liberal education" (Committee for the Study of Nursing Education 1923). In 1948, Esther L. Brown recommended that the term "professional" apply to nursing education that takes place in schools "able to furnish professional education as that term has come to be understood by educators." In 1951, Mildred L. Montag identified a *technical nurse* as one whose scope of practice is narrower than that of a *professional nurse* and broader than that of a practical nurse. Her study launched associate degree nursing education.

In 1965, the ANA House of Delegates adopted the position that "minimum preparation for beginning professional nursing practice …should be baccalaureate degree education in nursing and minimum preparation for beginning technical nursing practice should be associate degree education in nursing" (ANA 1965). In 1978, the ANA House of Delegates adopted a resolution that "by 1985, the minimum preparation for entry into professional nursing practice would be the baccalaureate in nursing and…ANA would work with state nurses associations to identify and define two categories of nursing practice by 1980" (ANA Commission 1979). In 1984, the ANA established a timeline for implementing their goal to establish the baccalaureate for professional nursing practice in 5% of the states by 1986, 15% by 1988, 50% by 1992, and 100% by 1995. Obviously, the timetable was not met.

In 1985, the ANA House of Delegates agreed that the term *registered nurse* be reserved for a professional nurse prepared with a baccalaureate degree and the term *associate nurse* be reserved for a technical nurse prepared with an associate degree (ANA Delegates 1985). That same year associate degree leaders organized the National Organization for the Advancement of Associate Degree Nurses to support the continued status of ADNs as professional nurses. In 1986, while many nursing organizations voted to support the ANA positions, the National Council of State Boards of Nursing (NCSBN) voted to take a neutral position regarding the educational requirements for entry into practice (Hartung 1986). In 1987, the NLN membership voted to postpone indefinitely resolutions concerning the issue of entry into practice. Since that time, nursing has focused on other issues, including advanced practice and national health care.

In 1987, North Dakota became the first state to change its nursing education rules to require that nurses have a bachelor's degree to apply for RN licensure and an assoicate degree to apply for LPN licensure (North Dakota 1986). By 1989, the nationwide shortage of nurses slowed the drive to make the BSN the minimum for "professional" practice, but efforts continued. That same year the Maine State Board of Nursing commissioned the NCSBN to conduct a job analysis of newly licensed, entry-level BSNs in order to create a supplemental licensure examination for BSNs. In 1993 the NCSBN published their report. They identified four roles (care provider, manager, leader, teacher) and three types of clients (individuals, families/small groups, communities) that are different for BSNs and ADNs (NCSBN Final Report 1993). Action on their findings has not been taken.

Controversial Issues

Whenever nurses consider changing criteria for entry into practice, several issues appear: titling, grandfathering, endorsement, scope of practice, and competencies.

Titling is perhaps the most controversial issue. Even though the ANA position statement calls for two levels of nursing, professional and technical, agreement has not been reached as to the titles each should use. Some suggested titles are professional/technical, registered/associate, registered/licensed practical, and nurse/nurse associate. The problem is that the term "registered nurse" is the traditional title, the one that commands the highest respect. No one wants to be downgraded from RN to anything else, least of all diploma and AD nurses who have passed the same basic licensing examination (NCLEX-RN) and who work as peers and even supervisors of BS nurses.

Grandfathering means allowing persons to continue to practice their occupation when new standards, which they do not meet, become law. Legally, licensing of occupational groups falls within the licensing power of the state to safeguard the health and welfare of citizens. When a new law is enacted, or if one is changed, a "grandfather clause" is included because the Fourteenth Amendment of the US Constitution guarantees that a state cannot deprive a person of life, liberty, or property without due process. The Supreme Court has ruled that a license to work is a property right as long as the licensee practices within the law. When applied to entry into practice, a grandfather clause guarantees that RNs with a diploma or an associate degree have the right to continue to be licensed and practice under the law (Waddle 1986). Although a grandfather clause protects a license, it does not guarantee job advancement or intangibles such as respect.

Endorsement for licensure between states becomes complicated if the states change their requirements one by one. Currently, nursing is one of the few occupations in which national examinations (NCLEX-RN and NCLEX-PN) are accepted by every state and territory. Both registered and practical nurses are able to move from state to state without having to retake and pass another examination. If one state requires a BSN for RN licensure, then those who move there without a BSN would not be able to practice as RNs. Whether or not the Fourteenth Amendment guarantees the right to an RN license in another state has not yet been tested in the courts.

Scope of practice refers to the legally sanctioned functions of a licensee. As nurses consider the implications of two categories of RNs, their scope of practice is a matter of great concern. It was of such importance to the ANA in 1985 that its House of Delegates charged a special task force to delineate the scope of practice for future professional and technical nurses. The group concluded that "nursing has but one scope of practice made up of four components: a core (diagnosed human responses to acute or potential health problems), a boundary (dynamic perimeters), intersections (interaction within nursing and between nursing and other health care professionals), and dimensions (characteristics: knowledge base of nurse, role of nurse, nature of clients, and practice environment)...differences between professional and technical nursing practice are found in all four dimensions" (ANA Task Force 1986). They did not delineate the differences.

Competencies are critical to the entry into practice issue. At present there are two recognized, clearly defined sets of competencies—one for registered nurses and one for practical nurses. The NCLEX-RN and

NCLEX-PN measure those competencies. Although many attempts have been made to define the competences of beginning ADN, diploma, and BSN nurses, no difference was found until the 1993 NCSBN study (NCSBN Final Report 1993).

The Two Positions

The issue of entry into practice is a complex one. Those committed to the ANA position believe a change in basic educational requirements for RNs is required if nursing is to achieve the status of a profession (Moloney 1992). Some even believe that nursing will not become a true profession until a doctorate is the entry-level degree. The first step, they maintain, is to raise the entry level to a baccalaureate degree. Those who oppose the ANA position believe a change in basic education requirements is unnecessary and disruptive. They cite the lack of objective evidence that BSNs score higher on the NCLEX-RN or perform better in clinical settings than do associate degree or diploma graduates. They note that ADN programs are cost-effective, community-based, and accessible; maintain high standards; and attract disadvantaged populations. They see a need for more registered nurses, not fewer. They propose that the present system continue and that additional education be recognized by certification.

In 1991, Margretta Styles and her colleagues proposed a means to achieve the goal of "higher standards of care, clear public recognition, accountability, roles, responsibilities, and rewards." They suggested awarding a national generalist certificate "to those with evidence of the baccalaureate degree in nursing and/or administration of an examination measuring the added dimensions of professional practice and/or other criteria. A title such as Certified Professional Nurse could attach to the certificate" (1991). They believe that this approach would achieve the goal of raising the standard of care and that nursing could thus "exit this quagmire before the 21st century" (1991).

◆ Continuing Education for Relicensure

One of the characteristics of a profession is *competence* (see Chapter 1). Nurses must continually update their knowledge, skills, and attitudes to be competent in their ever-changing field. To this end, nurses take brief courses, undertake independent study, and enter formal academic degree programs. "Continuing education in nursing," declared the ANA, "consists of planned, organized learning experiences designed to augment the knowledge, skill, and attitudes of registered nurses for the enhancement of nursing practice, education, administration, and research, to the end of improving health care to the public" (ANA 1978).

Continuing education (CE) is not a new idea. In about 1882 Nightingale wrote, "Nursing is, above all, a progressive calling. Year by year nurses have to learn new and improved methods as medicine, surgery, and hygiene improve" (1954). In 1899, Columbia University offered the first "postgraduate" nursing course of record in the United States. In the 1920s, nursing organizations began offering conferences and institutes. In 1967, the ANA published its first clear statement on continuing education. In 1973, the ANA established the Council on Continuing Education. By 1974, when the Council published *Standards for Continuing Education in Nursing,* most states had devised ways to recognize continuing education. The Council developed a system of accreditation, approval of continuing education courses, and a standard unit of measurement. One *continuing education unit* (CEU) equals ten hours of participation in an organized learning experience offered by a responsible sponsor, capable director, and qualified instructor (ANA *Facts about Nursing* 1985).

In 1987, the ANA established a system whereby organizations can seek accreditation as providers, approvers, or both. They defined a *provider* as an organization that is responsible for offering a course of instruction. An *approver* is an organization, such as state board of nursing or accrediting agency, that is responsible for recognizing courses.

Continuing education is mandatory for renewal of licensure for both registered and practical nurse licensees in about two-thirds of the states. Some states are moving toward mandatory continuing education for all licensed professionals, including physicians, lawyers, and nurses. Licensing boards of each state determine the number of required continuing education units, design a process to enforce the regulation, and set standards for approval of acceptable courses. Licensees are responsible for meeting the requirements of the state in which they seek license renewal.

◆ Nursing Literature

Nursing literature fills an important role in the transmission of knowledge. In 1885, Clara Weeks Shaw wrote the first US nursing text, *A Textbook of Nursing for the Use of Training Schools, Families, and Private Students.* In 1890, Lavinia Dock wrote *Materia Medica for Nurses.* Later she wrote the four-volume *History of Nursing* with M. Adelaide Nutting. Other early nursing authors were Isabel Hampton and Diana Kimber. By 1930, over 700 texts for nurses had been published in the United States (Donahue 1985). By 1992, more than 20,000 nursing texts had been published. The number continues to grow.

With so many texts, how do nurses choose what to read and what to buy? Here are some suggestions:

- Read book reviews and publisher advertisements in nursing magazines.

- Read the list of "Books of the Year" selected for the *American Journal of Nursing.*

- Browse through the bookstore and library of colleges that offer nursing programs.

- Ask nurse faculty members for suggestions; they receive review copies of many new texts.

- Consult *Books in Print*, a multivolume reference that lists books by title and author. It is available at most libraries and bookstores.

- Write to publishing companies for their catalogs of current offerings.

Textbooks are but one way to gain nursing knowledge. Periodicals are an important source of information about the ever-changing health care field. Perhaps the oldest nursing periodical in the United States is the *American Journal of Nursing*, first published on October 1, 1900. Today there are more than 80 nursing periodicals published. Among these are the official publication of nursing organizations; for example, the National League for Nursing's *Nursing and Health Care*, Sigma Theta Tau's *Image*, and the American Academy of Nursing's *Nursing Outlook.*

Libraries of college and universities with nursing schools subscribe to the most widely read periodicals and can obtain other periodicals by interlibrary loan. Often libraries subscribe to the *Cumulative Index to Nursing and Allied Health Literature* (CINAHL) and the *Index Medicus* (IM), which list articles, available both on line and in hard copy, by author and topic. Computer networks provide access to professional literature around the world. Ask your local reference librarian for information. Although not traditional "literature," audiovisual and computerized data are valuable sources of information for nurses. Many companies produce audiocassettes, videocassettes, and computer software. CINAHL and IM index these resources. Multimedia products are especially useful because they are convenient and interactive.

◆ Changing Roles for Nurses

Because nursing is theory-based, education is essential to the preparation of its practitioners. As the profession grows and expands, new roles and levels within those roles are emerging, each with its own educational requirements. It is important for nurses to learn about those roles and the preparation needed to fill them. Massive and rapid change in health care delivery is upon us. Opportunities for nurses in advanced practice are opening as never before. The rush for more education and certification is on. The challenge is to keep abreast of the times and seize opportunities as they appear.

◆ Preceptorships and Internships

Nursing education began as apprenticeship training, with task-based learning measured in months and years. When nursing education moved to universities and colleges, learning became concept-based, measured by achievement of learning objectives. Clinical hours shrank. Graduates of associate and bachelor's degree programs entered the work world with much less clinical experience than graduates of diploma programs. They could analyze, synthesize, and evaluate but had little experience applying their knowledge to practice. Even though Montag's original proposal for ADN education hinged on a period of clinical supervision for new graduates, that part of her plan has not been implemented. By 1970, the need to ease the transition from student to professional was obvious. Many schools and agencies began offering preceptorships and internships.

Preceptorships are learning periods for students nearing the end of a professional education program. Often preceptorships for nursing students are cooperative arrangements between a college and a health care agency. The college provides instructors to teach, organize, and monitor learning experiences, and the agency provides preceptors to model the role being learned. Some programs build preceptorships into the basic curriculum.

Internships are new employee programs provided by employers. They vary in length from a few days to several months. Often employers use an advisory support system, in which a neophyte is given a peer pal, sponsor, or mentor. Preceptor and intern programs benefit both new graduates and health care agencies. Staff morale increases, graduates adjust more easily, retention rates improve, standards of care rise, and performance standards rise. Unfortunately, many agencies drop internship programs when the applicant pool increases.

◆ Research in Nursing

Research in nursing focuses on building a body of knowledge about human responses to actual or potential health problems and about the effects of nursing actions on those responses. Research is basic to nursing practice, education, and administration. In 1986, the US Congress established the National Center of Nursing Research. In 1993, it became the 17th institute of the National Institutes of Health, changing its name to the National Institute of Nursing Research. If the knowledge gained by research is to be useful, it must be applied. To apply research, nurses must understand the research process, recognize ethical concerns, and learn to evaluate research reports.

The process of conducting research involves moving back and forth between ideas, hunches, existing knowledge, and observation (Wilson 1993). That process includes the following steps: (1) state the research question, (2) describe the purpose of the study, (3) review relevant literature, (4) formulate hypotheses and defining variables, (5) decide on a research design, (6) select a population, sample, and setting, (7) conduct a pilot study, (8) collect data, (9) analyze the data, and (10) communicate conclusions and implications in a written, standardized report.

Ethical concerns center on protecting clients' rights. Ethical considerations include: (1) physical, emotional, financial, and social safety, (2) full disclosure of the nature, duration, purpose, and method of data collection as well as the use of data, benefits that might result, inconveniences, side effects, alternatives to participation, identities of investigators and how to contact them, (3) freedom from coercion, (4) confidentiality and privacy, and (5) explanation of how these rights will be ensured.

Typically, research reports include (1) an abstract, or brief description of the study and its findings, (2) a statement of the purpose and of the hypotheses that were tested, (3) a review of pertinent literature, (4) a description of the method used to conduct the study, (5) a report of findings, (6) a discussion of the findings and their implications, and (7) references. Evaluating nursing research requires concentration and practice, but the benefits far outweigh the effort. As they become more adept in reading research reports, nurses find that the mystique dissipates and their ability to evaluate increases. This ability is critical if nurses are to build a scientific body of knowledge. It is the key to building a practice that is shaped by research rather than tradition, intuition, or habit. Investigative skills, regardless of the nurse's educational level, need to become a fundamental part of the set of skills all nurses possess.

◆ Theories of Nursing

True professions are theory-based (see Chapter 1). Before a profession can select a theory as its basis for practice, it must define its purpose. Medicine defines its purpose as diagnosing and treating disease. The theory that all disease is caused led medicine to adopt, though unconsciously, the "medical model." Nursing has defined its purpose as "diagnosing and treating human responses to actual or potential health problems" (ANA 1980).

Many scholars see nursing as too complex to be captured by the ANA definition. Their models and theories address human responses to health problems from different perspectives. Before we can compare some of these models, we need to define some terms:

- *Concepts.* Constructs or ideas, such as *person, goal,* and *health.*

- *Conceptual framework.* A set of concepts that fit together into a meaningful form, organizing information into a unique perspective or set.

- *Conceptual model.* A configuration that gives clear and explicit directions for nursing practice, education, and research with assumptions, a value system, and major units representing important features of the model.

- *Nurse theorists.* Nurses who systematically define the basis and principles of nursing practice by grouping together related concepts to describe nursing functions, components, and dimensions, in order to predict the effect of nursing actions.

- *Theory.* An abstract explanation for an observable fact that is more specific than a model or framework and consists of concepts, propositions, and hypotheses.

Theorists have developed many conceptual models of nursing practice. Unlike medicine, nursing has not chosen a single model. In fact, because of the nature of nursing, a single model may not be ideal. Table 2-1 compares some well-known models.

TABLE 2-1

Comparison of Selected Conceptual Models for Nursing Practice

Author	Central Theme	Definition of the Function of Nursing	Nursing Process
Imogene King (1981)	Goal attainment	A process of human interaction between nurse and client whereby each perceives the other and the situation. Through communication they set goals and explore and agree on means to achieve goals.	Human interpersonal process of action, reaction, interaction, and transaction between individuals and groups in social systems (interlocking circles)
Betty M. Neuman (1980)	Systems	Concerned with the variables affecting an individual's response to stressors; the nurse's function is to identify stressors and lines of resistance, and to help individuals to respond to stressors, using primary, secondary, and tertiary prevention strategies.	Assessment of lines of defense: • physiologic variables • psychologic variables • sociocultural variables • developmental variables • spiritual variables • environmental stressors (intra-, inter-, extrapersonal) Statement of problem Summary of goals Intervention plan Evaluation

TABLE 2-1 *(continued)*

Comparison of Selected Conceptual Models for Nursing Practice

Author	Central Theme	Definition of the Function of Nursing	Nursing Process
Dorothy Orem (1980)	Self-care: universal and health	A creative effort of one human helping another; the goal is to provide and manage self-care action on a continuous basis to help others sustain life and health, recover from disease or injury, and cope with the effects; to move the person toward responsible action, and family members toward increasing competence in making decisions about continuing care.	Interpersonal process; a cycle of assisting, checking, adjusting, and readjusting Step 1: Nursing diagnosis Step 2: Planning a system of nursing Step 3: Actions of nurse
Martha Rogers (1980)	Unitary man and life processes	A science and art, nursing seeks to promote symphonic interaction between humans and environment, to strengthen the coherence and integrity of the human field, and to direct and redirect patterning of the human and environmental fields for realization of maximum health potential.	Setting: life process and human field; nursing diagnosis; intervention; evaluation

TABLE 2-1 *(continued)*

Comparison of Selected Conceptual Models for Nursing Practice

Author	Central Theme	Definition of the Function of Nursing	Nursing Process
Callista Roy (1984)	Adaptation	A scientific discipline that is practice-oriented and concerned with humans as adaptive systems with cognator and regulator coping mechanisms that produce behavioral responses relative to the physiologic, self-concept, role function, and interdependence modes. The goal is to bring about an adaptive state in all four modes, thus contributing to the person's health, quality of life, and dignified dying.	Six steps: 1. Assessment in four modes of behaviors 2. Assessment in four modes of stimuli 3. Nursing diagnosis 4. Goal setting 5. Interventions 6. Evaluation

◆ Summary

Because nursing focuses on human responses to health problems rather than disease, its educational programs prepare caregivers at many levels. Historically, nurses were divided into two groups: practical and "trained." AD education for RNs blurred the division. In 1965, the ANA declared its support for the BSN as the minimum for entry into professional nursing practice, initiating a 30-year debate. The impetus for career-long learning brought innovative higher degree programs, mandatory continuing education, and advanced nursing practice. Literature and multimedia give nurses valuable learning tools; internships and preceptorships help the beginning practitioner; research provides the theory base for nursing practice.

Critical Thinking Questions

1. What assumptions are implied by the statement, "Hospital schools of nursing in the early 1890s developed programs to meet their service needs..."? Remember that an assumption is an idea or concept that we take for granted.

2. State your position on the debate about entry into practice. Give three reasons to explain why you hold this position.

3. State the position of someone who would disagree with you on the debate about entry into practice. What reasons might this person give to defend that position?

Learning Activities

1. Interview five registered nurses. Ask them at what level they began practicing nursing (nursing assistant, LPN, ADN, diploma, BSN), how their role has changed, and whether they plan to earn further degrees in nursing.

2. Survey nursing education in your community. Obtain specific program descriptions and compare entrance requirements, length, cost, accreditation, options for part-time study, completion degree or diploma.

3. From your community hospitals and clinics, obtain job descriptions and qualifications for generalist nurses, clinical nurse specialists, and nurse practitioners.

4. Discuss issues that relate to entry into practice as they affect your community. Include the issues of grandfathering, interstate endorsement, scope of practice, competency expectations, and titling.

5. What are the continuing education requirements of your state or territory? How do licensees prove they have met them? Who accredits courses?

6. Use CINAHL to search for articles published in the last three years on a topic of your choice.

7. Read a nursing research report. What parts did you understand, not understand? How did the research make sure human rights would be respected?

Annotated Reading List

Marriner-Tomey A. *Nursing Theorists and Their Work,* 3rd ed. Mosby, 1994.

This text gives a comprehensive picture of the history and development of nursing theory. The author discusses the process of theory development and the major nursing theorists. The book gives the reader the tools needed to analyze individual theories and make decisions about their application in clinical settings.

Boykin A (ed). *Living a Caring-Based Program.* National League for Nursing, 1993.

This little book proposes a comprehensive approach to creating a nursing education program from a caring perspective. It traces the history of the concept of caring and provides an organizational model that recognizes caring as the essence of nursing practice and education. The text suggests a way to facilitate the full participation of the faculty in integrating caring throughout the curriculum. It supports the notion that the time has come for student nurses to experience caring, even as they learn to care for others.

References

American Nurses Association. *Facts About Nursing '84 to '85.* ANA, 1985.

American Nurses Association. *First Position on Nursing Education. Am J Nurs* 65 (12):106–111 1965.

American Nurses Association. *Nursing: A Social Policy Statement.* ANA, 1980.

American Nurses Association. *Self-Directed Continuing Education in Nursing.* ANA, 1978.

American Nurses Association. *Twenty-Thousand Nurses Tell Their Story.* ANA, 1958.

American Nurses Association Cabinet on Nursing Education. *Education for Nursing Practice in the Context of the 1980's.* NE-11 5M4183, ANA, 1983.

American Nurses Association Cabinet on Nursing Education Task Force. *The National Plan to Implement ANA's Educational Goal.* ANA, 1985.

American Nurses Association Commission on Nursing Education. *A Case for Baccalaureate Preparation in Nursing.* Publ. No. NE-6 ANS, pp. 5–7. ANA, 1979.

American Nurses Association Task Force on Scope of Practice. *The Scope of Nursing Practice,* Draft II. ANA, 1986.

ANA delegates vote to limit RN title to BSN grad; "associate nurse" wins vote for technical level. *Am J Nurs* 1016–1017 1985.

Board of Registered Nursing. *Laws Relating to Nursing Education, Licensure-practice with Rules and Regulations.* Sacramento, CA: Department of Consumer Affairs, 1994.

Brown EL. *Nursing for the Future.* Russell Sage, 1948.

Committee for the Study of Nursing Education. *Nursing and Nursing Education in the US.* The Committee, 1923.

Culpepper MM, Adams PG. Nursing in the Civil War. *Am J Nurs* 88:981–984 July 1988.

Degree and certificate programs for registered nurses. Statewide Nursing Program, California State University, Dominquez Hills, Carson, CA, 1994.

Dock LL, Stewart IM. *A Short History of Nursing,* 4th ed. Putnam's Sons, 1938.

Dolan JA. Nursing in Society. *A Historical Perspective,* 15th ed. Saunders, 1983.

Donahue MP. *Nursing: The Oldest Art, An Illustrated History.* Mosby, 1985.

Gibbon JM, Mathewson MS. *Three Centuries of Canadian Nursing.* Macmillan of Canada, 1947.

Hartung D. Organizational positions on titling and entry into practice: A Chronology. In *Looking Beyond the Entry Issue: Implications for Education and Service.* No. 41-2173. 1986.

Johnston DF. *History and Trends of Practical Nursing.* Mosby, 1966.

King I. *A Theory for Nursing: Systems, Concepts, Process.* John Wiley, 1981.

Moloney MM. *Professionalization of Nursing and Nursing Education: Summary Report and Recommendations.* Lippincott, 1992.

Montag MM. *The Education of Nursing Technicians.* Putnam, 1951, p 70.

National Commission for the Study of Nursing and a Nursing Education: Summary, Report and Recommendations. *Am J Nurs.* 70:270-289 Feb 1970.

National Council of State Boards of Nursing. *Final Report Job Analysis Study: Newly Licensed, Entry-Level Registered Nurses with a Generic Baccalaureate Nursing Degree*. For the Maine State Board of Nursing, April 8, 1993.

Neuman BM. *The Neuman Systems Model: Application to Nursing Education and Practice*. Appleton-Century-Crofts, 1982.

New York Regents External Degree, Bachelor of Science (Nursing) Degree Description. U of NY Regents External Degree, 1994.

Nightingale F. Nursing the sick. In: Seymer LR. *Selected Writings of Florence Nightingale*. Macmillan, 1954.

North Dakota rule changes require associate, baccalaureate education. *Issues*, 7(2):1–3 1986.

Orem DE. *Nursing Concepts in Practice*, 2nd ed. McGraw-Hill, 1980.

Rogers M. *An Introduction to the Theoretical Base of Nursing*. FA Davis, 1970.

Roy Sr C. *Introduction to Nursing: An Adaptation Model*, 2nd ed. Prentice-Hall, 1984.

Stewart IM. *The Education of Nurses*. Macmillan, 1943.

Styles MM, Allen S, Armstrong S, Matsuura M, Stannard D, Ordway JS. Entry: A New Approach. *Nursing Outlook* 39:5, 200–203 Sept–Oct 1991.

Waddle FI. The grandfather concept: A simple process. *Oklahoma Nurse* Sept 1986.

Williams JK. Nursing Education: Why Students Choose ADN Programs. *Am J Nurs*, 89:386 Mar 1989.

Wilson HS. *Research in Nursing*. Addison-Wesley, 1993.

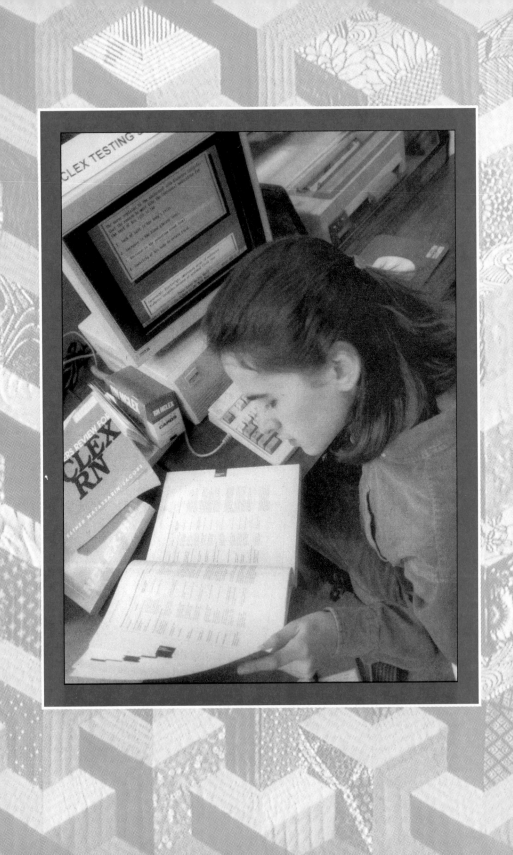

Credentialing: Licensure and Certification

3

◇ Learning Objectives

- Explain the difference between certificates and licenses.

- Describe the origin and current use of registration and licensure.

- Compare permissive and mandatory licensure.

- Describe the NCLEX-RN examination, including its content, the time and mode of administration, and the process for reporting results.

- State the purpose of nurse practice acts, rules, and regulations.

- Describe the requirements for licensure and the application process.

- Discuss the causes and consequences of disciplinary action by a board of nursing.

- Examine the purpose and process of certification.

- Discuss issues involved in creating a uniform credentialing system.

- Describe both the governmental and nongovernmental accreditation process.

Dana pored over the want ad section of the newspaper. "I don't see many jobs for beginning nurses like us. Everybody wants experience. How can you get experience if you can't get a job?" She fell silent for a minute, then asked, "What do you suppose all these initials mean: FNP, CEN, CNM, PHN, ACLSC?"

Dana's housemate, Sarah, looked up from the NCLEX-RN review book she was studying. "They're special credentials you've got to have to get those jobs."

"I know that, but what do they mean?"

"I don't know, but if you don't get busy and study for the state board examination, you won't need to know!"

"True, but I'd still like to know what they mean. My aunt used to tell me that if I got my RN degree I'd be set for life. But since I've been a student nurse, nobody ever mentions such a degree. They talk about associate degrees and bachelor's degrees, but not RN degrees. Maybe there is a degree I haven't heard about. I wonder if that's what these initials stand for. Are they degrees, licenses, or certificates? What are they?"

"They're just credentials, all kinds of credentials," Sarah replied impatiently. "Now please, if you're not going to study, you can at least be quiet and let me!"

Dana went back to searching the want ads. She didn't want to bother Sarah, but she felt even more perplexed. What were credentials? What was the difference between degrees, licenses, and certificates? Who awarded them? What did they mean?

◆ Credentials

Credentials are proof of qualifications, usually in writing, stating that an individual or organization has met specific standards. There are two types of credentials: certificates and licenses.

Certificates are credentials verifying that an individual or organization has met certain standards. They are issued by governmental, public agencies and nongovernmental, private agencies. Although both types of certificates have professional status, those issued by governmental agencies also have legal status. Examples of certificates include licenses, diplomas, college degrees, nurse practitioner certificates, and accreditation certificates.

Licenses are credentials issued by governmental agencies. Their purpose is to protect the health and safety of the public. They are enforced by the police power of the state. A license verifies that an individual or organization has met minimum standards. It gives the licensee permission to carry out prescribed functions. For example, a registered nurse (RN) license signifies that a person has met minimum entry-level requirements and may practice within the scope described by the nurse practice act (NPA) of a state or territory. A long-term care license verifies that a facility has complied with certain minimum requirements and may operate according to the prescribed conditions of the law governing long-term care facilities.

Institutional licensure of professionals is an alternative to individual licensure. Most governments issue licenses to health care facilities. These licenses grant permission to operate, and the issuing body holds the facilities responsible for such things as sanitation, fire safety, staffing, and equipment. Institutional licensure of individuals would give these facilities the added right to decide who is qualified to perform what tasks, and to award licenses to whom they see fit. Proponents of institutional licensure argue that it is reasonable to give these agencies such a right, since they are accountable for employee performance. Opponents argue that there would be no standard criteria between facilities and that employee mobility between facilities would be complicated, if not impossible. Furthermore, professional autonomy would be lost. Nursing organizations consider institutional licensure dangerous and an ongoing threat.

Registration is placement on an official roster of names of persons, places, or things that meet certain criteria. When requested, the registering agency verifies that a certain registrant has met the criteria necessary for inclusion on its roster. Where there are large numbers of registrants, the process can be cumbersome. Before licensure laws, graduates of nursing schools registered in official rosters, hence the term "registered nurse." Nowadays, except for employment registries, registration has been replaced by licensing and certification.

◆ Licensure

Historical Background

Credentials for nurses have not always existed as we know them today. In medieval times the public identified members of religious nursing orders by the design of their habit or the insignia displayed on their vestments. When the Nightingale school was established, its reputation for high standards spread throughout the world, but there was no credentialing system to verify the qualifications of individual graduates. Instead, the school wrote personal letters of recommendation attesting to their ability. When other schools of nursing began graduating nurses, they, too, wrote letters of reference. Eventually the schools replaced these letters with certificates of satisfactory completion: diplomas.

With the proliferation of schools in the United States during the late 1800s and early 1900s, standards of nursing practice and nursing schools varied widely. Programs differed in length from 6 to 36 months. Service, rather than education, characterized many schools. In 1896, to gain control over the profession and stem the growth of substandard schools, nursing leaders established the Nurses' Associated Alumnae of the United States and Canada. They saw licensure for nurses as the way to raise standards. However, hospitals opposed any form of regulation. Because of the publicity the brand-new publication, the *American Journal of Nursing,* gave to the issue, nursing leaders prevailed. In 1903, North Carolina passed the first nurse practice act in the United States. Canada passed its first nurse practice act in 1914. By 1923, all 48 states, the District of Columbia, and the territory of Hawaii had licensure laws.

Permissive Licensure

The first licensure laws could more accurately be called *nurse registration acts* than nurse practice acts. The term *registered nurse* was defined as a person who had graduated from an acceptable nursing program and passed an examination, rather than a person who engaged in a specific type of practice. These first laws provided for *permissive licensure*. That is, they offered a voluntary process by which nurses who met predetermined standards could obtain a license and have their names registered with the states. Those who did not meet the standards or did not bother to register could still practice nursing and call themselves nurses without legal consequences.

Mandatory Licensure

In 1938, New York became the first state to pass a *mandatory licensure law*, requiring a license of all persons who called themselves nurses. This law established two levels of nurses, registered and practical, restricting specific nursing functions to these two groups. For the first time this law defined the *scope of practice* for nurses. In 1955, the board of directors of the American Nurses Association (ANA) adopted model nurse practice acts for both professional and practical nursing. This action helped define nursing and fostered passage of mandatory nurse practice acts across the nation. In 1976, the ANA revised the model to reflect advanced practice roles in professional nursing, and in 1980, they revised it again (ANA 1990). In 1978, representatives of the states formed an independent National Council of State Boards of Nursing (NCSBN), with representatives from the 53 jurisdictions of the United States. In 1993, the NCSBN published a model nurse practice act, and in 1994 they published a model Administrative Rules for Nursing.

Licensure Examinations

By 1923, even though every state licensed nurses by examination, the tests varied widely. In 1945, the ANA formed the Council of State Boards of Nursing. It assumed responsibility for developing a uniform examination. By 1950, all states used the same test, which had been prepared by the National League for Nursing (NLN) Testing Division. That first examination was divided into five subject areas: medical, surgical, obstetric, pediatric, and psychiatric nursing.

In 1980, the newly formed NCSBN developed a new test plan using the steps of the nursing process. The Testing Division of the NLN prepared the first test. Soon thereafter, the NCSBN called for competitive bids for the creation of the examination. CTB Testing Service, a subsidiary of McGraw-Hill Publishing Company, won the contract.

They prepared the February 1983 examination and continue to prepare examinations to this day. Besides preparing and scoring the test, the company furnishes a statistical analysis of test results for the NCSBN, state licensing boards, and individual schools. In 1987, the test was revised to reflect the findings of a study that analyzed the tasks of entry-level RNs (NCSBN 1987). In 1994, after extensive field-testing, the NCSBN initiated computer-adaptive testing (CAT) for registered and practical nurses. They continue to develop clinical simulation testing (CST), in which client situations appear on the computer screen and test-takers determine appropriate actions.

National Council Licensure Examination for Registered Nurses

The name of the current test for registered nurses is the *National Council Licensure Examination for Registered Nurses* (NCLEX-RN). The test includes two components: nursing process and client needs. See Table 3-1. To help students prepare for the examination, the NCSBN offers a booklet entitled *Specific Nursing Behaviors to Be Measured in NCLEX-RN (Detailed Test Plan)*. To obtain a copy, write to the National Council of State Boards of Nursing, 625 North Michigan Avenue, Suite 1544, Chicago, IL 60611.

Under contract with the NCSBN, CTB Testing Services administers both the NCLEX-RN and NCLEX-PN in Sylvan Technology Centers (STC). These testing centers are located in convenient sites, with at least one in every state and territory. Candidates submit an application to take the test to their board of nursing. After the application is approved, the candidate receives an authorization to test and an informational pamphlet describing the testing process. When candidates are ready to take the test, they call the STC of their choice to schedule an appointment. Testing is available 15 hours a day, six days a week and on Sundays when needed to meet peak demand (NCSBN 1993).

In computer-adaptive testing, multiple-choice questions appear on the computer screen. The program contains a bank of questions, and although individuals are given different questions, all tests are equal. As the candidate answers the questions, the program computes the score and chooses an appropriate next question. The examination ends when all components of the test plan have been tested and enough questions have been answered to give a definitive

TABLE 3-1

NCLEX Test Plan Percentages

Nursing Process	
Assessment:	17–23%
Analysis:	17–23%
Planning:	17–23%
Implementation:	17–23%
Evaluation:	17–23%
Client Needs	
Safe, effective care environment	15–21%
Physiologic integrity	46–54%
Psychosocial integrity	8–16%
Health promotion/maintenance	17–23%

From: Changes Incorporated into NCLEX-RN™ Test Plan: New Test Plan to be Implemented in October 1995, *Issues*, Vol. 15 No. 4. National Council of State Boards of Nursing, Inc., 1995.

pass or fail score. The test takes a maximum of 5 hours, with some candidates completing it much sooner. Within 48 hours, test center personnel send test results to the authorizing board of nursing. The board notifies candidates of test results and issues licenses to successful candidates.

Nurse Practice Acts and Rules and Regulations

A *nurse practice act* is a law made by a state or territorial legislature that regulates nursing practice to protect the public. Each NPA authorizes an administrative body, usually called a board of nursing, to implement the provisions of the NPA. The board writes a set of *rules and regulations* (R&Rs) that become administrative law (see Chapter 8). The police power of the state enforces both nurse practice acts and rules and regulations. Every nurse should know the provisions of these statues and can obtain a copy of them from their state licensing board. See Appendix A for current addresses.

Although both the ANA and NCSBN have published model nurse practice acts, no two acts are exactly the same. Some jurisdictions

Definition of Nursing from the American Nurses Association Model Nurse Practice Act of 1990

The "practice of nursing" means the performance of services for compensation in the provision of diagnosis and treatment of human responses to health or illness;

"Professional nursing practice" encompasses the full scope of nursing practice and includes all its specialties and consists of application of nursing theory to the development, implementation, and evaluation of plans of nursing care for individuals, families, and communities. Professional nursing practice requires substantial knowledge of nursing theory and related scientific, behavioral, and humanistic disciplines. Professional nursing practice includes, but is not limited to:

(1) assessment, diagnosis, planning, intervention, and evaluation of human responses to health or illness;

(2) the provision of direct nursing care to individuals to restore optimum function or to achieve a dignified death;

(3) the procurement, coordination, and management of essential client resources;

(4) the provision of health counseling and education;

(5) the establishment of standards of practice for nursing care in all settings, including the development of nursing policies, procedures, and protocols for a specific setting;

(6) the direction of nursing practice, including delegation to those practicing technical nursing;

➤

have a single act for both registered and practical nurses; others have two separate acts. Some acts are broad in scope, leaving specifics to the rules and regulations. Others are detailed, requiring legislative action for minor changes. Regardless of their differences, nurse practice acts and rules and regulations address similar issues, as follows.

Definition of Nursing

To clarify meaning, legislative acts begin with a definition of terms. Perhaps the most important is the definition of nursing. In 1990, the ANA revised their model nurse practice act and definition of nursing practice to reflect their position that the bachelor's degree should be the minimum requirement for entry into professional nursing practice. In the model they define both professional and technical nursing practice but do not address practical nursing practice. See the accompanying box.

(7) the supervision of those who assist in the practice of nursing;

(8) collaboration with other independently licensed health care professionals in case finding and the clinical management and execution of intervention as identified to be appropriate in a plan of care; and

(9) the administration of medication and treatments as prescribed by those professionals qualified to prescribe under the provision of (*cite state statute[s]*);

"Technical nursing practice" includes the skilled application of nursing principles in the delivery of direct care to individuals and families within organized nursing services. Technical nursing practice requires the study of nursing within the context of the applied sciences. Technical nursing practice includes, but is not limited to:

(1) participation in the development, evaluation, and modification of a plan of care;

(2) the provision of direct care to individuals to restore optimum function or to achieve a dignified death;

(3) patient teaching;

(4) the supervision of those who assist in the practice of nursing;

(5) the administration of medications and treatments as prescribed by those professionals qualified to prescribe under the provisions of (*cite state statute[s]*).

Excerpted from: American Nurses Association. (1990). *Suggested state legislation: Nursing practice act, nursing disciplinary diversion act, prescriptive authority act*, © 1990 by American Nurses Association. Reprinted with permission.

Scope of Practice

The *scope of practice* is a statement clearly defining a range of duties. Although the wording differs from state to state, most nurse practice acts refer to the nursing process, specialized knowledge of nurses, and performance of service for compensation. Several states include some reference to treating human responses to actual and potential health problems. About half of the nurse practice acts describe advanced practice roles for nurses.

Titling

Nurse practice acts make it illegal for persons to represent themselves by the title registered nurse (RN), licensed practical nurse (LPN), or licensed vocational nurse (LVN) if they do not meet stipulated requirements. Some nurse practice acts also protect other titles such as nurse midwife, nurse anesthetist, and nurse practitioner.

Administrative Board

The administrative board, often called the *board of nursing,* is the body legally empowered to carry out the intent of a nurse practice act. The number, makeup, and term of board members vary from state to state. The number of board members ranges from 7 to 17 members. Some nurse practice acts stipulate membership according to occupation, for example: 5 employed nurses, 1 nurse educator, 1 physician, and 2 public members. The governor appoints board members in every state and territory except in North Carolina, where licensees elect board members. In all but six states there is a combined board for registered nurses and licensed practical nurses. In those six states there are two separate boards. While all boards function within their own state government, they all are represented in the NCSBN and cooperate with the NLN and ANA.

All boards of nursing hire an executive director who is responsible for administering the work of the board and seeing that the nurse practice act and rules and regulations are followed. The ANA recommends that boards of nursing (1) govern their own operation and administration; (2) approve or deny approval to schools of nursing; (3) examine and license applicants; (4) review licenses, grant temporary licenses, and provide for inactive status for those already licensed; (5) regulate specialty practice; and (6) discipline those who violate provisions of the licensure law.

Requirements for Licensure

Because granting licenses is not a function of the federal government, nurses must meet the requirements of the state or territory where they practice. Nonetheless, no state or territory may make age, residence, or citizenship a licensure requirement. Such restrictions have been judged unconstitutional. Typical licensure requirements include:

- *Education.* Applicant must complete an educational program in a state-approved school of nursing and receive a diploma or degree from that program. There are exceptions. For example, California allows persons who have completed certain courses in the bachelor of science in nursing (BSN) programs to apply for licensure even though they have not yet earned a degree. North Dakota requires a BSN degree for an RN license and an associate degree in nursing (ADN) for a PN license. North Dakota issues temporary licenses to nurses from other states, giving RNs four years, and PNs two years, to earn the required degrees. Some states also require evidence of high school education.

- *Examination.* The applicant must pass the NCLEX-RN or NCLEX-PN.

- *Health.* Some states require evidence of physical and mental health.

- *Moral character.* Many states require a statement that the applicant is of good moral character as determined by the licensing board. In practice, this means that applicants who have been convicted of a felony must submit, with their licensure application, a description of the offense, the penalty, and evidence of rehabilitation.

- *Payment of fees.* Applicants pay fees for processing and administering the NCLEX-RN and NCLEX-PN, for interim work permits, and for temporary licenses.

Application Procedure

Boards of nursing develop their own application forms, which they send to nursing programs before the end of the school year. If graduates wish to begin practicing in another state or territory, they should send for forms from that jurisdiction. (See Appendix A for addresses.) Application forms give information about fees, transcripts needed to verify nursing education, and court records if the applicant has had a felony conviction.

Exemptions from Licensure

In what is termed an *exception clause*, nurse practice acts and rules and regulations include provisions to allow people who are licensed in one jurisdiction to practice nursing in another. Because every exemption from licensure weakens mandatory aspects of the law and reduces public protection, exemptions must be justified by overriding factors. Exemptions usually include (1) students enrolled in nursing programs, (2) unpaid people caring for friends or family members, (3) caregivers who conduct religious rites and who do not claim to be RNs or LVN-LPNs, (4) RNs and LVN-LPNs licensed in one state and temporarily passing through another state who work for clients in that state, (5) RNs and LVN-LPNs working for the Red Cross during a disaster, and (6) RNs and LVN-LPNs practicing in a federal agency such as a military hospital. Some states also exempt attendants working under the supervision of licensed nurses and physicians, although organized nursing opposes this exception.

Interim/Temporary Permits

An *interim/temporary permit* is a full and unrestricted license to practice professional or practical nursing in the jurisdiction issuing the permit, pending verification of some detail. Usually such permits are limited to specific time periods and require payment of a fee. Persons with interim permits may not call themselves RNs or LVN-LPNs, but may identify themselves as permittees. They are subject to the same disciplinary action of the law as licensees. In some states a temporary license is issued to RNs under special circumstances, such as excusable delays in meeting licensure requirements or in completing license renewal applications.

Endorsement and Reciprocity

Endorsement is the granting of a license without requiring reexamination. Because boards of nursing use the same standardized examination and cooperate with one another, nurses in the United States have greater mobility than many other licensed professionals. With the few exemptions from licensure listed above, nurses must be licensed in the state or territory where they practice. However, if they fulfill requirements for licensure, submit proof that the license they possess in another state is in good standing, and pay an endorsement fee, they are granted a license by endorsement without having to retake the examination.

Reciprocity is not the same as endorsement. Reciprocity means acceptance of the licensees of one jurisdiction by another as a result of a mutual agreement between the two jurisdictions. It is not available to RNs or LPN-LVNs in the United States.

Foreign Nursing School Graduates

Nurses who have graduated from nursing schools in foreign countries and want to practice as RNs in the United States must meet the requirements of the state or territory in which they reside and must pass the NCLEX-RN. These requirements are spelled out in the state nurse practice act. To prevent exploitation of foreign graduates who come to the United States to practice nursing but fail to pass the licensing examination, the ANA and NLN sponsor an independent organization called the Committee on Graduates of Foreign Nursing Schools (CGFNS). The organization administers an examination to foreign-educated nurses in various locations in the United States and throughout the world. The examination tests proficiency in both English and nursing and helps foreign nurses assess their chances of passing the NCLEX-RN. There is no CGFNS test for practical nurses. Foreign nurses who pass the CGFNS examination receive a certificate from CGFNS that allows them to obtain a work permit from the US Labor Department or a nonimmigrant preference visa from the US Immigration and Naturalization Service. In 42 states at the present time, foreign-educated nurses must have a CGFNS certificate to apply to take the NCLEX-RN. In 1993, the CGFNS started a Credentials Evaluation Service to evaluate credentials of foreign nurses who apply to states and territories that do not require a CGFNS certificate (*New FNG Credentials Service Is Launched 1993*).

Disciplinary Action

Every licensee and holder of a certificate awarded by a board of nursing may be disciplined for unprofessional conduct. Nurse practice acts vary, but the ANA lists the following acts as unprofessional: (1) fraud in gaining a license, (2) conviction of a felony, (3) addiction to drugs, (4) harm to or defrauding of the public, and (5) willful violation of a nurse practice act (LeBar 1984). Disciplinary action may take the form of license revocation, suspension for a period of time, or restrictions on practice. Such action must respect individual constitutional rights and must be based on criteria stated in the law.

The disciplinary process begins with a report filed with the board of nursing charging a nurse with an unlawful act. A representative of the board investigates the charge. If the investigator finds substantial evidence that the charge is true, the board notifies the nurse of the charges and gives the nurse time to prepare a defense. The board sets a hearing date and issues a subpoena to appear. The nurse has the right to be represented by counsel, and the counsel has a right to cross-examine witnesses. The board acts as the judge and jury, and decides what disciplinary action, if any, is appropriate.

Although boards of nursing must protect the health and safety of the public, many recognize *diversion programs*, which are designed to rehabilitate nurses whose competency may be impaired because of substance abuse or mental illness. These programs are independent from licensing boards and are designed to treat substance abuse and mental illness. No nurse is forced to enter a diversion program, and any nurse may enroll, whether or not the nurse has been charged with an offense. If charges have been filed and the nurse decides to enter a program, the board is notified only if the nurse fails to complete the program. All information divulged by a nurse during the course of treatment is confidential and not subject to discovery or subpoena. Diversion programs include assessment, development of a rehabilitation plan, referral for treatment, monitoring of participation and compliance, and referral to a support network. Disciplined nurses are responsible to make periodic reports to the board. When they have met the conditions of discipline and rehabilitation, they may apply to the board for reinstatement of the license (California Board of Registered Nursing 1989).

Educational Programs in Nursing

Only graduates of accredited/approved nursing programs may take the examination to become licensed nurses. An important function of nurse practice acts is to regulate educational programs to make sure they meet certain standards. Nurse practice acts give this responsibility to the administrative board, which hires consultants to examine educational programs. If they find that a program meets board-established criteria, the board issues a certificate of accreditation or approval. The accreditation process of educational institutions is discussed later in this chapter.

Advanced Practice

Some nurse practice acts provide for advanced practice for nurses such as clinical nurse specialists, nurse practitioners, and nurse midwives. Often nurse practice acts have their own detailed advanced practice requirements. Others require certification by professional organizations such as the American College of Nurse Midwives and the ANA. Still others do not regulate advance practice at all. As the health care delivery system changes and greater numbers of nurses engage in advanced practice, it is likely that more states will regulate their practice. Not all nursing groups agree that advanced practice should be regulated by state law. Many believe that the states should regulate only minimum safe practice and that specialty boards should regulate advanced practice, as they do in medicine. They point out that nurse practice acts, as laws, are rigid and less responsive to change and that many boards of nursing include persons from non-nursing occupations. By placing advanced nursing practice under the control of non-nurses, the power to regulate nursing is shifted to others.

Continuing Education

Many states require evidence of *continuing education* (CE) before the license is renewed. Their rules and regulations stipulate the number of required educational units, the process for verifying units, and the standards for measuring the quality of the continuing education. Because these requirements differ from state to state, nurses need to find out exactly what the requirements are before renewing licenses. See Chapter 2 for a discussion of continuing education.

◆ Certification

Certification is a form of credentialing that has both professional and legal status. Generally, it indicates a level of competence above minimum criteria for licensure. Certification verifies that an individual or organization has met certain standards of preparation and performance. Both private, nongovernmental agencies and public, governmental agencies issue certificates to individuals and groups.

Certification of Individuals

Certification documents proof of the specific qualifications of RNs who provide professional nursing care in a defined area of practice. A certificate awards the person the right to use the title conferred by the certificate. For example, the Emergency Nurses Association awards a certificate to RNs who meet its qualifications. Those persons may use the title certified emergency nurse (CEN) and write "CEN" after their names.

Nongovernmental Certification

American Nurses Association Certification. The ANA established its certification program in 1973 to "provide tangible recognition of professional achievement in a defined functional or clinical area of nursing." The program is administered by the American Nurses Credentialing

American Nurses Association Certification

Generalist Certification

Requirements: RN license in US; effective 1996, BSN; current clinical practice in specialty; authorized designation RN,C.

General nursing practice

Medical-surgical nurse (plus continuing education in medical-surgical nursing after 1996)

Gerontologic nurse (plus continuing education in gerontological nursing)

Pediatric nurse (plus continuing education in pediatric nursing)

Perinatal nurse (plus continuing education in perinatal nursing)

College health nurse (plus BSN)

School nurse (plus BSN, academic course work, practicum)

Community health nurse (plus BSN)

Psychiatric-mental health nurse (plus access to clinical consultation, letter of reference, continuing education)

Nursing continuing education/staff development (plus BSN)

Home health nurse (plus BSN)

Cardiac rehabilitation nurse (plus BSN, advanced cardiac life support [ACLS] certified, continuing education in cardiac rehabilitation)

Nurse Practitioner Certification

Requirements: RN license in US; effective 1998, masters degree in nursing; current clinical practice in specialty; education in specialty; authorized designation NP.

Adult nurse practitioner

Family nurse practitioner

Center (ANCC) and is "reserved for those nurses who have met requirements for clinical or functional practice in a specialized field, pursued education beyond basic nursing preparation, and received the endorsement of their peers" (American Nurses Credentialing Center 1994). The ANCC offers four categories of certificates: generalist, nurse practitioner, clinical specialist, and nursing administration. See the accompanying box. Applicants submit evidence of education and nursing practice and take an examination in a specific clinical area. Membership in the ANA is not required, and certificates are valid for 5 years. Renewal entails proof of continued education and related clinical practice. For the *Certification Catalog*, write to the American Nurses Credentialing Center, P.O. Box 92820, Washington, DC 20090-2820.

School nurse practitioner
Pediatric nurse practitioner
Gerontologic nurse practitioner

Clinical Specialist Certification
Requirements: RN license in US; effective 1998, masters degree in area of
    specialty; current clinical practice; authorized designation RN,CS.
Clinical specialist in gerontologic nursing
Clinical specialist in medical-surgical nursing
Clinical specialist in community health nursing
Clinical specialist in adult psychiatric & mental health nursing (plus consulta-
    tion/supervision)
Clinical specialist in child and adolescent psychiatric & mental health nursing
    (plus consultation/supervision)

Nursing Administration Certification
Requirements: RN license in US; BS degree; effective 1996, continuing
    education in nursing administration or masters degree in nursing admin-
    istration.
Nursing administration (plus current experience as nurse manager or execu-
    tive; authorized designation: RN,CNA)
Nursing administration, advanced (plus MS degree; effective 1996, continuing
    education in nursing administration or masters degree in nursing admin-
    istration; current experience as nurse executive; authorized designation:
    RN,CNAA)

From: American Nurses Credentialing Center. (1994). *Certification Catalog*. Washington, DC.

Specialty Nursing Organization Certification. Many specialty nursing
organizations offer certification to individuals. The box on page 80
shows a sampling of these organizations and their certificates. Qualified nurses may secure these certificates whether they are members
of the organization or not. Often a related but separate agency actually confers the certificates. This action is taken to avoid what the
Federal Trade Commission ruled was illegal restraint of trade. The
ruling prevents organizations from monopolizing credentials by
requiring membership of applicants.

Governmental Certification

Some states and territories award certificates for advanced practice in
nursing on the basis of specific educational and practice criteria set up

A Sampling of Specialty Organization Certification*

American Association of Critical Care Nurses (AACN)
    Certified critical care nurse (CCRN)
American Association of Occupational Health Nurse (AAOHN)
    Certified occupational health nurse (COHN)
American Association of Nurse Anesthetist (AANA)
    Certified registered nurse anesthetist (CRNA)
American College of Nurse Midwives (ACNM)
    Certified nurse midwife (CNM)
American Society of Post-Anesthesia Nurses
    Certified post-anesthesia nurse (CPAN)
Association of Operating Room Nurses (AORN)
    Certified nurse operating room (CNOR)
Association for Practitioners in Infection Control (APIC)
    Certified in infection control (CIC)
Association of Rehabilitation Nurses (ARN)
    Certified rehabilitation registered nurse (CRRN)
Emergency Nurses' Association (ENA)
    Certified emergency nurse (CEN)
International Association for Enterostomal Therapy (IAET)
    Certified enterostomal therapy nurse (CETN)
National Association of Pediatric Nurse Associates/Practitioners (NAPNAP)
    Certified pediatric nurse practitioner (CPNP)
National Association of School Nurses (NASN)
    Certified school nurse (CSN)
Oncology Nursing Society (ONS)
    Oncology certified nurse (OCN)
The Organization for Obstetric, Gynecologic, & Neonatal Nurses (NAACOG)
    Reproductive nurse certified (RNC):
        Ambulatory women's health care
        High risk obstetric nurse
        Inpatient obstetric nurse
        Low risk neonatal nurse
        Maternal newborn nurse
        Neonatal intensive care nurse
        Reproductive endocrinology/infertility nurse
    Neonatal nurse practitioner (NP)
    Ob/Gyn nurse practitioner (NP)
    Women's health care nurse practitioner (NP)

* Certificates may be awarded by closely related, but separate and independent organizations.

by their board of nursing. They also may recognize certificates awarded by private specialty organizations. Certificates issued by governmental agencies assume legal status because they are enforced by the police power of the state. For example, a state may recognize the certificate issued by the American College of Nurse-Midwives (ACNM) and restrict the title certified nurse midwife (CNM) to persons who meet the ACNM criteria for that certificate. The states authorize a variety of titles for advanced practice nurses, including advanced registered nurse (ARN), nurse practitioner (NP), advanced registered nurse practitioner (ARNP), specialized registered nurse (SRN), independent nurse practitioner (INP), and certified registered nurse (CRN).

A Uniform Credentialing System

Ideally, a system of credentialing for individuals applies universally and communicates qualifications clearly. By 1975, a great many specialty organizations were awarding various certificates reflecting diverse educational requirements. It became apparent to nursing leaders that the system lacked uniformity and consistency. To address the problem the ANA funded a major research study on credentialing in cooperation with 47 specialty groups. Researchers at the University of Wisconsin, Milwaukee School of Nursing guided by an ANA-appointed committee, conducted the study. They assessed all types of credentialing mechanisms, including licensure, certification, and granting of degrees. In the 1978 final report, the researchers suggested various ways to increase the effectiveness of credentialing and a means to implement the proposed changes (ANA 1978).

The major recommendation of the study was that nursing establish a centralized, independent center for credentialing. The authors of the study believed such an independent center would provide the checks and balances necessary to preserve equity for every part of the system. It would be an efficient, cost-effective service that would avoid duplication of efforts and provide geographic mobility for nurses. In 1988 the ANA established just such a center, called the American Nurses Credentialing Center, consolidating all of its credentialing activities. The ANA invited other credentialing organizations to join. Some did, but most did not, choosing instead to retain their independence.

In 1991, eight national nursing certification programs established a new organization, the American Board of Nursing Specialties (ABMS).

They represented the American Nurses Credentialing Center of ANA, American Board for Occupational Health Nursing, American Board of Neuroscience Nursing, Association of Rehabilitation Nurses, Council on Certification of Nurse Anesthetists, National Board of Nutritional Support Certification, Nephrology Nursing Certification Board, and Orthopaedic Nurses Certification Board (Specialty Certification Groups Form Organization 1991). Together, ABMS represents some 150,000 nurses, or about half of all certified RNs (Hurley 1994). The association may eventually lead to a single credentialing center for all advanced practice credentials as recommended in the 1978 study.

Certification of Organizations (Accreditation)

Certification of organizations is called *accreditation*. Much like certification of individuals, accreditation is documented validation that an organization has met certain standards. Both private, nongovernmental agencies such as the NLN, and public, governmental agencies such as boards of nursing, award certificates of accreditation to organizations. They grant the award when the organization demonstrates that they have met specific criteria.

Nongovernmental Accreditation

Educational Institution Accreditation. Both regional and specialized accrediting agencies offer accreditation to educational institutions. Regional accrediting agencies evaluate entire educational institutions. Currently, there are six regional associations for universities and colleges in the United States: (1) New England Association of Schools and Colleges, (2) Middle States Association of Schools and Colleges, (3) North Central Association of Colleges and Secondary Schools, (4) Southern Association of Colleges and Schools, (5) Western Association of Schools and Colleges, and (6) Northwestern Association of Secondary and Higher Schools.

The accreditation process begins with intensive self-evaluation followed by a site visit of peers to confirm the evaluation. An accrediting panel reviews the self-study and report of the visiting team. If the school meets the criteria, the agency awards accreditation for a specific period of time. When a school is accredited, its courses are honored and its graduates are respected by other institutions.

Specialized accrediting agencies evaluate particular programs within educational institutions. The NLN is the designated accrediting agency for all educational programs in nursing. It is nationally recognized by both the nursing profession and the US Office of Education. The NLN continually revises evaluation criteria for nursing programs. Currently, it evaluates programs in five areas: (1) organization and administration, (2) students, (3) faculty, (4) curriculum, and (5) resources, facilities, and services. The process of accreditation consists of a self-study report, a site visit by two or more peers, and scrutiny by a board of review. The board of review grants or denies accreditation, with or without recommendations. Because most graduate programs in nursing require a BSN from an NLN-accredited program, BSN programs seek NLN accreditation.

Health Care Institutional Accreditation. Nongovernmental accreditation of health care institutions is provided by the Joint Commission on Accreditation of Healthcare Organizations (JCAHO) and by state medical associations. As in other accreditations, the process begins with an intensive self-study, followed by a site visit of an evaluation team. Hospitals seek accreditation because it makes them eligible to receive funds from state and federal sources and from insurance companies.

Governmental Accreditation

Governmental accreditation of institutions of higher learning is unusual. However, accreditation of specialized programs within educational institutions is common, especially where the state is responsible for public safety, or for public money. For example, state boards of nursing oversee nursing programs and accredit/approve them for specific periods of time. Boards maintain control by stipulating that only graduates of accredited/approved programs may take the licensure examination.

The accreditation process by boards of nursing is patterned after the NLN model. A board identifies criteria in specific spheres, such as (1) philosophy; (2) policies and procedures; (3) physical space, budget, and personnel; (4) faculty qualifications and roles; (5) curriculum; (6) evaluation plan; (7) clinical facilities; and (8) student involvement. Well before their current accreditation expires, educational programs engage in intensive self-study and write a detailed report. Then, board-appointed evaluators visit the school to verify the report, document their findings, and report them to the board. The board grants or denies accreditation, with or without recommendations, for a specific period of time.

Governmental accreditation of health care institutions varies considerably from state to state. In many jurisdictions, state agencies such as the Department of Health accredit or license health care facilities. In other jurisdictions, state agencies accept accreditation by JCAHO as adequate public protection and do not conduct their own evaluation. When nurses consider employment in a health care facility they should consider the accreditation status of the facility. It is an important indicator of quality of care.

◆ Summary

Credentials, as proof of the qualifications of individuals and groups, take many forms: individual registration, licenses, certificates, and institutional accreditation. The first licensure laws for nurses were really registration acts, with permissive, rather than mandatory licensure. Today, all states and territories have nurse practice acts and administrative boards that regulate registered and practical nursing practice. Their boards of nursing are members of the Council of State Boards of Nursing, the organization that oversees the NCLEX-RN and NCLEX-PN. Professional nursing organizations and licensing boards offer certification of nurses for advance practice roles and accreditation of institutions.

Critical Thinking Questions

1. An argument is a line of reasoning in which certain statements (reasons) are given in support of another statement (the conclusion). For example:

   Reason: Intact skin is the body's first line of defense against pathogens.

   Reason: A surgical incision is a break in this defense.

   Conclusion: Therefore, clients who have had surgery are at increased risk for infection.

   State the argument for institutional licensure. State the argument against institutional licensure.

2. What is your position on specialty certification for nurses? Are you for or against it? How might personal values influence your position?

3. What evidence is there that the ANA is truly committed to a centralized credentialing center? Could this evidence be interpreted in any other way?

Learning Activities

1. Obtain a copy of the nurse practice act and rules and regulations in your state; identify the definition of nursing, licensure requirements, provisions for interim permits, and procedures for disciplinary action.

2. Find out if there is a diversion program for nurses with chemical dependency or mental illness in your state. If so, interview the consultant who oversees the program; ask how it is administered and its success rate. If not, what does the board of nursing do for these nurses?

3. Attend a public meeting of your state board of nursing. Write a paper describing the number of members on the board, their occupations, the role of the executive director and consultants, the issues discussed, and your reactions to the experience.

4. In a group, discuss the advantages and disadvantages of including advanced nursing practice in the nurse practice acts.

5. In an interview with someone in the personnel department of your hospital, find out what certificates are required to hold various nursing positions. Is there a pay differential? Write a report.

6. Debate the advantages and disadvantages of a single certifying agency for nurses.

Annotated Reading List

National League for Nursing. *Policies and Procedures of Accreditation for Programs in Nursing Education,* 6th ed. NLN, 1990.

This informative little book is a definitive guide to the NLN's education accreditation program, its goals and philosophy, and its development of accreditation policies, procedures, and criteria. It offers details of the six stages of the accreditation process: eligibility, application, self-study and report, site visit, evaluation by the Board of Review, and continuing self-evaluation. The book is divided into two sections, the accrediting program and the accrediting process.

Saxton DF, Nugent PM, Pelikan, PK. *Mosby's Comprehensive Review of Nursing,* 14th ed. Mosby, 1993.

This extensive resource prepares graduates to take and pass the NCLEX-RN in the United States and the comprehensive licensure examination in Canada. Reflecting changes in the NCLEX-RN, all content review questions are "stand alone" questions, independent of situations. The text integrates the five-step nursing process in content reviews. It supplies high-quality sample questions, answers with rationales, and two 375-question practice examinations.

References

American Nurses Association. *Suggested State Legislation: Nursing Practice Act, Nursing Disciplinary Diversion Act, Prescriptive Authority Act.* ANA, 1990.

American Nurses Association. *The Study of Credentialing in Nursing: A New Approach.* Vol 1, *The Report of the Committee.* ANA, 1978.

American Nurses Credentialing Center. *Certification Catalog.* 1994.

California Board of Registered Nursing. *Registered Nurses in Recovery.* Diversion Program, 1989.

Hurley ML. The Push for Specialty Certification. *RN.* 36-44, June 1994.

LeBar C. *Statutory Requirements for Licensing of Nurses.* ANA, 1984.

National Council of State Boards of Nursing. *Test Plan of the National Council Licensure Examination for Registered Nurses.* NCSBN, 1987.

National Council of State Boards of Nursing. *The Model Nurse Practice Act*. NCSBN, 1982.

National Council of State Boards of Nursing. The NCLEX Development Process. *Issues*, NCSBN, 1993.

National Council of State Boards of Nursing. Walk-through of the Computerized Testing Experience. *Issues*, NCSBN, 1993.

New FNG Credentials Service is Launched. *Amer J Nurs* 81, November 1993.

Specialty Certification Groups Form Organization. *Am Nurs* 23(4):20, 1991.

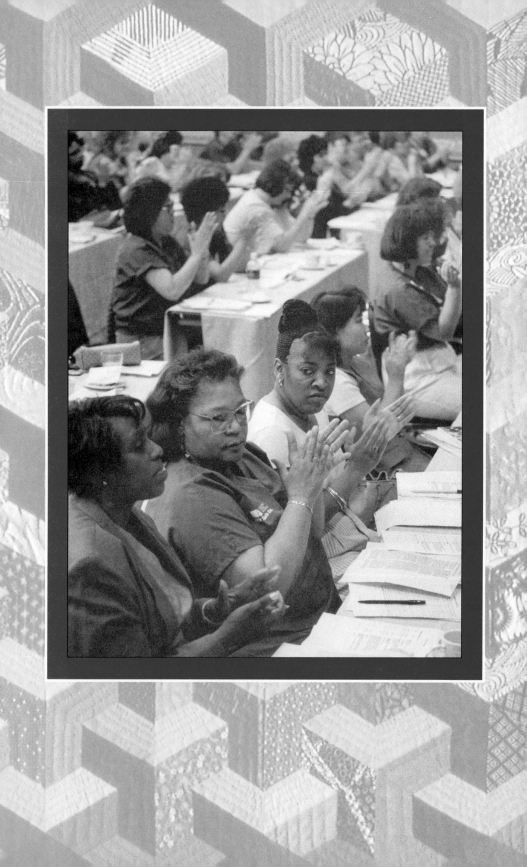

Nursing Organizations

◆ Learning Objectives

- Describe the origin, membership requirements, organizational structure, purposes, and activities of an alumni association.

- Recount the origin, membership provisions, organizational structure, and activities of the American Nurses Association (ANA).

- Describe the membership requirements, organizational structure, and major activities of the National Student Nurses Association (NSNA).

- Explain the relationship of the stated purposes and functions of the National League for Nursing (NLN) to its historical beginnings.

- Compare the membership requirements and organizational structure of the ANA and NLN.

- State the purposes, functions, and membership of the International Council of Nurses (ICN).

- State the frequency and next scheduled dates of the conventions/congress of the ANA, NLN, NSNA, and ICN.

- Explain the increasing membership of specialty organizations in the past 20 years.

- Discuss the importance of government and health-related organizations to the nursing profession.

- Name the official publications of the ANA, NLN, NSNA, and ICN.

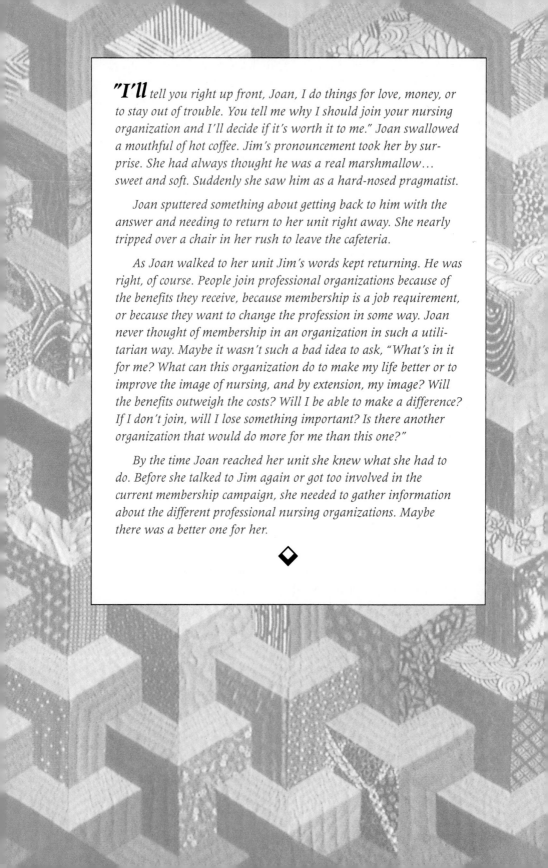

"*I'll* tell you right up front, Joan, I do things for love, money, or to stay out of trouble. You tell me why I should join your nursing organization and I'll decide if it's worth it to me." Joan swallowed a mouthful of hot coffee. Jim's pronouncement took her by surprise. She had always thought he was a real marshmallow… sweet and soft. Suddenly she saw him as a hard-nosed pragmatist.

Joan sputtered something about getting back to him with the answer and needing to return to her unit right away. She nearly tripped over a chair in her rush to leave the cafeteria.

As Joan walked to her unit Jim's words kept returning. He was right, of course. People join professional organizations because of the benefits they receive, because membership is a job requirement, or because they want to change the profession in some way. Joan never thought of membership in an organization in such a utilitarian way. Maybe it wasn't such a bad idea to ask, "What's in it for me? What can this organization do to make my life better or to improve the image of nursing, and by extension, my image? Will the benefits outweigh the costs? Will I be able to make a difference? If I don't join, will I lose something important? Is there another organization that would do more for me than this one?"

By the time Joan reached her unit she knew what she had to do. Before she talked to Jim again or got too involved in the current membership campaign, she needed to gather information about the different professional nursing organizations. Maybe there was a better one for her.

◆

An important function of a professional organization is to enhance the personal identity of the members as a group, their "profession-hood" (Styles 1982) and to "shape the profession and make a difference" (Bower 1994). Through their many activities, these organizations benefit both individual nurses and the profession as a whole. They provide professional and public education, support the economic welfare of nurses, set standards, grant scholarships, give recognition, supply opportunities for networking, support research, take political action, and work with other organizations to solve health problems.

There are a great many nursing organizations. Each year the *American Journal of Nursing* publishes a *Directory of Nursing and Health-Related Organizations*, reproduced in part in Appendix B. Although the number and variety is immense, these organizations can be grouped into five categories: alumni, general interest, special interest, government, and health-related.

◆ Alumni Organizations

Description and History

Alumnae organizations were the first professional organizations for nurses. *Alumna* is the female form of the word; *alumnae* is the plural female form. Those early organizations were called alumnae organizations because only women were admitted to and graduated from schools of nursing. Today, with both men and women graduates, the correct name is the plural form of *alumnus*, or *alumni*.

The oldest alumni organization in United States was organized in 1889 by graduates of the Bellevue Hospital Training School in New York. Others followed, including the Illinois Training School in 1891, Johns Hopkins Hospital Training School in 1892, and Massachusetts General Hospital School in 1895. In 1897, representatives of ten alumnae associations established the National Associated Alumnae of United States and Canada. When the association sought incorporation, it found that New York law prohibited foreign membership. Thus, "and Canada" was removed from the name. In 1911 the name was changed to the American Nurses Association (ANA). In 1908, Canadian nurses formed the Provisional Organization of the Canadian National Association of Trained Nurses. In 1924 they changed the name to Canadian Nurses Association (CNA) (Donahue 1985).

Even though the ANA in the United States and the CNA in Canada became the consolidated voices for nursing, individual alumni organizations across the United States and Canada continued to thrive.

Membership and Organizational Structure

Membership in alumni organizations traditionally is open to graduates, faculty, and individuals the school wants to honor. The organizational structure of alumni associations varies from school to school. Some are independent organizations. Others are subgroups of larger alumni organizations, a common arrangement for university schools of nursing.

Purpose and Activities

Regardless of the organizational structure, alumni organizations provide a lifelong link between the school and its graduates. Alumni groups offer numerous mutual benefits. They provide a pool of committed graduates to whom schools look for advice on current nursing practice, assistance with recruitment, fund-raising for scholarships and research, and service as mentors and role models to students and new graduates. Alumni groups help members maintain a personal commitment to and identification with the ideals graduates first encountered as students. They provide continuing education and a channel for networking with others in the nursing profession. Alumni organizations offer a means of maintaining a special personal and professional bond between members. They furnish a focus for membership pride and an opportunity to display loyalty to the nursing profession. Usually dues are minimal and time commitments are optional. Regardless of what other professional memberships nurses maintain, they reap lifelong benefits from membership in alumni associations.

◆ General-Interest Organizations

General nursing organizations serve a wide spectrum of nurses and engage in a variety of activities. The most notable of these organizations are the American Nurses Association, National Student Nurses Association, National League for Nursing, and International Council of Nurses. Although Sigma Theta Tau International is an honorary society, we have included it in the general-interest group because it engages in a variety of professional activities and is the second largest nursing organization in United States.

◆ American Nurses Association

Description and History

The American Nurses Association (ANA) is the largest professional organization for registered nurses in United States. It is composed of three constituent member groups: state nurses associations, multi-state nurses associations, and US nurses' overseas associations (ANA 1993). These constituents include over 900 regional associations serving nurses at the local level.

As related earlier, the ANA grew out of the Nurses' Associated Alumnae of United States and Canada. Since its founding in 1897 and subsequent renaming in 1911, the ANA has undergone many changes. Through them all it has remained the leading voice for professional nursing.

Membership and Organizational Structure

Membership in ANA is open to all registered nurses. Individuals become members through a constituent association, such as a state nurses association (SNA). Figure 4-1 shows the organizational structure of ANA as amended in 1993.

At the national level the organization is managed by an executive director and a professional staff headquartered at 600 Maryland Avenue SW, Suite 100 West, Washington DC, 20024. The executive director is hired by the Board of Directors, who are elected by the House of Delegates to carry out their directives. The House of Delegates is made up of representatives from the constituent members. It meets annually and is the top policy-making body of the organization. Elections occur at national conventions held in even-numbered years at various cities throughout the United States.

The ANA Board appoints members to its committees and congresses, holds official membership in the International Council of Nurses, maintains a relationship with the National Student Nurses

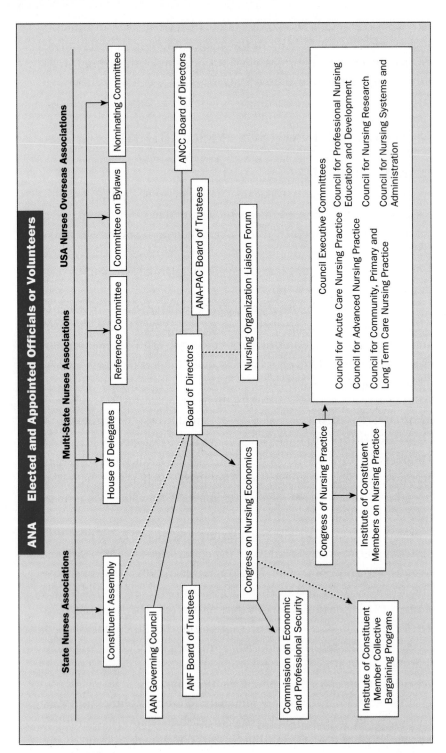

Figure 4-1 Organizational structure of the American Nurses Association (1994).

Association, is sole stockholder of the American Journal of Nursing Company, sponsors the American Nurses Credentialing Center, constitutes the membership of the American Nurses Foundation, and is the ANA liaison with other health-related agencies.

In ANA, a *congress* is an "organized deliberative body that focuses on long-range policy development essential to the mission of the association" (ANA 1993). There are two congresses: the Congress on Nursing Economics and the Congress on Nursing Practice. Each 15-member congress is accountable to the Board of Directors and reports to the House of Delegates. The Congress on Nursing Economics assigns specific duties to its Commission on Economic and Professional Security and Institute of Constituent Members Collective Bargaining Programs. The Congress on Nursing Practice assigns specific duties to its Institute of Constituent Members on Nursing Practice and Councils.

The *councils* are the units through which members participate in improvement or advancement of a specialized area of nursing practice or interest. They are designed to meet the same needs of practitioners that independent specialty organizations meet. Membership in a council is open to individual ANA members who meet the qualifications of that council. Currently there are 12 councils: continuing education, nurse researchers, computer applications in nursing, nursing administration, clinical nurse specialists, psychiatric and mental health nursing, medical-surgical nursing practice, gerontologic nursing, community health nurses, primary health care nurse practitioners, maternal-child nursing, and cultural diversity in nursing.

Purposes and Functions

The purposes of the ANA are to: "(1) work for the improvement of health standards and the availability of health care services for all people, (2) foster high standards of nursing, and (3) stimulate and promote the professional development of nurses and advance their economic and general welfare...unrestricted by considerations of age, color, creed, disability, gender, health status, lifestyle, nationality, race, religion, or sexual orientation" (ANA 1993). The functions of the ANA are to: "(1) establish standards of nursing practice, education, and services, (2) establish a code of ethical conduct for nurses, (3) ensure a system of credentialing in nursing, (4) initiate and influence legislation, governmental programs, national health policy, and international health policy, (5) support systematic study, evaluation, and research in nursing, (6) serve as the central agency for the collection, analysis and dissemination of information relevant to nursing, (7) promote and protect the economic and general welfare of nurses, (8) provide leadership in national and international nursing, (9) provide for the professional development of nurses, (10) conduct an affirmative action program, (11) ensure a collective bargaining program for nurses, (12) provide services to constituent members, (13) maintain communication with constituent members through official publications, (14) assume an active role as consumer advocate, and (15) represent and speak for the nursing profession with allied health groups, national and international organizations, governmental bodies, and the public" (ANA 1993).

Activities

To fulfill its stated functions, the ANA carries on many activities, including certification, political action, publishing, research, collective bargaining, recognition giving, and international participation.

Certification of Individuals

Certification of individuals engaged in advanced nursing practice assures the public and other health care providers that a nurse possesses distinct knowledge and ability in a specialized field. Certification is offered by the American Nurses Credentialing Center in many clinical specialties, at both the generalist and clinical specialist level. The process of certification entails meeting education and practice requirements and passing a written examination. (See Chapter 3.) Detailed requirements for each ANA certificate are published annually in the *Certification Catalog,* available without cost from American Nurses Credentialing Center, 600 Maryland Avenue, SW, Suite 100 West, Washington, DC 20024-2571.

Political Action

The ANA is actively involved in political action through ANA-PAC (Political Action Committee). This is a voluntary, nonpartisan organization that works to meet the legislative objectives of ANA. Its major functions are education and political action. At both the national level and at state and local levels, registered lobbyists and volunteers speak on behalf of nursing and work with legislators on health-related issues.

Publications

The *American Journal of Nursing* (*AJN*) is the official journal of the ANA. It is published monthly by the American Journal of Nursing Company in New York City and is wholly owned and controlled by the ANA. In 1900 the *AJN* became the first nursing journal in the United States to be owned, operated, and published by nurses. ANA also publishes *Nursing Research, MCN: American Journal of Maternal-Child Nursing* and *International Nursing Index*.

The *American Nurse* is the official mouthpiece of the association. Published every other month, it contains official announcements of the association and news relevant to nurses and other healthcare providers. The American Nurses Publishing Company publishes books and pamphlets on many topics. *ANA Publications Catalog* is available without cost by writing to ANA Marketing Services, Box 2244, Waldorf, MD 20604. *AJN* also produces a variety of audiovisual and computer simulation products described in the *AJN Multimedia Catalog*, available without cost from AJN Company, 555 West 57th Street, New York, NY 10019.

Research Support

The American Nurses Foundation (ANF) was established in 1955 as a tax-exempt, nonprofit corporation for the purpose of supporting research related to nursing. The board of directors of the ANA makes up the membership of the ANF. The purpose of the ANF is to conduct analyses of specific problems, to provide information needed to make policy decisions, to develop a group of nurse scholars who are active in such areas as journalism and public policy, and to support the research and educational activities of ANA.

Collective Bargaining

As part of its goal to promote the economic welfare of nurses, an important activity of ANA is to support collective bargaining. These efforts occur at the regional level. They focus not only on financial gains for nurses but also on the rights of nurses to participate in decisions about client care and working conditions. (See Chapter 12.)

Giving Recognition

To recognize the significant contributions of individuals to nursing, the House of Delegates voted to establish the American Academy of

Nursing (AAN) in 1966. The organization is an independent body that reports annually to the Board of Directors of the ANA. The original members were chosen by the Board in 1973. Candidates for membership must be sponsored by at least two members and elected by a majority. An inducted member is designated a Fellow of the American Academy of Nursing and is entitled to use the initials FAAN after his or her name.

National and International Participation

Through its Nursing Organization Liaison Forum (NOLF), the ANA works with a number of United States organizations on issues of concern to the nursing profession. In addition, the ANA collaborates actively with the National Student Nurses Association.

The ANA is the official United States representative to the International Council of Nursing. As such, the ANA speaks to the world for all the nurses in United States. Its delegates attend the quadrennial international congress and participate in other ICN activities.

◇ National Student Nurses Association

Description and History

The National Student Nurses Association (NSNA) is the largest independent health professional student organization in the United States and the only one for nursing students. It was founded in 1953 and incorporated in New York in 1959. It is composed of constituent associations made up of school chapters and state associations. Although the NSNA is a completely independent organization, it works closely with the American Nurses Association and the National League for Nursing to give and receive information and points of view.

Membership and Organizational Structure

Membership in the NSNA is open to all students in programs for registered nurses and to students taking prenursing courses in colleges offering nursing programs. There are four categories of members: active, associate (prenursing majors), sustaining (non-student, interested individuals or organizations), and honorary. If membership is

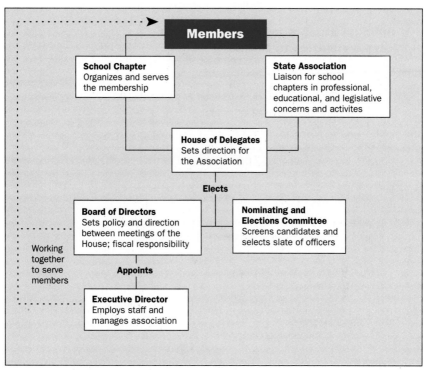

Figure 4-2 Organizational structure of the National Student Nurses Association.

not available through a local or state association, eligible students may join the NSNA as individual members.

Members have representation in the House of Delegates through school and state associations (constituents). The House of Delegates is the major decision-making body of the NSNA, meeting annually in cities throughout the United States. The House sets the direction of the association and elects members of the Board of Directors and the Nominating and Election Committee (NSNA 1993).

The Board of Directors is composed solely of student nurses. Between meetings of the House, it sets the policy for the NSNA, has fiscal responsibility, and directs the activities of the association. The Board maintains liaison with the ANA, the NLN, state boards of nursing, and Congress and constitutes the membership of the NSNA Foundation, a separate corporation providing scholarships for nursing students. The Board appoints an Executive Director who, with a professional staff, manages the association from the national headquarters at 555 W. 57th Street, New York, NY 10019. See Figure 4-2.

National Student Nurses Association Responsibilities to Members

Communication

Provide communication mechanisms for constituents
Develop guidelines and evaluation tools
Produce and distribute publications
Publish magazine/newsletters
Serve as a clearinghouse for resources and referral information
Public relations

Education

Provide leadership training for self-governance activities
Liaison with appropriate state and national associations
Liaison with state boards of nursing
Liaison with schools of nursing
Develop guidelines
Plan programs to train students for participation in curriculum committees
Provide consultation services
Provide educational programs

Finances

Manage finances
Seek funding: contract/grants
Provide financial consultation
Serve as a clearinghouse for scholarships, traineeships, and loan
  information
Develop guidelines
Provide fund-raising information

Legislation

Political education
Voter registration campaign

Purposes and Responsibilities

The purposes of NSNA are to "assume responsibility for contributing to nursing education in order to provide for the highest quality health care, provide programs representative of fundamental and current professional interests and concerns, and aid in the development of the whole person, his/her professional role, and his/her responsibility for the health care of people in all walks of life" (NSNA 1993).

Liaison with legislators on certain legislation
Liaison with legislative organizations
Liaison with government agencies
Develop legislative positions as needed
Monitor legislation
Develop guidelines
Distribute information

Membership services

Process membership
Distribute membership cards
Gather statistics and keep records
Provide benefits and services
Assist in recruitment and retention of members

Recruitment into nursing and career counseling

Liaison with faculty, deans, and directors of nursing schools
Liaison with hospital recruiters
Career counseling services
Develop and distribute materials
Promote Breakthrough to Nursing Project

Relationships with other organizations

Liaison with appropriate national and international associations
    eg, ANA, NLN
Liaison with appropriate student health associations
Represent NSNA members' views

Student rights and grievance information

Disseminate the Bill of Rights and Responsibilities for
    Nursing Students

From: *Getting the Pieces to Fit Together 1993/94.* NSNA, 1993.

To clarify its obligation, the NSNA publishes a list of its responsibilities to members. See the accompanying box. It also publishes lists of reciprocal responsibilities to help constituent state associations and school chapters understand their specific functions.

The NSNA fulfills its purposes by promoting and encouraging participation in community affairs and activities; representing students to consumers, institutions, and other organizations; promoting collaborative relationships with other nursing and health organizations; influencing the educational process; and promoting and encouraging students' participation in interdisciplinary activities and recruiting efforts, regardless of race, color, creed, lifestyle, sex, national origin, age, or economic status.

Activities

Some of the most significant activities of the NSNA are in the areas of networking, political action, scholarship, recruitment, publishing, and community service.

Networking

At the annual convention, mid-year conference, and many other national, state, and local gatherings, members have the opportunity to meet other nursing students from many geographic areas and backgrounds. The resulting collegial network provides support and encouragement, serving individuals long after graduation.

Political Action

One of the important activities of the NSNA is political action, whereby it takes positions on a wide range of subjects, including collective bargaining, education, health care, and the environment. Once the House of Delegates votes to take a position on some issue, the officers and members may promote that position in the name of the NSNA.

Scholarships

Each year the NSNA Foundation gives thousands of scholarship dollars to nursing students. These tax-deductible funds are donated by various individuals and organizations and distributed according to criteria approved by the Board of Directors. Scholarships are available to both NSNA members and nonmembers.

Recruitment

Since 1965, the NSNA has actively supported Project Breakthrough to Nursing, an undertaking aimed at recruiting nurses from minority groups, such as African Americans, Hispanics, and Native Americans. NSNA members gather information about nursing programs in their geographic area. Then they go out into the community to speak to minority groups, encouraging them to consider a career in nursing.

Publications

The official journal of the NSNA is *Imprint*, which is published four times during the academic year and sent to all members. The *NSNA News* contains news of the organization. It is published six times a year and sent to state officers and school presidents. The NSNA also publishes many useful pamphlets on such topics as guidelines for planning meetings, career planning, and taking legislative action.

Community Service

At the local level, members of the NSNA participate in many types of community service. They set up and assist with such things as health fairs, hypertension screening, activities focused on the prevention of child and elder abuse, and immunization drives. By so doing, members of the NSNA enhance the image of nursing, gain valuable experience, and provide needed services.

◇ National League for Nursing

Description and History

The National League for Nursing (NLN) was formed in 1952 from the merger of seven national organizations: the National League of Nursing Education, the National Association of Collegiate Schools of Nursing, the Association of Collegiate Schools of Nursing, the Joint Committee on Practical Nurses and Auxiliary Workers on Nursing Service, the Joint Committee on Careers in Nursing, the National Committee for the Improvement of Nursing Services, and the National Nursing Accrediting Services (NLN 1991).

With the formation of the NLN, two large nursing organizations, each with a different emphasis, were available to nurses: the ANA, focusing on the needs of individual nurses and the profession, and the NLN, focusing on nursing education and nursing service. In 1989, the NLN created the Community Health Accreditation Program to accredit community health agencies and the National League for Health Care, Inc., to sponsor for-profit projects.

Membership and
Organizational Structure

There are four classes of members in NLN: individual, agency, allied agency, and honorary. Individual membership is open to anyone who is interested in "fostering the development and improvement of nursing services or education" (NLN 1991). There are three types of individual members: student, retired, and life. Agency membership is open to any organization that provides nursing service or conducts an educational program in nursing. Category I agency members have 10 votes, category II have 5 votes. Allied agency membership is open to organizations that do not provide nursing service or conduct educational programs in nursing. Allied agency members have no vote. Honorary membership is conferred by the Board of Governors on "persons whose position or special interest in the League and its objectives qualifies them for such honor" (NLN 1991). Honorary members pay no dues and do not vote or hold office. Members participate at the community level in Constituent Leagues and in the special interest councils of their choice.

At the national level, the NLN is governed by a Board of Governors and managed by a chief executive officer and staff, headquartered at 350 Hudson Street, New York, NY 10014. The Board meets at least once in even-numbered years and just before and after the biennial convention, held in odd-numbered years. Five advisory standing committees formulate policy proposals and programs, including the Committee on Constitution and Bylaws, Finance, Nominations, Accreditation, and Education and Practice.

The councils are open to all members and represent the special interest of members. They meet at least once a year and are created or dissolved according to need. Currently, councils exist in these areas: Nurse Executives, Nursing Centers, Nursing Informatics, Nursing Practice, Research in Nursing Education, Associate Degree Programs, Baccalaureate and Higher Degree Programs, Community Health Services, Constituent Leagues, Diploma Programs, and Practical Nurse Programs.

Purpose and Functions

The purpose of the NLN or "League," as it is fondly called, is "to foster the development and improvement of hospital, industrial, public health, and other organized nursing service and of nursing education through the coordinated action of nurses, allied professional groups, citizens, agencies, and schools to the end that the nursing needs of the people will be met" (NLN 1991). As a consequence, the NLN and ANA, together with the American Association of Colleges of Nursing and the National Organization of Nurse Executives, formed the Tri-Council. This organization provides expert testimony for committees and commissions that are considering health-related legislation.

The functions of NLN are to "identify the nursing needs of society and to foster programs designed to meet these needs; develop and support services for the improvement of nursing service and nursing education through consultation, continuing education, testing, accreditation, evaluation, and other activities; work with voluntary, governmental, and other agencies, groups, and organizations for the advancement of nursing and toward the achievement of comprehensive health care; and to respond in appropriate ways to universal nursing needs" (NLN 1991).

Activities

The League engages in numerous activities that help it fulfill its stated functions, including consultation and accreditation, testing and evaluation, information and continuing education, publishing, and research.

Accreditation and Consultation

Accreditation is a voluntary self-study process whereby a school or agency measures aspects of its program or service against a set of criteria. When the self-study is completed, peer reviewers visit the school or agency to verify the findings of the study. If they find that the school or agency meets the criteria, the NLN issues a certificate of accreditation for a specific period of time. (See Chapter 3.)

The NLN is designated by the US Office of Education as the official accrediting body for all nursing education programs. Members of the education councils from accredited schools develop specific criteria, which the NLN publishes. It provides workshops and other opportunities for schools to discuss the accreditation process. In addition, schools may employ a League consultant for special help to meet accreditation standards. The accreditation process is carried out by peer reviewers: faculty members and administrators from similar schools.

The Community Health Accreditation Program (CHAP) provides accreditation for community and home care agencies throughout the United States (NLN April 1994). The process is similar to the model used for accrediting schools of nursing.

Testing and Evaluation

The NLN pioneered testing and evaluation services in nursing and supervised the first licensure examinations. Although it does not currently produce the licensing tests, it provides a wide variety of tests for practical and registered nurses, including pre-entrance, achievement, and proficiency tests. Schools across the US use these tests to help students and faculty evaluate learning. Catalogs describing these tests are available from NLN headquarters.

Information and Continuing Education

The NLN Career Information Service publishes lists of accredited schools, scholarships, and loans for prospective students and others. The NLN Office of Public Affairs collects data in broad areas of nursing concerns. Consequently, it serves as a source of information for legislative hearings on nursing education. The NLN offers continuing education workshops and conferences throughout the nation on topics selected in consultation with the councils.

Publications and Multimedia

The official mouthpiece of NLN is the monthly publication *Nursing and Health Care*. It focuses on educational and administrative concepts, theories, methods of health care delivery, research, and other broad issues that affect nursing. The NLN offers numerous pamphlets, books, and audiovisual products in a wide range of topics. In 1994, NLN began offering various publications on "e-book" Internet Bookstore and on CD-ROM (NLN May 1994). These materials are described in the annual *Book & Video Catalog*, available without cost by writing to NLN, 350 Hudson Street, New York, NY 10014.

Research

The Division of Research collects statistical data about nurses, nursing education, and nursing service, publishing it in the annual *Nursing DataSource*. It also publishes an annual "blue book" about state-accredited schools of nursing, and conducts other useful studies.

◆ International Council of Nurses

Description and History

The International Council of Nurses (ICN) is the oldest international professional organization in the health care field. It is a federation of nurses' associations from around the world, banded together to improve nursing service and education and to address professional ethics. Through its member associations, ICN represents about a million nurses. It was one of the first health care organizations to adopt a policy of nondiscrimination on the basis of nationality, race, creed, color, politics, sex, or social status.

The ICN began as an idea among nursing leaders at the Columbia Exposition in Chicago in 1893. A provisional committee laid the groundwork in 1899. At a meeting of the International Council of Women in London, ICN was founded. In 1900, the constitution was adopted, with nurses from England, United States, Canada, New Zealand, Australia, and Denmark listed as founding members (Bridges 1967). By 1994, there were 114 members ("A Real Look 'Inside'" 1994).

Membership and Organizational Structure

The membership of ICN is composed of one national nurses' association from each member country. The ANA is the constituent member from the United States, and the Canadian Nurses Association the member from Canada. The governing body of the ICN is the Council of National Representatives (CNR), composed of the president of each member association. It meets every two years and operates on a one-country-one-vote principle.

The Board of Directors of ICN consists of the president, three vice-presidents, seven area representatives, and four members-at-large. Representatives are elected from seven regions of the world: Africa, Eastern Mediterranean, Europe, North America, South and Central America, Southeast Asia, and Western Pacific. The Board makes decisions for the ICN between meetings of the CNR, recommends action to the CNR, appoints committees, and governs the Florence Nightingale International Foundation, an endowed trust established to advance nursing education. The Professional Services

Committee and Socioeconomic Welfare Committee consider trends and problems relative to nursing education, practice, service, and the socioeconomic welfare of nurses.

An executive director and staff manage ICN from the headquarters at 3 place Jean-Marteau, CH-1201, Geneva, Switzerland. The ICN maintains an official relationship with many international organizations, including the World Health Organization (WHO), United Nations Educational, Scientific, and Cultural Organization (UNESCO), International Labour Organization, United Nations International Children's Emergency Fund (UNICEF), Economic and Social Council, and International Committee of the Red Cross.

The official journal of the ICN is the *International Nursing Review*, published bimonthly in English, French, and Spanish. The ICN produces many other publications, such as *Guidelines for Public Policy Development Related to Health, Cost-Effectiveness in Health Care Services, Guidelines for Nursing Research Development*, and *Caring for the Carers*.

Purposes

The purposes of ICN are "to promote the development of strong national nurses associations, assist national nurses associations to improve standards of nursing and competence of nurses, assist national nurses associations to improve the status of nurses within each country, and serve as the authoritative international voice for nurses and nursing" (ICN 1993).

Activities

The activities of the ICN reflect the broad range of interests and needs of its international membership. These interests include education, nursing practice and service, legislation, research, economic welfare of nurses, and cooperation with other health professions. At any given time, the ICN is involved in 30 to 40 projects. These include regulating nursing practice, revising and updating the ethical code for nurses, conducting educational programs in various cities throughout the world, making policy statements on health and social issues, offering legislative seminars, administering the annual 3M Nursing Fellowship Programme awards, and staging the Quadrennial Congress, next scheduled in 1997 in Vancouver, Canada.

A recent project of immense importance to nursing is the creation of an International Classification of Nursing Practice. It will establish a common language about nursing practice; describe nursing care; enable comparison of nursing data across clinical populations, settings, and time; project trends; stimulate nursing research; and provide data about nursing practice to influence health policy decisions (Clark & Lang 1992).

As individuals, nurses are not eligible for membership in ICN. However, as members of the ANA they are a part of the worldwide voice of nursing and can participate in ICN activities. The ICN keeps nurses informed of international opportunities, educational programs, and scholarships available to individuals.

◇ Sigma Theta Tau International Honor Society of Nursing

Description and History

Sigma Theta Tau International Honor Society of Nursing was founded in 1922 by six nursing students at Indiana University. The founders chose the name from the initials of the Greek words *storga, tharos,* and *tima,* meaning love, courage, and honor. The society is the second-largest nursing organization in United States. By 1994 it had more than 200,000 inducted members, 60% of whom held graduate degrees, and 345 chapters in 58 countries. Chapters are located in colleges and universities with bachelor's or higher degree programs in nursing. The society is managed by an executive officer/editor and headquartered at 550 West North Street, Indianapolis, Indiana 46202.

Membership and Organizational Structure

There are two types of members, regular and honorary. Regular membership is by election to a local chapter. Candidates must demonstrate superior scholastic achievement, evidence of professional leadership potential, and/or marked achievement in a field of nursing. They may be community nurse leaders or students enrolled in bachelor's and master's degree accredited nursing programs. Honorary membership is awarded by the Governing Council to persons who are not eligible for regular membership but are nationally recognized in nursing or other fields that contribute to nursing. Honorary members are inducted at the biennial convention.

Ultimate power rests with the House of Delegates. This body consists of two delegates from each chapter, elected officers, standing committee chairpersons, regional coordinators, the editor of the official journal, and regional coordinators. The House meets biennially to elect officers and address other issues of concern to the society.

Purposes

The purposes of Sigma Theta Tau are to recognize superior achievement, foster high professional standards, recognize the development of leadership qualities, encourage creative work, and strengthen commitment to the ideas and purposes of the nursing profession.

Activities

Sigma Theta Tau sponsors theory and research conferences, seminars for writers, special conferences, and programs focusing on nursing and health issues. The society encourages professional development and recognizes achievement through many awards, including the Founder's Awards, Regional Media Awards, Research Utilization Award, Information Resources Technology Awards, Honorary Memberships, Distinguished Lecturer Recognition, Public Service Awards, and the Baxter Foundation Episterme Award for a highly significant single research accomplishment. Sigma Theta Tau supports research with grants to qualified applicants and sponsors of the Nursing Knowledge Series, Research Utilization Series, and Writers Grantswriting Series. The Society publishes *Image: Journal of Nursing Scholarship*, *Directory of Nurse Researchers*, *Online Journal of Knowledge Synthesis for Nursing*, monographs on research findings, and its official mouthpiece, *Reflections*. It maintains the International Nursing Library, a comprehensive focal point for nursing research. This state-of-the-art electronic library is designed to assist nurses with the development, utilization, and dissemination of nursing research findings to the public.

◆ Special-Interest Organizations

Description and History

As nursing practice diversified and nurses began to specialize, they felt a need for personal and professional support. They formed local groups, such as the Industrial Nurses Club, established in 1915, and the Nurses Christian Fellowship, begun in 1936. As other nurses heard of these clubs, they formed their own groups, and these combined into larger groups. As a result, from 1965 to 1985 the number of special-interest nursing organizations increased dramatically, and the number of nurses actively supporting the ANA decreased. In an effort to stem the tide and meet the needs of individual nurses, the ANA instituted councils in areas such as gerontologic nursing, maternal-child nursing, and nursing administration. As a means to increase communication between itself and the specialty organizations, the ANA formed the Nursing Organization Liaison Forum.

In 1973, a group of specialty organizations formed the National Federation of Specialty Nursing Organizations to provide a formal network between their organizations. In 1981 the name was changed to the National Federation for Specialty Nursing Organizations. Its purpose is to foster excellence in specialty nursing practice by providing a forum for communication and collaboration and to support activities that contribute to the recognition of specialty nursing practice.

Types

Special interest nursing organizations fall into five groups: clinically related, educational, political action, honorary, and minority. Clinically-related organizations make up the largest group of specialty organizations. These include such organizations as the American Association of Occupational Health Nurses, Inc., and the Association of Operating Room Nurses. Educational groups include such organizations as the American Association of Colleges of Nursing and the National Association for Practical Nurse Education and Service. Political action groups include the Nurses Coalition for Action in Politics (N-CAP) and others whose primary purpose is to influence legislative bodies. Honorary organizations include such organizations as the American Academy of Nursing and Sigma Theta Tau International. Minority organizations include such groups as the National Black Nurses Association, Inc., and the Lesbian and Gay Nurses Alliance.

Purposes and Activities

The specific purposes of special interest organizations vary, but in general they promote the personal and professional growth of members and support their collective concerns. To carry out their purposes, specialty organizations engage in a wide variety of activities, including sharing information; providing educational seminars, workshops, and conferences; publishing; lobbying; and networking. Volunteers run many of these organizations from modest headquarters. As a result, dues are low and participation of members is high. These factors contribute to the success of specialty organizations. Membership in these organizations enhances professional satisfaction but should not prevent membership and participation in the ANA and NLN.

◆ Government Agencies

Nurses are members of a variety of agencies of the US government, especially those whose primary focus is health, such as the US Public Health Service, and those whose policies indirectly affect nursing and health, such as the Office of Personnel Management. Because of the numbers of agencies and volume of information available about them, they are not described in detail in this chapter. However, complete information about them is available by writing to the agency in question. Addresses of some agencies are listed in Appendix B.

◆ Health-Related Organizations

There are many health-related organizations of particular interest to nurses, such as the American Heart Association, the American Cancer Society, Planned Parenthood, and the like. Most are not-for-profit corporations that provide direct client care, fund research, and offer professional education and public information. Nurses can contribute a great deal to these organizations and can gain much in return. Their contribution may be to raise funds, lobby legislatures, give direct client services, teach, hold office, serve as spokespeople, function on committees, and lend reputation and expertise. Nurses benefit from these groups by developing new skills, obtaining additional education, participating in research projects, acquiring a network of personal and professional colleagues, and finding satisfaction in working in an area of intense personal interest.

◇ Summary

One of the criteria of a profession is that it maintain its own professional organizations. Nurses can experience their "professionhood" by becoming officially identified with one or more of these organizations. These groups can be classified as alumni, general-interest, special interest, government, and health-related. They perform many important activities: providing education, setting standards, giving recognition, supporting economic welfare, and contributing to research. By active involvement in these organizations, nurses have a part in shaping and advancing their profession and informing the public of its achievements.

Critical Thinking Questions

1. Practice insightful thinking (refer to the box "Questions That Stimulate Effective Thinking" in Chapter 5). Given the stated purposes of the ANA, how can you account for the relatively small percentage of nurses who are members?

2. Given the strict criteria for membership in Sigma Theta Tau, what would you cite as the primary reason it continues to grow and prosper?

3. Relevant information is information that pertains to the issue at hand. Before you decide to join a nursing organization, what relevant information do you need? State one piece of information about a nursing organization that would not be relevant to your decision about joining.

1. To a group of beginning nursing students, present the history, organizational structure, and activities of a nursing school alumni association.

2. Visit the office and attend a meeting of a region or state nurses' association.

3. Debate the assertion: Membership in the ANA is the mark of a true professional.

4. Write a comparison of the ANA and NLN regarding the following: types of members, purposes, policy-making body, activities, publications, and national convention dates.

5. Present the benefits of membership in the NSNA, its organizational structure, and primary activities to a group of nursing students.

6. Present the purposes, membership requirements, and benefits of membership of several specialty organizations to a discussion group.

7. Write a list of government and health-related agencies whose services may help the following: sexually active teenager, homeless schizophrenic, veteran, caregiver of an aged, disoriented client.

8. Review copies of the official publication of the ANA, NLN, and NSNA. Note the types of articles, editorial slant, and special features.

Annotated Reading List

American Nurses Association. *ANA Bylaws*, as Amended June 18, 1993. ANA, 1993.

The actual bylaws of an organization provide uncluttered, factual information and make surprisingly interesting reading. It is particularly valuable to see how the philosophical position of the ANA is reflected in its bureaucratic structure.

National League for Nursing. *NLN Bylaws*. NLN, 1991.

The NLN bylaws are unexpectedly brief. The bureaucratic structure and even the writing style of the NLN reflect its philosophy. Worthwhile reading!

Moloney MM. *Professionalization of Nursing, Current Issues and Trends*, 2nd ed. Lippincott, 1992.

This text examines the concept of professionalism and "nursing's journey toward its current state of professionalism." It describes the development of nursing's scientific knowledge base as well as the issues of autonomy and control of nursing education and practice by the nursing profession. The text is comprehensive, realistic, fact-filled, and highly readable.

References

American Nurses Association. *ANA Bylaws,* as amended June 18, 1993. ANA, 1993.

A Real Look "Inside." *Int Nurs Rev* 41,3,66, 1994.

Bower F. Personal communication. 1994.

Bridges DC. *History of the International Council of Nurses, 1899–1964, the First 65 Years.* Lippincott, 1967.

Clark J, Lang N. An Internal Classification for Nursing Practice. *Int Nurs Rev* 39,4,109-112, 1992.

Donahue MP. *Nursing, the Finest Art.* Mosby, 1985.

National Student Nurses Association. *Getting the Pieces to Fit Together 1993/94.* NSNA, 1993.

International Council of Nursing. *ICN Bylaws.* 1993.

National League for Nursing. *NLN Bylaws, June 1991.* NLN, 1991.

NLN News. CHAP is Here to Stay. *Nurs & Health Care* 15:4 205 April 1994.

NLN News. President Carol Lindemann Briefs NLN Council Executive Committees. *Nurs & Health Care* 15:5, 266-268 May 1994.

Styles M. *On Nursing: Toward a New Endowment.* Mosby, 1982.

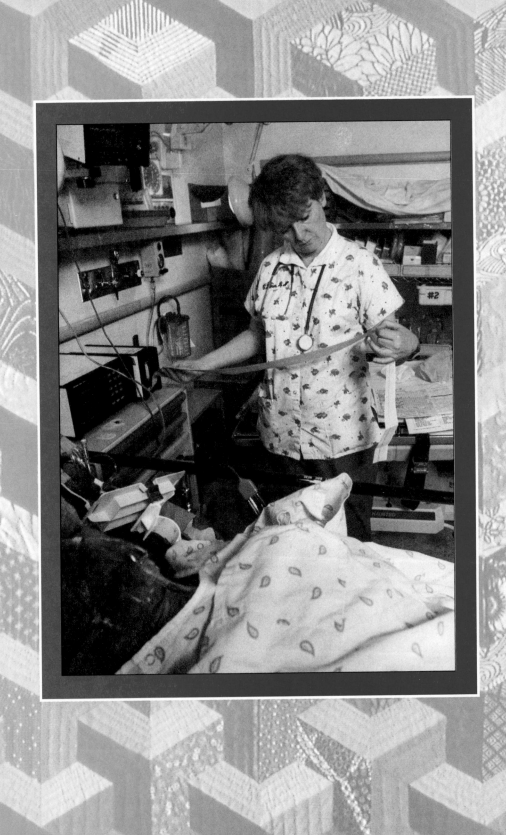

Critical Thinking, Cultural Competence, and Caring

◆ Learning Objectives

- Compare various definitions of critical thinking.

- Describe the characteristics of critical thinkers.

- Compare factual, imaginative, rational, and evaluative thinking.

- Discuss ways to apply critical thinking skills in nursing practice.

- Explain the relevance of culture to nursing practice.

- Explain the characteristics of culture.

- Discuss how nurses can become culturally competent practitioners.

- Compare the various definitions of caring.

- Explain and illustrate each of Leininger's tenets of the culture care theory.

- Describe qualities of power associated with caring.

Claire *came home from her first day in the emergency department. Her body ached from stress. Traumatic images filled her
mind. As a senior student she had looked forward to ED, but today
was unreal! With anger she remembered the young bride from
North Africa who had been circumcised as a child. A prearranged
marriage brought her to the United States. On her wedding night,
when the groom's specially-grown fingernail could not tear open
her vagina, he used a knife. That was a week ago. When his bride
became too feverish and weak to stand, the husband brought her
to the hospital. Claire remembered how respectfully the ED nurse
asked the husband's permission to examine his wife. She thought
of how the nurse protected her privacy and gently examined the
terrified, but silent woman. Claire shuddered and closed her eyes.*

*Other images flooded Claire's mind . . . the baby someone found in
a garbage can, its cord attached, but its heart still beating . . . the
Vietnamese immigrant with horrible burns on his face from a
grease fire in the kitchen where he worked . . . the teenager shot in
the back by a random bullet. In each situation the ED nurses
rapidly assessed and analyzed client conditions, making crucial
decisions based on knowledge and experience. They demonstrated
respect for the diverse values and beliefs of their clients, and they
displayed immense kindness and sensitivity. Claire admired them
and wanted to become as capable as they. She realized how much
more she needed to know about critical thinking, cultural competence, and caring.*

◆

In 1915, Anne Goodrich wrote, "Nursing imbues the simplest acts with importance and instills a desire for the utmost skill and accuracy in their performance. Beyond all other drives [nursing] commands devoted service, ... a broad perspective, ... rigorous analyses, close association with scientific findings, fine perceptions, and enduring tolerance born of understanding" (1964, p. 62). If Anne Goodrich were alive she might use the terminology of the day and say, "Nursing commands, beyond all other abilities *critical thinking*, *cultural competence*, and *caring*." Each of these abilities is necessary for a professional nurse in the twenty-first century, for each contributes to a richer understanding of the other and to a wider perspective of the future of nursing practice.

◆ Critical Thinking

You may ask, "What is critical thinking? How do I know when I am thinking critically? How can I use critical thinking in nursing practice?"

Critical thinking has been defined in many ways. Paul (1990, p. 2) said it was "a disciplined, intellectual process of applying skillful reasoning as a guide to belief or action." The nursing faculty of the University of Missouri defined critical thinking as "the systematic use of reflective reasoning to solve problems and make effective decisions (1992, p. 117)." Bandman and Bandman (1988, p. 5) said it as "the rational examination of ideas, inferences, assumptions, principles, arguments, conclusions, issues, statements, beliefs, and actions." Chaffee (1990, p. 37) said critical thinking "makes sense of our world by carefully examining the thinking process in order to clarify and improve understanding," and Strader (1992, p. 226) described it as "the process of examining underlying assumptions about current evidence and interpreting and evaluating arguments for the purpose of reaching a conclusion from a new perspective."

Kozier et al (1995, p. 185) said, "*critical* means requiring careful judgment and *thinking* means having an opinion, reflecting, pondering, calling to mind, remembering, forming a mental picture, and reasoning. Therefore, critical thinking is a purposeful mental activity in which ideas are produced and evaluated, plans made, and desired conclusions determined."

Some definitions of critical thinking include the idea of *creative thinking*. This is because creative thinking is more likely to occur in people with well-developed thinking skills. Creative thinking is the ability to form new combinations of ideas to meet a need. Marzano (1988 p. 17) said "the difference [between critical thinking and creative thinking] is not of kind, but of degree and emphasis." Paul and Bailin (1988) contend that distinguishing clearly between critical thinking and creative thinking is not possible because "all good thinking involves both qualitative assessment and the production of novelty."

From considering these definitions you can see that there are many ways to think about thinking. The *Teaching for Thinking Project* (TTP) of the Minnesota Community College System developed one of the clearest perspectives. It uses the acronym FIRE to describe four aspects of critical thinking: **F**actual, **I**nsightful, **R**ational, and **E**valuative. The TTP says that thinking, like cooking a meal, requires all four "burners on the stove," as follows:

Factual thinking is detailed thinking concerning observations and factual claims. It is used to gather factual information and apply it to a given problem in a manner that is relevant, clear, comprehensive, and conscious of possible bias in the information selected.

Insightful thinking is big-picture thinking, drawing on insight and imagination. It is used to imagine and seek out a variety of possible goals, assumptions, interpretations, or perspectives that can give alternative meanings or solutions to given situations or problems. Creative solutions develop in this aspect of critical thinking.

Rational thinking is logical thinking focused on reasoning and structure. It is used to analyze logical connections among the facts, goals, and implicit assumptions relevant to a problem or claim and to generate and evaluate the implications that follow.

Evaluative thinking is reflective thinking that draws out underlying values and feelings. It is used when one recognizes and articulates the value assumptions that underlie and affect decisions, interpretations, analyses, and evaluations (Peterson & Stacks 1994).

All four areas of critical thinking are of equal importance. In fact, it is the ability to weigh, balance, and sort these dimensions of thinking that improves the capacity of people to learn, solve problems, and make decisions.

Characteristics of Critical Thinkers

People who think critically exhibit a number of personal attributes. Facione (1992) found that people who are critical thinkers have similar traits or dispositions. Those with a *strong critical thinking disposition* will probably agree with statements such as

> *"I really enjoy trying to figure out how things work."*

> *"People should have reasons if they disagree with someone's view."*

> *"I always do better on tests that require thinking (or application), not just memorization."*

> *"I hold off making decisions until I've thought through my options."*

> *"I try to see the merits in another's opinion, even if I reject it later."*

> *"Coming to intelligent decisions is more important than winning arguments."*

People with a *weak critical thinking disposition* will probably agree with statements such as

> *"When I'm reading, I'm easily distracted."*

> *"Open-mindedness is overrated."*

> *"I'll look something up only if I absolutely can't avoid it."*

> *"I hate it when teachers discuss problems instead of just giving the answers."*

> *"All your evidence is irrelevant if my belief is sincere."*

> *"I'll give whatever reason people want to hear to get them to agree with me."*

Table 5-1 lists the characteristics (habits of mind) of critical thinkers identified by Peterson and Stacks (1994). The accompanying box lists the characteristics (personal dispositions) of critical thinkers identified by Facione and Facione (1992).

TABLE 5-1

Habits of Mind for Effective Thinking

Factual Thinking: *detailed thinking concerning observations and factual claims*

Factual clarity, accuracy, and fairness

Observational detail, reliability, and scope

Effective record and recall strategies

Alertness for patterns

Insightful Thinking: *"big-picture" thinking drawing on insight and imagination*

Seeking the larger context

Seeking alternative perspectives

Seeking similarity and difference; relating the known to the unknown

Seeking alternative means of expression

Using questions as probes

Applying learning to self-understanding

Drawing lessons from experience

Rational Thinking: *logical thinking focused on reasoning and structure*

Identifying structure and order

Formulating hierarchies and rules governing patterns

Identifying and evaluating arguments

Constructing arguments

Working with rules in order to reach goals

Judging strength of evidence

Awareness of thinking strategies (metacognition)

Evaluative Thinking: *reflective thinking which draws out underlying values and feelings*

Sensitivity to values—individual and collective

Applying values to problems

Respect for individual and collective differences

Willingness to risk and commit

Valuing your individual and collective self

From: Peterson J, Stack C. *The Teaching for Thinking Project.* Minnesota Community College System, St. Paul MN, 1994.

Personal Dispositions of Critical Thinkers

Truth-seeking: Courageously desires the best knowledge, even if that knowledge fails to support or undermines self-interest or preconceived beliefs.

Open-mindedness: Exhibits tolerance of divergent views; monitors oneself for possible bias or prejudice.

Analyticity: Diligently applies reason. Demands evidence and watches for problematic situations, anticipating the consequences of action.

Systematicity: Values organization. Focuses on and diligently approaches problems of all levels of complexity.

Inquisitiveness: Eagerly acquires knowledge and explanations, even when applications of that knowledge are not apparent.

Maturity: Exhibits prudence in making, suspending, or revising judgment; understands that multiple solutions can be acceptable yet appreciates the need to reach closure even in the absence of complete knowledge.

Self-confidence: Sees oneself as a clear thinker; trusts one's own reasoning skills.

Adapted from: Facione PA, Facione NC. *The California Critical Thinking Disposition Inventory Test Manual,* California Academic Press, 1992.

Critical Thinking Skills

Effective thinking is more than metacognition (thinking about thinking while we are thinking). It is the result of a deliberate thinking process. People who think critically interpret, analyze, evaluate, make inferences, explain, and regulate themselves. Table 5-2 expands this list of skills. For example, when you encounter a situation in nursing, you use all of these abilities to intervene effectively, just as the emergency department nurses did in the vignette.

Critical Thinking in Nursing Practice

Because nursing decisions affect the lives of clients and their families in such significant ways, critical thinking in nursing practice is essential. Nurses must be able to think clearly, define and describe accurately, and make unbiased judgments. They use critical thinking to create new information and ideas, to make reliable observations, to draw sound conclusions, to evaluate lines of reasoning,

TABLE 5-2

Critical Thinking Skills

Interpretation:	Categorization (grouping similar ideas)
	Decoding sentences (comprehending the meaning)
	Clarifying meaning
Analysis:	Examining ideas
	Identifying arguments
	Analyzing arguments
Evaluation:	Assessing claims
	Assessing arguments
Inference:	Querying evidence (questioning alleged facts)
	Conjecturing alternatives (considering various options)
	Drawing conclusions
Explanation:	Stating results
	Justifying procedures
	Presenting arguments
Self-regulation:	Self-examination
	Self-correction

From: Facione PA. Critical Thinking: A Statement of Expert Consensus for Purposes of Educational Assessment and Instruction. *The Delphi Report*. California Academic Press, 1990.

and to improve their own self-knowledge. Critical thinking is so important that it is one of the required outcome measures for program accreditation of schools of nursing by the National League for Nursing (1992). In Canada, where the Canadian Provincial Nursing Associations set the standards for nursing education, critical thinking is becoming a required part of the approval process of schools of nursing.

How can nurses use critical thinking in clinical practice? What tools are available to help them think critically? The accompanying box gives a list of questions you can ask yourself as you go about providing nursing care.

Questions That Stimulate Effective Thinking

The factual thinker gathers factual information and applies it to a given problem in a manner that is relevant, clear, comprehensive, and conscious of possible bias in the information selected.

- What are the relevant facts?
- What evidence can you give to support your claims?
- What evidence might undermine your claims?
- Can the evidence be interpreted in any other way?
- How reliable is the evidence?
- Are any of the key terms unclear or ambiguous?
- In what ways might errors have entered into the observations?
- What other information is important to attaining full understanding?
- How can the information be displayed or recorded most effectively?
- Does the information suggest the existence of underlying patterns?

The insightful thinker imagines and seeks out a variety of possible goals, assumptions, interpretations, or perspectives that can lead to alternative meanings or solutions to given situations or problems.

- What is the larger context, the "big picture" within which this problem or situation resides?
- What other broad contexts or interpretations of the problem or situation can you imagine or discover?
- Can you relate the unknown aspects of this problem to the known aspects of more familiar problems?
- What alternative means or media can you use to depict or explain the present problem or situation?
- What new insights arise from depicting the problem or solution in alternative ways?
- What open-ended questions for further reflection and investigation arise from this situation?
- What insights into your own thinking and understanding can you gain from considering the problem?

The rational thinker analyzes logical connections among the facts, goals, and implicit assumptions relevant to a problem or claim and generates and evaluates the implications that follow.

- What are the major components or necessary sequences that structure this problem or situation?

➤

- What rules or hierarchy appears to govern the order?
- What assumptions are logically implied by your view and others' views of the problem or situation?
- What are the implications that follow from your solution or view of the problem or claim?
- What arguments are can be made about the problem or claim?
- How good are the various arguments that can be made about the problem or claim?
- Can you construct an argument of your own to prove a point or raise an issue about the problem?
- Given a set of procedures or rules, can you manipulate them effectively to reach a desired outcome?
- Given conflicting evidence, can you defend judging evidence on one side as stronger than evidence on the other?
- What process did you use in approaching this problem?
- What alternative strategies did you consider in approaching this problem?
- Why did you choose the strategy you chose?
- What changes in strategy would make you more effective next time?

The evaluative thinker recognizes and articulates the value assumptions that underlie and affect decisions, interpretations, analyses, and evaluations made by ourselves and others.

- What feels most important to you in this problem or situation? Why?
- Are your own feelings of what is important here related to the feelings of others on this issue? How?
- How do your own values and feelings about what is important apply to the present problem?
- Do you have difficulty respecting those who hold views opposed to yours on this issue? Explain.
- Does anything hold you back from taking risks and making commitments in this situation or problem?
- How does your work on this problem make you feel about yourself? Is this feeling personal or is it shared?
- Are you pulled in different directions by conflicting values or feelings about the issue? If so, how? Which seems most important?

Adapted from Peterson J, Stack C. Probes for Effective Thinking, *Teaching for Thinking Project.* Minnesota Community College System, 1994.

◆ Cultural Competence

When Anne Goodrich defined nursing as demanding "fine perceptions and enduring tolerance born of understanding," she had no way of anticipating the changes that would occur in American society by the twenty-first century. However, nursing leaders of today echo her call, declaring that nurses need to become culturally competent. Leininger (1994b, p. 254) said, "providing culturally congruent care should be one of the highest priorities of nursing organizations and educational institutions as they plan for universal health care reform and function in a multicultural world."

Indeed, as we enter the twenty-first century, dramatic changes are taking place in the population. The 1990 US census revealed that between 1980 and 1990 the number of Hispanics rose 53%; Asians, 108%; and Native Americans, 38%. Statisticians predict that by the year 2000 one-third of the population of the United States will be nonwhite (New Face of America 1993). These demographic changes affect every institution in the nation, especially those that provide health care. Nurses must prepare to care for multicultural populations. They must become culturally competent.

Just what is cultural competence? *Cultural competence* is a combination of knowledge and attitudes: knowledge of the values, beliefs, and practices of various cultures, and attitudes about those cultures. To appreciate these issues, nurses must understand the terms used to discuss culture—the characteristics of culture and specific information about various cultures—and must recognize their own beliefs and values.

Culture

Culture is the values, beliefs, and practices that are shared by people and passed down from generation to generation. Culture includes the objects that are unique to a group of people, such as dress, art, and religious artifacts, and the ways these things are used. Culture also includes the beliefs, customs, language, and social institutions of a group of people. *Race* refers to the physical traits people inherit from their parents, such as hair color and curliness, skin pigmentation, and bone structure. *Ethnicity* refers to a state of belonging to a specific ethnic group and sharing a unique cultural and social heritage that is passed from generation to generation. *Enculturation* is the process of learning a culture over a period of time, as children do in their family of birth. *Acculturation* is the process of adopting the culture of another people. *Ethnocentrism* is the belief that one's culture is superior to all others. *Stereotyping* is the assumption that all members of a culture are alike.

Characteristics of Culture

Cultures have four basic characteristics. They are (1) learned from birth through the processes of language acquisition and socialization, (2) shared by all members of the same cultural group, (3) adapted to specific conditions related to environmental and technical factors and to the availability of natural resources, and (4) dynamic and ever-changing (Barkauskas 1994, p. iv). Nurses need to take these characteristics into consideration as they consider the effect of culture on nursing practice.

From birth on, people learn to accommodate their behavior to the people around them. Besides a language, they learn beliefs, values, and practices that affect every area of their lives, including right and wrong behavior (moral values), social roles, artistic and musical expression, religious customs, bodily functions, and health practices. Culture influences the lives of people—their way of knowing and their behavior—so deeply that it is like a tinted lens through which they view reality. The lens colors every aspect of their lives. Because this view becomes part of the self, it is relatively constant and exceedingly difficult to change. Furthermore, because all people have a basic need to feel safe and secure, they view people of other cultures as threats to their safety and security. Thus, they seek to annihilate, or at least isolate, foreign cultures. For this reason, cultural sensitivity has not always been valued, nor is it easily attained. However, if nurses are to meet the needs of clients in a pluralistic society, they must learn about client beliefs, values, and practices.

Knowledge of Other Cultures

There are many ways for nurses to gain knowledge about other cultures. Some nurses use formal educational approaches, taking courses in foreign languages, anthropology, cross-cultural psychology, and comparative social science. A number of schools of nursing offer transcultural nursing courses, and some base the entire curriculum on transcultural theories. Many schools offer short-term, intensive courses, whereas others offer master's and doctoral programs in transcultural nursing. Nurses who prefer self-directed learning may choose to read books, journals, and research in cultural diversity. There is a wide array of fiction and nonfiction literature about other cultures on library and bookstore shelves. Some nurses seek to enrich their understanding of other cultures by working in ethnic communities at home and by serving in distant lands as traveling nurses, as Peace Corps volunteers, or in the military. These nurses find that nothing broadens their perspective and expands their knowledge like living and working in another culture.

The most readily available information about other cultures, however, comes from the clients nurses find right in their home towns. When nurses show respect, warmth, and genuine interest, they may be surprised to find how willing people are to share their values and beliefs because everyone wants to be understood and respected. A word of warning: guard against stereotyping; remember that every person is an individual and every family a unique entity.

Attitudes about Cultures

To become culturally competent, nurses need to recognize their own beliefs and values. This chapter begins with the story of Claire, who looked with horror on the practice of female circumcision, judging both the woman and her husband. The ED nurse, by contrast, was able to give them sensitive care without allowing her own personal prejudice to interfere.

Prejudice is a term that many people use but few examine carefully. Prejudice serves many functions. It is a way of discriminating, a means to an end, a method of thinking, and a mode of emotional release. As a means to an end, it is used to bolster one's feeling of confidence or to remove a threat. As a way of thinking, prejudice generalizes and simplifies life; it strips individuals of their personhood, blurs their faces, and makes them into objects. As a mode of emotional release, prejudice provides a focus for a range of emotions, from blind acceptance to paralyzing fear. Regardless of its function, prejudice generalizes and subverts rational thought (Hamilton 1992).

To avoid prejudice, nurses must adopt a stance of cultural relativism. *Cultural relativism* is a point of view that describes the behav-

Eleven Ways to Become Culturally Competent

1. Gain an understanding of your own values and beliefs.

2. Recognize that your own culture conditioned your point of view.

3. Develop a perspective of cultural relativism; view other cultures as unique solutions to a societal problem.

4. Appreciate that cultural values are ingrained and therefore difficult to change.

5. Look at people as individuals, not as members of an amorphous group.

6. Seek information from your clients, including beliefs and practices about family roles, the meaning of health and illness, and healing practices.

7. Give safe, effective care to all clients regardless of their culture or diagnosis.

8. Be willing to modify health care delivery to accommodate the culture of a client.

9. Beware of stereotyping; all members of a cultural group may not behave in the same way as other members.

10. Embrace other caregivers from other cultures; learn from their perspective.

11. Allow caring to guide your every act.

iors, beliefs, and values of people but does not evaluate them as good or bad. Instead, those behaviors, beliefs, and values are seen as a workable solution to the problem of living in a particular situation at a particular time. Such a point of view helps remove the threat other cultures present and helps one look at people as individuals instead of members of an unfamiliar group.

How to Develop Cultural Competence

Because cultural competence is a combination of knowledge and attitudes, nurses can take a number of actions to develop this capacity. The box above lists 11 ways to become culturally competent.

◇ Caring

Throughout history the idea of nurturance and kindness have held a place of honor in nursing. However, during the 1950s, 1960s and 1970s, many nursing leaders believed that the profession would gain greater recognition if it emphasized its scientific base rather than its art and humanity. The worldwide transcultural research of Leininger and her associates challenged that belief and found that science does not displace caring in nursing; it enhances it. Her research led to the culture-care theory of nursing. The theory defines nursing as "that body of knowledge generated through systematic research methods (qualitative and quantitative) that is focused on assistive, supportive, facilitative, enabling, and other expressions of caring modes to individuals, groups, institutions, cultures, or societies to improve their services to humanity" (American Academy of Nursing 1990, p. 19). These researchers confirmed the relevance and importance of caring to nursing, conclusively joining it to science and culture. They declare that caring is the "central and dominant domain of nursing" (Leininger 1994a, p. 3).

Definitions of Caring

Most nurses have their own definition of caring. They define it by using such terms as comforting, showing compassion, concern, empathy, involvement, kindness, nurturance, tenderness, and trusting. Unfortunately, these terms are subjective and do not describe objective, specific behaviors. In her research among various cultures of the world, Leininger found that although caring occurs universally, its expression varies widely. What people expect from caregivers also differs. For instance, cultures that perceive illness mainly as an internal bodily experience caused by physical or genetic stressors are more apt to view those who provide therapy as caring. Cultures that perceive illness as due to extrapersonal forces are more apt to view those who ward off harm as caring. Leininger suggests that the goal of health care personnel should be to understand the values, beliefs, and lifestyle of individuals and to provide culture-specific care. She described caring in her Ten Tenets of Culture Care Theory (see the box on page 132).

Besides differences in clients' views of what constitutes a caring individual, there are differences in caregivers' views of what behav-

Leininger's Ten Tenets of Culture Care Theory

1. Care is essential for development, growth, and survival of human beings.

2. Generic and professional care meanings, expressions, patterns, and action modes vary transculturally, with some culturally universal features.

3. Care is the essence of nursing and the distinctive feature explaining nursing.

4. A culture's care-meanings and action-patterns are largely embedded in its worldview, social structure, cultural values, language, and environment.

5. The use of generic and professional care knowledge is a powerful means of promoting health, well-being, and recovery from illness or disability, or of helping clients and families during the dying process.

6. Ethical-moral care values and practices have differences and similarities in Western and non-Western cultures.

7. Emic (within the culture) and etic (view of the culture by outsiders) care-knowledge are important differential aspects of care in determining and providing culturally congruent care to clients.

8. Human beings may exist without curing, but not without caring.

9. Cultural, social, and physical environmental contexts give meaning and structure to assessing and guiding professional care practices and policies.

10. The goal of professional care is to provide culturally congruent care to people of diverse cultures.

From: American Academy of Nursing. *Knowledge About Care and Caring.* 1990

iors demonstrate caring. In a study of white and black caregivers, Leininger found that white American nursing personnel viewed care and caring as (1) alleviating stress, (2) providing health education, (3) teaching strategies for self-care, and (4) using complex technology. In contrast, a sample of black American caregivers viewed caring as (1) showing concern for family members, (2) using presence and touch in specific ways, and (3) getting into the client's world in order to understand and be effective (Leininger 1994a).

Henderson describes a caring nurse as one who "gets under the skin of each of her patients in order to know what he or she needs"

(1964, p. 64). Nodding describes caring as a reciprocal process between the "one-caring" and the "cared-for" (1984). She says that human caring and the memory of being cared for form the foundation for ethical behavior.

MacPherson and colleagues say that caring involves stepping out of one's own personal frame of reference into another's. "When we care, we consider the other's point of view, his objective needs, and what he or she expects of us. Our attention, our mental engrossment is on the cared for, not on ourselves. Our reasons for acting, then, have to do both with the other's wants and desires and with the objective elements of his problematic situation" (1991, p. 29).

Mayeroff says, "We sometimes speak as if caring did not require knowledge, as if caring for someone were simply a matter of good intentions or warm regard.... To care for someone, I must know many things. I must know who the other is, what his powers and limitations are, what his needs are, and what is conducive to his growth" (1971, p. 13).

In this day of high technology and cost containment, Watson's (1985) ten carative factors seem especially pertinent. She says nurses demonstrate caring when they

1. Form a humanistic-altruistic system that values caring.

2. Instill faith and hope in clients to supplant discouragement and despair.

3. Cultivate sensitivity to human feelings in oneself and others.

4. Develop a helping-trusting relationship with clients.

5. Express positive and negative feelings and encourage clients to do the same.

6. Use a creative problem-solving caring process.

7. Promote interpersonal teaching-learning, thus shifting responsibility for wellness to clients.

8. Provide a supportive, protective, or corrective mental, physical, sociocultural, and spiritual environment.

9. Assist with the gratification of human needs by attending to physical, emotional, social, and spiritual needs of clients.

10. Become sensitive to existential-phenomenologic-spiritual forces, thus, demonstrate acceptance.

The ethicist Carol Gilligan (1982) studied how girls and women learn, think, and make ethical decisions. She came to the conclusion that caring is the highest form of moral development. "Those operating within a morality of responsibility and care, primarily women, reject the strategy of blindness and impartiality. Instead, they argue for an understanding of the context for moral choice, claiming that the needs of individuals cannot always be deduced from general rules and principles and that moral choice must also be determined inductively from the particular experiences each participant brings to the situation" (Belenky et al 1986, p. 8).

Caring in Nursing Practice

You may ask, when nurses exhibit caring behaviors in their practice, what results can they expect? Benner and Wrubel examined the relationship of caring, stress, coping, and health and found that caring was most important. They declare that caring means "that persons, events, projects, and things *matter to people*" (1989, p. 1). They add that such "mattering" is central to human expertise, to curing, and to healing in three ways:

1. *Because caring sets up what matters to a person, it also sets up what counts as stressful, and what options are available for coping.*

2. *Coping based on caring [may not abolish loss and pain but it] allows for the possibility of joy and the satisfactions of attachment.*

3. *Caring sets up the possibility of giving and receiving help. A caring relationship sets up the conditions of trust that enable the one cared for to appropriate the help offered and to feel cared for (Benner & Wrubel 1989, pp. 1–4).*

Patricia Benner observes that expert nurses offered glimpses of the nature of the power that resides in caring. These nurses use caring "to empower their patients—not dominate, coerce, or control them" (1984, p. 209). She identifies six qualities of power associated with caring:

1. *Transformative power* whereby nurses help clients gain a sense of control by helping them realize they have choices.

2. *Integrative caring* whereby nurses help clients continue with meaningful life activities despite the limitations a disability might impose.

3. *Advocacy power* whereby nurses act on behalf of clients to remove obstacles and enable them.

4. *Healing power* whereby nurses mobilize hope; find acceptable understandings; locate emotional, social, and spiritual support; and use internal and external resources.

5. *Participative/affirmative power* whereby nurses experience pain and loss along with clients yet in the process give clients strength and affirmation.

6. *Problem solving* whereby nurses use a "caring-involved stance," a sensitivity to cues that allows them to search for solutions and even to recognize solutions when they are not directly looking for them" (Benner 1984, p. 215).

We see, then, that caring is empowerment: empowerment for clients, for nurses, and for the nursing profession.

As we move into the twenty-first century, Anne Goodrich's words seem especially relevant: "Beyond all other drives, nursing commands devoted service, a broad perspective, rigorous analyses, close association with scientific findings, fine perceptions, and enduring tolerance born of understanding [critical thinking, cultural competence, and caring]." Each of these abilities contributes to a richer understanding of the other and to a wider perspective for the future of nursing practice.

◆ Summary

Because nursing decisions affect the lives of clients and their families in such significant ways, critical thinking in nursing practice is essential. Critical thinking has many definitions. It is factual, insightful, rational, and evaluative thinking. Cultural competence is more than being sensitive to cultural differences. It consists of knowledge of and attitudes about the values, beliefs, and practices of various cultures. Nurses can take many actions to increase their cultural competence. Caring has been described, defined, and studied by many researchers.

Leininger and others identified ten tenets of their culture-care theory of nursing; Watson listed ten carative factors, and Benner identified six qualities of power associated with caring. All agree that caring is the essence of nursing practice.

Critical Thinking Questions

1. What new insights about the thinking process have you gained from reading this chapter?

2. Critical thinkers avoid ambiguous, general, imprecise, and non-specific descriptions. Identify any of the key terms used to describe cultural competence that are unclear or ambiguous. What would you need to know to clarify them?

3. What are the relationships among critical thinking, cultural competence, and caring? Describe the line of reasoning you used to arrive at these conclusions.

Learning Activities

1. Analyze the critical thinking characteristics in yourself, using the box on page 123, "Personal Dispositions of Critical Thinkers," and Table 5-1, "Habits of Mind for Effective Thinking."

2. Lead a group discussion of classmates about a clinical problem using the list in the box on page 125 and 126, Questions That Stimulate Effective Thinking.

3. Write a journal entry describing your feelings about clients from cultures, lifestyles, generations, economic circumstances, and races that are different from your own.

4. Interview a person you consider very different from yourself. Describe the values and beliefs that you see as different and those that are similar to your own.

5. With your classmates create a reading list of the best examples of books that help you "pull yourself out of your shoes and place your feet in your client's."

6. In a small group discussion, compare and contrast the concepts of critical thinking, cultural competence, and caring. How do these concepts complement each other?

Annotated Reading List

Galanti G. *Caring for Patients from Different Cultures, Case Studies from American Hospitals.* University of Pennsylvania Press, 1991.

This engaging text is a collection of anecdotes and stories of culturally insensitive blunders collected from medical anthropology students. The author categorizes the areas of misunderstanding between cultures as (1) communication and time orientation, (2) religion and beliefs, (3) family, (4) men and women, (5) birth, and (6) folk-medicine practices and perspectives. The book offers valuable information and insights for nurses.

Leininger M. *Transcultural Nursing: Concepts, Theory, Research and Practice,* 2nd ed. McGraw Hill & Greyden Press, 1994.

This is the definitive text about caring as it applies to transcultural nursing.

New Face of America, special edition, *Time* 1993; 142:21.

This special issue of *Time* magazine provides a journalistic account of the changing ethnic face of the United States. Its wonderful pictures and graphics provide an immediacy and reality that only photographs can give.

Wilkinson J. *Nursing Process in Action: A Critical Thinking Approach.* Addison-Wesley, 1992.

This innovative, step-by-step text uses concrete examples and hands-on exercises to help the reader clearly understand and apply the five steps of the nursing process. There is a separate chapter on critical thinking. Critical thinking is incorporated in each step of the nursing process.

References

American Academy of Nursing. *Knowledge About Care and Caring*. Kansas City, 1990.

Bandman E, Bandman B. *Critical Thinking in Nursing*. Appleton & Lange, 1988.

Barkauskas VH. *Quick Reference to Cultural Assessment*. Mosby, 1994.

Belenky M, Clinchy B, Goldberger N, Tarule J. *Women's Ways of Knowing: The Development of Self, Choice, and Mind*. Basic Books, 1986.

Benner P. *From Novice to Expert: Excellence and Power in Clinical Nursing Practice*. Addison-Wesley, 1984.

Benner P, Wrubel J. *The Primacy of Caring: Stress and Coping in Health and Illness*. Addison-Wesley, 1989.

Chaffee J. *Thinking Critically*, 3rd ed. Houghton-Mifflin, 1990.

Facione PA. Critical Thinking: A Statement of Expert Consensus for Purposes of Educational Assessment and Instruction. *The Delphi Report*. California Academic Press, 1990.

Facione PA. *Critical Thinking: What It Is and Why It Counts*. The California Academic Press, 1992.

Facione PA, Facione NC. *The California Critical Thinking Disposition Inventory Test Manual*. California Academic Press, 1992.

Gilligan C. *In a Different Voice: Psychological Theory and Women's Development*. Harvard University Press, 1982.

Goodrich A. The Nature of Nursing. *American Journal of Nursing* 1964; 64:62–68.

Hamilton PM. *Realities of Contemporary Nursing*. Addison-Wesley, 1992.

Henderson V. The Nature of Nursing. *American Journal of Nursing* 1964; 64:62–68.

Kozier B, Erb G, Blais K, Wilkinson W. *Fundamentals of Nursing*, 5th ed. Addison-Wesley, 1995.

Leininger M. *Transcultural Nursing; Concepts, Theory, Research and Practice*, 2nd ed. McGraw Hill & Greyden Press, 1994a.

Leininger M. Transcultural nursing education: A worldwide imperative. *Nursing & Health Care* 1994b; 15(5): 254–257.

MacPherson K, Neil R, Watts R (eds). *Caring and Nursing: Explorations in Feminist Perspectives*. National League for Nursing, 1991.

Marzano RJ. *Dimensions of Thinking: A Framework for Curriculum & Instruction*. ERIC Clearinghouse, 1988.

Mayeroff M. *On Caring*. Harper & Row, 1971.

National League for Nursing. *Accreditation Guidelines*. National League for Nursing, 1992.

New Face of America, special edition, *Time*. 1993; 142:21.

Nodding N. *Caring: A Feminine Approach to Ethics and Moral Education*. University of California Press, 1984.

Paul R. *Critical Thinking: What Every Person Needs to Survive in a Rapidly Changing World*. Center for Critical Thinking and Moral Critique, Sonoma State University, 1990.

Paul R, Bailin S. The Creatively Critical and Critically Creative Thinker. In Marzano RJ. *Dimensions of Thinking*. ERIC Clearinghouse, 1988.

Peterson J., Stacks C. *The Teaching for Thinking Project*. Minnesota Community College System, St. Paul MN, 1994.

Strader M. Critical Thinking. In Sullivan EJ, Decker PJ. *Effective Management in Nursing*, 3rd ed. Addison-Wesley, 1992.

University of Missouri School of Nursing. *Accreditation Report for the National League for Nursing*. University of Missouri, 1992.

Watson J. *Nursing: Human Science and Human Care*. Appleton-Century-Crofts, 1985.

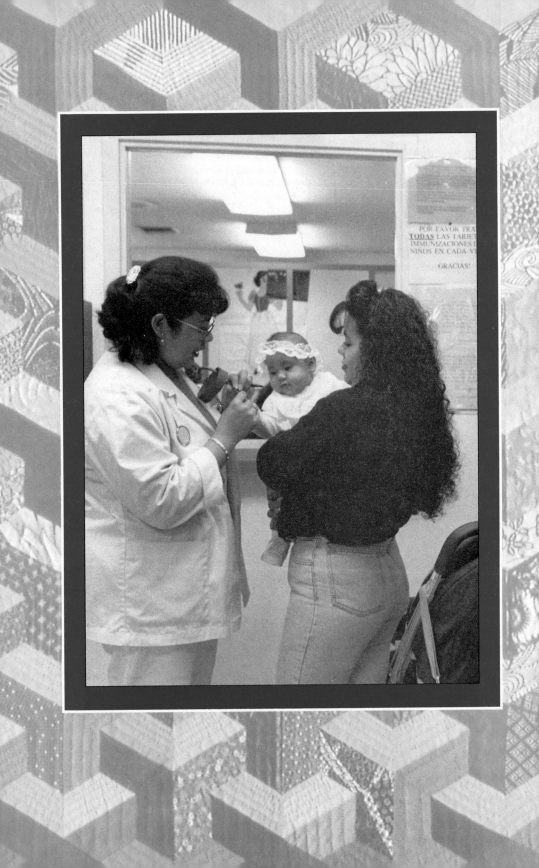

Health Care Systems

6

◇ Learning Objectives

- Discuss the influence of political and economic forces on health care systems.

- Discuss effects of standards and regulations on health care.

- Trace the history of the US health care system.

- Describe the purpose and composition of the US health system.

- Discuss how the principles of shared sovereignty and separation of powers affect the US health care system.

- Discuss the various methods of financing health care in the United States.

- Explain the importance of the Social Security Act of 1935 to US health care.

- Explain the health care coverage provided by Medicare, Parts A and B, and Medicaid.

- Compare various managed care plans in terms of access to and payment for care.

- Discuss how health policy affects access to care and what services are offered.

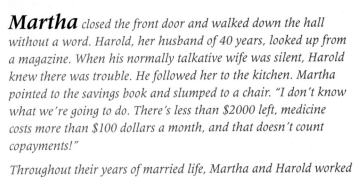

Martha *closed the front door and walked down the hall without a word. Harold, her husband of 40 years, looked up from a magazine. When his normally talkative wife was silent, Harold knew there was trouble. He followed her to the kitchen. Martha pointed to the savings book and slumped to a chair. "I don't know what we're going to do. There's less than $2000 left, medicine costs more than $100 dollars a month, and that doesn't count copayments!"*

Throughout their years of married life, Martha and Harold worked for a chemical factory; he on the plant floor, she in the office. A lifetime smoker, Harold lost his health insurance when he retired at age 65 with emphysema. Now, his only health insurance is Medicare, which pays just 80% of approved charges. He cannot purchase supplemental insurance because of his preexisting health condition. Martha, age 60, had to retire because of heart disease, complicated by diabetes. When she left her job, she lost her health insurance. Because of her health condition, Martha cannot afford the cost of private health insurance, but she is not yet eligible for Medicare. They must pay all out-of-pocket medical costs for such things as medicine. Their retirement income barely meets their expenses. If Martha needs any major medical care before she is eligible for Medicare, they may lose their home. Fortunately, their family physician accepts whatever reimbursement Medicare allows, but as their savings dwindle, Harold and Martha are caught in a downward spiral.

Why must access to health care be tied so closely to employment? Why do insurance companies have the right to deny health insurance to people with preexisting conditions? In a free-market economy, is comprehensive health care possible?

◆ Purpose and Influences

Although the purpose of all health care systems is to provide citizens with health care, economic and political forces profoundly affect every system. Roemer (1991, volume 1) used these forces to describe the organizational types of health care systems throughout the world. He measured the economic factor by the gross national product per capita, that is, the value of all goods and services produced in a nation during the year. He classified countries as: industrialized and affluent, or developing/transitional and very poor. He measured the political factor by the extent of government involvement in the health system and classified countries as (1) entrepreneurial and permissive, (2) welfare oriented, (3) comprehensive, and (4) socialist. These are not precise definitions, but general descriptions.

Using Roemer's terms, we can characterize the United States economy as affluent and industrialized and the political climate as entrepreneurial and permissive. The private health care market is strong, and government involvement is minimal. Some affluent countries, such as Canada, have welfare-oriented systems in which the government intervenes in the private health care market by financing health care, not by changing conventional delivery patterns. Other affluent industrialized countries, such as Great Britain, have universal and comprehensive systems that provide equal access to care for all citizens without charge. In socialist countries, such as the People's Republic of China, a centrally planned system prevails, with human and physical resources collectivized under direct government control. It is interesting to note that all socialized countries have some free-market health care in which physicians accept patients who pay them privately. Because this chapter focuses on US health care, we will discuss only the entrepreneurial permissive system.

In the permissive system of the United States, with a free-market economy, the health care system is expected to make a profit or at least balance income with expenses. This philosophy of freedom includes not only the economy, but every aspect of life. Thus, individuals have the right to choose any lifestyle they wish, whether or not it is healthy, as long as it does not interfere with the rights of others. Each state has the right to regulate delivery of health care within its political jurisdiction without regard to citizen needs. Personal and public freedom is highly valued. Thus, the health care system is marked by tension and compromise between the private, for-profit health care sector, serving individuals who are insured or otherwise able to afford health care, and the tax-supported health care sector, serving the poor or uninsured. This permissive approach has created a system where health care is unevenly distributed among the people.

While the political and economic system of a country influences the distribution of health care, the prevailing definition of health and illness influences what type of care is given and who provides it. Traditionally, biomedical science has defined health and medical care in terms of diseases of the body. This definition does not address factors that promote health, such as social and family support, safe neighborhoods, housing, education, and employment options. Social science and policy planners are concerned about these factors. Many nurses and other health professionals believe that if the health of individuals and communities is to be improved, social science must begin to influence the health care system, at least to the same degree that biomedical science influences it.

Composition

Health care systems are composed of the resources, functions, controls, and organization needed to deliver health care to populations (Roemer 1991, volume 2). As an integral part of all health care systems, nurses work to promote health, prevent and treat injury and disease, and foster rehabilitation. By gaining an understanding of the composition of a system and how it works, nurses can support broader social and psychologic aspects of health, using the system to benefit the people they serve.

Resources

Resources include facilities and personnel.

Facilities The resources of health care systems consist of health care facilities and personnel. Facilities are the settings where health care providers work. These settings are centers of authority, service, and training where initial health care, preventive care, and rehabilitation and terminal care are given. See the accompanying box on page 145. Persons who do not have a source of primary care usually seek treatment in a more costly secondary or tertiary facility, such as a hospital emergency room (Jonas 1992). A lack of available and accessible pri-

Types of Health Service Facilities

Primary care (care to foster health and prevent disease)

- Community health centers
- Day-care centers
- Employee health centers
- Health maintenance organizations
- Neighborhood health centers
- Offices of physicians and advance practice nurses
- Preferred provider organizations
- Prison health services
- Public health clinics
- School of health services
- Self-help support groups, eg, Alcoholics Anonymous

Secondary care (care to treat acute illness and prevent disease complications)

- Ambulatory care centers
- Free-standing emergency care centers
- Home health-care agencies
- Hospitals:
    acute, short-stay: less than 30 days
    long-term: more than 30 days
- Hospital special care units: neonatal, coronary, burn centers, etc.
- Physicians' offices: extended care, intermediate care, nursing homes

Tertiary Care (care that is supportive and rehabilitative)

- Adult day care
- Hospice services
- Long-term care facilities
- Rehabilitation

mary providers, especially for the poor, adds to the overall high cost of health care in the United States.

Until recently, hospitals were the center of the US health care system, employing the majority of workers and accounting for the greatest proportion of health care costs (Hull 1994). Rising costs and reduced federal reimbursement lowered occupancy rates, causing hospital closures, mergers, and acquisitions. To meet the need for services yet control costs, the industry created more efficient, specialized agencies such as surgicenters, clinics, home health agencies, mental health clinics, extended care facilities, pharmacies, and free-standing laboratories, as well as a network of emergency vehicles and specially equipped vans and taxis to transport disabled persons. The type, number, and location of these facilities depend on the payment method and the degree to which the system is centralized under government control or localized in the private sector.

Even in a permissive health-care system like the United States, there are programs so crucial to the well-being of the population that some central planning is required. For example, most state and local governments provide funds to maintain pure food, air, and water; waste disposal; and immunization against infectious disease. The extent of these programs depends on the wealth of the country and its willingness to allocate a portion of the budget for the health of citizens.

In health systems based on a free-market economy, health care facilities are built to compete for health care dollars available through private insurance or programs funded by federal and state governments. In these systems, populations are served on the basis of ability to pay, not necessarily on need. The existence of a program to pay for medical care is not a guarantee of its availability. For example, in United States, physicians may refuse to accept patients sponsored by a state or federal financing system.

Availability of health care restricted by ability to pay is reflected in the health of the people. A sensitive indicator of such health is the infant mortality rate (number of infant deaths during the first year of life per 1000 infants born in a given year). This indicator reflects access to a number of vital health services such as prenatal care, intrapartal care, nutrition, pure food and water, education, immunizations, and well-child care. Table 6-1 gives infant mortality rates in four countries. It shows that the political and social organization of a health care system is as important in reducing infant mortality as is the relative wealth of the country.

It is important to remember that availability of health care resources is influenced by cultural values, employment options, housing standards, and literacy. Table 6-2 shows how these issues affect infant mortality rates in several US states. Regardless of the state, African-American infants are more likely than others to die in their first year of life. These birth outcomes cannot be attributed to

TABLE 6-1

Infant Mortality Rate by Economic Level and Political Control of Health Care in 1993

Country	Per capita gross national product in US dollars[1]	Political control of health care[2]	Economic status	Infant mortality rate[3,4]
United States	$23,120	Entrepreneurial/ Permissive	Affluent	8.3
United Kingdom	$17,760	Universal/ Comprehensive	Affluent	6.6
Nigeria	$320	Universal/ Comprehensive	Poor	87.0
China	$380	Socialist/ Centrally planned	Poor	31.0

[1] An indicator of economic development, determined by the total number of hours worked by a nation's labor force and the average value of goods and services produced per hour of work.

[2] Roemer MI. *National Health Systems of the World.* Vol. I, *The Countries.* Oxford University Press, 1991, pp. 83–99.

[3] Infant deaths under 1 year of age per 1000 live births.

[4] Population Reference Bureau. *World Population Data Sheet,* 1994.

TABLE 6-2

Infant Mortality Rate[1] by Selected States and Race in the United States in 1990[2]

	African-American	Other	Total
California	14.2	7.6	7.9
Illinois	21.5	7.7	10.7
New York	17.3	7.7	9.6
Kansas	15.4	7.7	8.4
Mississippi	16.1	8.5	12.1
Georgia	18.0	9.1	12.4

[1] Infant deaths under 1 year of age per 1000 live births.

[2] US Census Bureau. *Statistical Abstract of the United States,* 113th ed. 1993.

biologic differences. They would seem to arise from social and economic barriers to health care.

Personnel All countries have similar categories of health personnel such as nurses and physicians. However, the number, type, distribution, and use of health professionals vary with the degree of government control and the wealth of the country. In the United States, there are about 700 categories of health care workers, including those who provide support services for health care facilities, such as janitorial and food service personnel. About 7% of workers are physicians, or about 144 per 100,000 population. This ratio is expected to rise to 176 per 100,000 by the year 2000. The private sector employs about 96% of physicians, two-thirds of whom practice in offices in urban areas. Fewer than 40% of physicians are in general or family practice, internal medicine, obstetrics, or pediatrics—services most likely to focus on health promotion and illness prevention (Grumbach & Lee 1994).

In developing countries the supply of all types of health personnel is lower than in affluent countries. In 1986, there were, on average, 51 physicians per 100,000 population in developing countries, defined as those with a GNP per capita of less than $3000 per year (Roemer 1994, volume 2, pp. 9–11). Yet, developing countries with centralized health care systems have a higher ratio of all types of health workers-to-population than developing countries with private enterprise systems. In countries with centralized systems, ministries of health decide how many and what type of physicians, nurses, or other health workers are needed, how many to educate, and where to send them when educated, thus assuring a balance of primary and specialty providers throughout the country (Roemer 1994, volume 2, pp. 9–11). Thus, education and employment are maximized, costs are reduced, and return on educational dollars is increased. Factors other than cost, including the business interests of medical associations, competition among physicians, and satisfaction of the public with nurses as primary health care providers, influence a country's decision about the number of health personnel to educate and the ratio of physicians to nurses and other workers.

Although there is no centralized planning of health care in the United States, nurses are as crucial to the system as they are in centralized systems. In the United States there are three times as many nurses as physicians, or about 726 registered nurses per 100,000 population. Over 66% are employed by hospitals, 7% in nursing homes,

6.6% in community health, 5.7% in physician and dentist offices, 3.7% in education, and the remainder in other settings (Department of Health & Human Services 1994a). Several thousand nurses now work in areas of advanced clinical practice as nurse practitioners and clinical specialists, providing services to children, adults, and the aged.

Unfortunately, advanced practice nursing in the United States is restricted by legal constraints and liability insurance. In spite of extensive literature on client satisfaction, safety, and cost containment, physician groups have pressured state legislators to pass laws requiring physician supervision. Such pressure is exerted ostensibly to protect clients; however, many observers believe the true reason is to protect physician control of health care, chiefly the monies they generate. Liability insurance limits advanced nursing practice because of the reluctance of insurance companies to provide coverage for self-employed nurses at reasonable rates, especially nurse-midwives. Problems with liability insurance affect the ability of all health care providers to be protected from malpractice claims. These problems are due to liberal laws that favor plaintiffs, profits gained by lawyers in malpractice litigation, lack of self-discipline by the medical community, and business practices of insurance companies. As a result, most advanced practice nurses work in hospitals and agencies where their insurance is paid for by the institution or practice (Stafford & Appleyard 1994).

Functions

Health care functions consist of the services the health system provides, ranging from health education to disease treatment. They are classified as primary care and specialty care.

Primary care is the service patients receive at their first point of contact with the health care system (Jonas 1992). It includes health promotion, prevention, diagnosis, treatment, and referral to specialty care when required. Everyone needs access to a source of primary care. Providers may be physicians in general practice, family practice, internal medicine, pediatrics, and sometimes obstetrics. They may be nurses in family, pediatric, and school health practice; midwives; or physician assistants. Because of the development and growth of advanced practice roles for nurses and physician assistants, more people can now receive primary care.

Community-oriented primary care is a modification of personal primary care. This type of care links the techniques of individual primary care to public health practice such as epidemiology, demography, biostatistics, health services planning, and program evaluation. Individuals are viewed as members of a community. Practitioners use demographic data to describe communities in terms of the age range of the population, sex distribution, access to health services, and payment for health services. The population of communities is further described by its need for health services. For example, health service needs of an elderly population are different from the needs of young families or single college students.

The World Health Organization places particular emphasis on primary care as a means to achieve its goal of health for all by the year 2000. In 1978, at a conference in Alma Ata, USSR, member nations were urged to cooperate in allocating national health care resources to achieve universally accessible and affordable primary health care systems. These systems would rely on both health workers and traditional healers for routine health care and use a referral system for specialty services. They would establish relationships with national programs for agriculture and employment. By so doing, they would foster economic prosperity, an important factor in the physical and mental health of individuals and communities.

Specialty care is given by health care providers who specialize in a particular area of medicine. Except for emergency care, most specialty care is provided on referral after clients enter the health care system by way of primary care. Specialty care is *secondary care* in that it may prevent complications of disease and injury. It may also be *tertiary care*, providing supportive and rehabilitative care. Specialty care developed as a result of the growth in medical knowledge to the point where no individual practitioner could master the knowledge and skill of every medical specialty. Beginning in 1913 with the founding of the American College of Surgeons, specialty societies were formed to verify the competence of members practicing in these areas. Nurses patterned their specialty practice after medical societies, but in areas appropriate to nursing. In 1955, nurse midwives organized a professional certifying body, the American College of Nurse Midwives. In the 1970s the ANA established a program to certify other nursing specialties, as described in Chapter 3.

In countries with centralized health systems, specialty services usually are found in hospital settings. In entrepreneurial/permissive systems, specialty care is available in private and public settings affiliated with medical schools, teaching hospitals, or private charitable institutions. Such care is offered by private providers on a fee-for-service basis. Supporters of this system believe that free-market forces balance the supply of specialists with demand for their services. Yet, when similar institutions compete for clients, uneconomical duplication may occur. The medical establishment may encourage people to use the more expensive specialties, not because of need, but to increase income for the service.

Controls

Controls include standards and regulations.

Standards The controls of the health care system are the standards and regulations created to ensure that resources are used safely and effectively. Standards for the health care system specify the scope of professional practice and set criteria. They do not have the force of law but serve to protect the health of people indirectly. Standards influence what a community expects from a health care system in areas of scientific excellence and humanitarian concern. They fulfill the obligation of a profession to improve the quality of care and serve as a basis for job descriptions, educational programs, and certification. Standards reflect the current state of knowledge in a specific field and characterize, measure, and provide guidance for quality. Public and private health care payment systems, such as insurance companies and federal health care programs, set standards for health care. If an individual provider or agency fails to meet standards for minimum safety, the system imposes sanctions. These penalties usually require withholding part or all of the payment for the service. (Jonas 1992, Mitchell 1994).

In the United States, the Cabinet on Nursing Practice of the American Nurses Association sets standards for the nursing profession. To date, the cabinet, through its councils and specialty task forces, has published standards for 23 areas of nursing practice, including medical-surgical, maternal and child health, geriatrics, and psychiatric-mental health with their subspecialties (ANA 1987). In addition, the cabinet has set standards for hospital nursing practice areas, primary health care, and health services in home, school, and correctional facilities. Other professional groups publish standards to guide individual practitioners in specific health care settings. The American Public Health Association has several sets of standards for water, food, and dairy products; ambulatory, maternal, and child health; family planning services; and health services in correctional institutions (APHA 1993–94).

Regulations The laws that govern the licensing of health care providers and practice settings are intended to protect the population from unsafe practices by regulating such things as the education of health professionals, drugs, treatments, products, and the environment of health care settings. Governmental regulations impose controls on rates and quality, and licensure laws restrict entry into practice.

Certification is a type of regulation that signifies expertise in a specialty area of medicine or nursing practice. Although certification is not a requirement for basic licensure, employers may specify certification for advanced clinical practice as a prerequisite for a specific position (Bulechek & Maas 1994). Through the accreditation process, specialty boards and professional societies exert control over educational programs. In other countries, licensure examinations for health professionals are not uniformly required. Graduation from a government-approved educational program is sufficient for licensure without additional examination. In nations with cooperative or socialist health care systems, individuals are registered by a ministry of health or its equivalent on completion of prescribed education. In these countries professional societies have less influence on both licensure and certification than they have in the United States.

In a study conducted by the International Council of Nurses (ICN), researchers found that credentialing nursing is difficult because "nursing" has no universal definition of functions or standards of education and practice. Laws regulating nursing differ widely. "A common finding for all countries is that the legal definition of the scope of nursing practice is generally more restrictive than the performance ability of nurses" (Styles 1986, p. 28). In response to these findings ICN adopted several principles for professional regulation, including the principle that there should be two categories of nursing personnel: nurse and nurse auxiliary and that nurses should be licensed and regulated, as are other professionals.

Organization

The organization of health care involves planning and administration. Planning is required to ensure appropriate allocation of human and material resources to meet priorities. Administration is necessary to monitor activities and evaluate outcomes, including use of services, cost of care, and client health status. Planning and administration of health programs are attempts to make the best use of facilities, personnel, and funds for the purpose of achieving an equitable and cost effective system of health care. Blum (1981) points out, however, that planning may be reduced to a technical exercise. He defines health as a biologic, social, and psychologic state of well-being and says that without a balanced view of what health is, the allocation of resources may promote only the special interests of powerful business and professional groups.

Planning Health planning requires several steps, beginning with assessment. The individual or group responsible for health planning asks, "Is there a problem?" For example, are pregnant women finding prenatal care in a timely way, and are they able to complete the required number of visits before delivery? Health planners seek to answer these questions. They obtain data identifying pregnant women who may be at special risk because of lack of access to prenatal care, such as homeless women and those in rural areas or without health insurance. To ensure comprehensive coverage of the population in question, planners divide a country, state, or local region into units. They collect data from each unit by such means as individual interviews, group discussions, and review of patient records and documents. Researchers seek data about the socioeconomic status, education level, and income of pregnant women who are not receiving early and continuous prenatal care. They also gather data about the availability and accessibility of prenatal care services, the cost of services, and the health outcomes of infants born to mothers with late or fewer than recommended prenatal visits.

Following a careful definition of a health problem, health planners identify overall goals and specific objectives. They then design and implement a program to correct the identified problem. Measures to evaluate the effectiveness of a program include such factors as calculating the percentage of change in women entering prenatal care during a certain time period. When a program is implemented and shown to be working well, health planners then ask if the program is efficient. Evaluation of efficiency gives information about relative benefits compared to costs. Because health care resources are limited and programs compete for available funds, administrators must know if benefits equal costs and if the same benefits can be obtained for less cost. Unfortunately, such a study may not demonstrate a relationship between lower costs and improved health, because it may assess only short-term benefits.

Program Areas of State Health Agencies

Alcohol and drug abuse

Chronic disease screening

Communicable disease control

Dental health

Environmental health

Health education

Health professions licensure

Health resources management

Laboratory

Maternal and child health

Mental health

Mental retardation

Services for children with special health care needs

Administration Administration of the healthcare system in the United States is influenced by two constitutional principles: shared sovereignty between the states and federal government, and separation of power among the executive, legislative, and judicial branches of government (Jonas 1992). The states have primary responsibility for planning and administering health care services. This responsibility is based on their authority to enact and enforce laws to promote and protect public safety. The accompanying box lists typical program areas within state health agencies. Agencies responsible for health services vary from state to state and may be shared by more than one branch of government. The legislative branch enacts the legal framework for public and private health services, allocating funds for these services. The judiciary protects the rights of individuals, addressing controversial issues in the courts, such as access to abortion. The executive branch of state governments implements health legislation, provides for education and professional licensure, and supports research.

Health administration at the federal level is also subject to the checks and balances of the legislative, judicial, and executive branches of government. The federal government, acting through its health planning and administrative agencies, gives money to the states for health care and professional education. A variety of federal programs administer and set standards for the states. The states are free to participate in federally recommended health programs and may or may not accept federal funding to supplement state health care budgets. This same process of setting policy, recommending programs, and funding them goes on between state and local health jurisdictions. The box on pages 156 and 157 shows selected planning and administrative agencies of the federal government.

The Department of Health and Human Services (DHHS) is the principal health agency in the United States. The two major financing programs for health care services, Medicare and Medicaid, are located in this agency under the Health Care Financing Administration. Within the DHHS is the United States Public Health Service, the administrative center for major policy decisions and research for public health in the United States. These federal agencies are linked to both private and public health care sectors by revenue-sharing and grants for health training, health care demonstration projects, and research.

Planning and administration for health in the United States is decentralized to the states and local communities, but with continued support by the federal government in the form of funds and technical expertise. In this decentralized system people have the right to demand accountability for the way their health care dollars are spent. Citizen activity greatly influences what kinds of programs are supported by state legislatures and the United States Congress. The Children's Defense Fund is an example of a citizen lobby. It continually monitors the needs of poor, handicapped, and minority children and attempts to influence the United States policy for child health.

Planning and administration in other countries varies with the degree of centralization of the health care system. When planning is centralized in the government, a potential for a more equitable distribution of health services exists. However, Roemer (1991) notes that administrative officials who plan health care are not necessarily appointed because of technical expertise. Political considerations and favoritism have a strong role, with voluntary health groups and citizens playing a relatively minor part in planning. The former Soviet Union, with a highly centralized health care system, permitted data to be released on some failures of central planning (Schultz & Rafferty 1990). These data revealed that both male and female life expectancy in the Soviet Union was about 10 years less than in the United States and had been declining for 20 years. Infant mortality had risen to 2.5

Selected US Health Administration and Planning Agencies

Department of Agriculture

Concerned with animal, human, and plant health; establishes minimum daily food requirements and food safety regulations; Women, Infants, and Children (WIC) feeding program; National School Lunch Program; food stamp program

Department of Commerce

Conducts the decennial census; provides a wide variety of US population and statistical data on people and the economy

Department of Defense

Concerned with comprehensive health planning, education, and medical care of military personnel and their dependents

Department of Education

Support for special education and rehabilitation services to reduce dependency, increase self-reliance and productive capability of children with disabilities.

Department of Energy

Ensures compliance with environmental health and safety regulations, including nuclear energy.

Department of Health and Human Services

Principal federal agency concerned with health, includes:
1. Health Care Financing Administration: Responsible for financing the two major treatment service programs: Medicare and Medicaid
2. United States Public Health Service:
   a. Office for the Assistant Secretary of Health: Responsible for programs in disease prevention and health promotion, family planning, smoking and health, international health, President's Council of Physical Fitness and Sports, National Center for Health Statistics, and National Center for Health Services Research
   b. Centers for Disease Control
   c. Food and Drug Administration
   d. Agency for Toxic Substances and Disease Registry
   e. Alcohol, Drug Abuse, and Mental Health Administration
   f. National Institutes of Health, the major national force in biomedical research
   g. Health Resources and Service Administration: Responsible for primary health care, health professions, Maternal and Child Health
   h. Indian Health Service
3. Administration on Aging
4. Social Security Administration: Administers Social Security Program

5. Administration for Children and Families
   a. Administers Aid to Families with Dependent Children (AFDC)
   b. Assists states in enforcement of child-support obligations owed by absent parents
   c. Administers community service block grant and refugee resettlement program
   d. Administers adoption assistance, foster care, and child welfare service
   e. Administers the Social Services Block Grants
   f. Administers Head Start, a preschool program
6. Administration on Developmental Disabilities

Department of Housing and Urban Development

Assists families to become home owners; provides rental assistance; lead-based paint abatement and poisoning prevention

Department of Interior

Bureau of Indian Affairs

Department of Justice

Offices of Civil Rights, Prisons, Immigration, Drug Enforcement, Juvenile Justice and Delinquency Prevention, Victims of Crime

Department of Labor

Occupational Safety and Health Administration

Department of Transportation

Provides for safe and efficient transportation through the US Coast Guard and maritime, aviation, highways, and railroad

Department of Veteran's Affairs

A medical care program including medical centers, nursing homes

ACTION

Provides opportunities for voluntary service through Foster Grandparents, Senior Companions, Volunteers in Service of America (VISTA)

Consumer Products Safety Commission

Protects against unreasonable risk of injury from consumer products; develops uniform safety standards, investigates product-related deaths and injuries

Environmental Protection Agency

Concerned with air and water quality; control of radiation hazards, pollution, and toxic substances; solid waste disposal; and pesticide regulation

---

Source: Office of the Federal Register, National Archives and Record Administration. *The United States Government Manual 1993/94,* US Government Printing Office, 1993.

times that of the United States and ranked 50th in the world. Prior to the dissolution of the Soviet Union, the leadership made a commitment to increase the share of gross national product for health care from 3.9% to 6% by the year 2000. They also expected to gradually introduce private enterprise in the form of staff-owned, cooperative clinics that would rely on patient fees for operating expenses. Although Russia is moving to a capitalistic system, no one knows what effect the change will have on its centralized health care system or the access people will have to care.

◆ United States Health Care System

Health care in the United States evolved as a result of historical and cultural influences. Its financing is a complex mix of private and public financing.

Historical and Cultural Influences

Health care in the United States began as a private business. In the 1700s and 1800s, people viewed physicians as tradesmen who relied on their patients to pay for service. Private philanthropies provided for the poor in ambulatory settings that became outpatient departments of teaching hospitals. Medical schools operated as commercial enterprises, charging tuition and conferring diplomas. Some schools offered only lectures with no clinical experience. Although New York City passed the first licensing law in 1760, it did not mandate licensure or require graduation from medical school (Myers 1986). Licensing of physicians was not widely accepted until after 1900.

The Flexner Report of 1910 was a turning point in medical education. It exposed a serious lack of uniformity and standards in many schools. As a result, schools with higher standards, such as those found in colleges and universities, received financial grants, and schools with lower standards closed. Admission criteria rose, and curricula began to reflect the scientific discipline that characterizes medical education today.

During the years that medicine was developing into a regulated, scientific discipline, nursing also was changing. Curricula of nursing schools were modeled after the Nightingale School in England. By the turn of the century, nursing leaders founded the precursor organizations of the American Nurses Association and National League for Nursing. By 1923, 48 states had licensure laws (Henderson & Nite 1978). Just as medical and nursing education were self-regulated, so, too, was the health care industry. Prior to 1900, the only health service provided by the federal government was for seamen and members of the armed forces. After that time, the government became increasingly involved in health care.

Mental Health Care

Care of the mentally ill followed a different path from that of general health care. Whereas general health care was built on private practice, mental health care began as a government responsibility, preceding its involvement in general health care by 50 years. State hospital systems became alternatives to the abusive or nonexistent care in local communities. However, these systems isolated psychiatry from mainstream medicine. Conditions in state mental hospitals were far from ideal. Private psychiatric practice and its teaching in medical schools were not common until the 1930s (Gruenberg 1986). The reform movement of the early 1900s was sparked by the publication of *A Mind that Found Itself,* an account of the experience of Clifford Beers, a patient in a mental hospital. In 1909, Beers founded a voluntary association, the Association of Mental Hygiene, initiating interest in preventive mental health and improved care for the mentally ill. During World War II, the federal government became involved in the treatment and research of psychiatric disorders among military personnel. Since 1946, the National Mental Health Act has made funds available to the states for mental health research, training, and community service centers.

Community Responsibility for Health

Health as a community concern came about as a result of the increasing knowledge of bacteriology and communicable disease of the late 1800s. Early efforts to promote public health included the provision of clean milk at "milk stations" in metropolitan areas and physical examination of school children. Nurses actively participated in these programs, providing care and education in clinics, schools, and homes. The first evidence of federal acceptance of responsibility for child health came in 1912 with the founding of the Children's Bureau in the Department of Labor. It may seem strange to find an agency devoted to children in the Department of Labor. The major threat to child health in that day was their employment in hazardous industries such as mines and mills. Ironically, child labor did not end in United States until the economic depression of the 1930s. It ended then, not because of society's concern for child safety and education, but because children took jobs from unemployed men.

Social Security Act of 1935

A survey conducted by the Children's Bureau contributed to passage of the Social Security Act of 1935. This act provided for income support and health care. Income supports were of two types: insurance (old age, survivor's, disability, and unemployment) and assistance (aid to families with dependent children). Health care, embodied in Title V of the act, consisted of maternal and child health and crippled children services. The act also included a provision for grants to state public welfare agencies to establish and extend services for homeless and neglected children.

The Social Security Act involved the federal government in the health and welfare of individuals as never before. Its passage represented a national desire to prevent a recurrence of the Great Depression and the efforts by humanitarian groups to improve the conditions of families and children. It gave federal assistance to states in areas of health and welfare, even though such assistance meant loss of some control by states over those programs.

With the passage of the Social Security Act, some members of Congress considered a compulsory national health insurance program. Two major reasons halted such action: (1) the zeal with which the American Medical Association argued against any proposal that might take the practice of medicine out of private hands and (2) the expansion of private health insurance, leading the public to believe that there was no need for a government program (Laham 1993). Even so, the Social Security Act has served as a major vehicle for health and welfare legislative amendments ever since its passage.

Increasing Federal Involvement

Following World War II, the federal government increased its role in health care. Research and training in mental health were strengthened by the National Mental Health Act of 1946. That same year the

Hill-Burton Act provided funds for the construction of hospitals, improving access to hospital care (Myers 1986). Government involvement with health care reached new heights with passage of the 1965 amendments to the Social Security Act: Medicare and Medicaid, major programs providing care for the aged, indigent, and disabled.

Over time, legislation has modified Medicaid to increase benefits or offer new programs for eligible persons. In 1972, health personnel developed the Early Periodic Screening Diagnosis and Treatment Program to provide preventive health services for eligible children. In 1984, the act was amended to require states for the first time to cover single women who were pregnant and women who were pregnant in two-parent families with an unemployed breadwinner. In 1989, Congress raised income eligibility for Medicaid benefits for pregnant women and children under six years to 133% of the federal poverty index and mandated increased reimbursement by states for pediatric and obstetric care providers.

The *poverty index* is based on a determination by the Department of Agriculture that families spend approximately one-third of their incomes on food. The *poverty level* is therefore set at three times the cost of an economy food plan that includes specific amounts of meat, vegetables, and other commodities. As of March 1994, a family of four meets the family guideline stated as 100% of poverty if their annual income is $14,800 (Department of Health & Human Services 1994b).

Regional Health Planning

In the 1960s and 1970s, as federal direct payment and revenue sharing programs for health care grew, interest increased in monitoring programs and avoiding duplication of services. In 1974, Congress passed the National Health Planning and Resource Development Act. It enabled state planning boards to regulate health care facilities, determining if new construction, programs, or modification of facilities were in the public interest (Shonick 1986). The act divided the nation into 212 local planning agencies that were to carry out population-based health planning. This program no longer exists, but other plans are being tried at the federal and state level to control health care costs while making care available to everyone. Other health care reform proposals will be discussed in the section on health care financing.

Categorical Programs

The trend in federal-state relations from about 1945 to 1975 was for the federal government to play an increasing role in planning health services and in directing how states spent federal money. Such control required a large bureaucracy in Washington, DC. Some saw this bureaucracy as a valuable source of technical assistance. Others viewed it as a costly and unwelcome interference in affairs that rightfully belonged to the states. Most controversial were the increasing numbers of categorical programs for distinct populations. Funds for such programs were limited to narrowly defined services and channeled through special grantees, usually universities. State and local health departments had no power to determine the need for a program or to alter the use of funds in any way. Limitation and duplication of services resulted. Some categorical programs authorized by 1965–1967 amendments to the Social Security Act include maternity and infant care projects, children and youth projects, neonatal intensive care, family planning, and dental care. Although these programs were recognized as excellent, federal funds supporting them could not be used for any other purpose, even though other needs might be more pressing.

Block Grants

A profound change in federal health policy followed the 1980 presidential election. The administration initiated a block grant method of funding. The Omnibus Reconciliation Act of 1981 consolidated more than 50 categorical grants for health promotion and care. Funds formerly allocated to categorical programs were given to the states in block grants, increasing state control and decreasing federal oversight of program quality. Such freedom from federal regulation seemed too good to be true. It was. With program consolidation came funding reduction. In 1981, the states received about 25% fewer federal health care dollars for programs consolidated under the maternal and child health block grant (General Accounting Office 1984). Lobbying for health programs moved to states and local communities, where decisions about the use of block grant funds were made. A lack of national standards resulted in wide disparities in programming. The Omnibus Reconciliation Act of 1989 (Public Law 101-329) corrected some of the problems resulting from the 1981 law by increasing federal oversight of state planning to better meet the needs of the public.

Financing Health Care in the United States

Sources of private funds

1. Individuals
2. Blue Cross Blue Shield
3. Commercial insurance
4. Self-insurance (corporations)
5. Health maintenance organizations
6. Contributions of philanthropic organizations
7. Employee health services

Programs supported by public funds

1. Federal health programs
   a. Medicare
   b. Native Americans
   c. Federal employees
   d. Merchant marines
   e. Members of armed forces and dependents
   f. Veterans
2. Federal and state revenue-sharing programs
   a. Medicaid
   b. Other programs
      1. Workers' compensation
      2. Family planning
      3. Food assistance
      4. Immunization
      5. Injury control
      6. Children with special health-care needs
      7. Vocational rehabilitation

Source: Kovner AR. *Health Care Delivery in the United States*, 4th ed. Springer, 1990, pp. 247–250.

Financing Health Care

The United States is the only advanced industrial democracy without national health insurance. The population has access to health care only through diverse and complex private and public methods of payment. Understanding these methods is crucial for nurses working in the system and trying to make informed decisions as voters on health care reform proposals. The accompanying box lists the principal sources of private funds and the major programs supported by public funds in the United States.

Private Funds

Private sources of funding for health care come from private health insurance, self-insurance, health maintenance organizations, contributions to philanthropic health services, employee health services, and individuals (out-of-pocket costs). If the health care dollar is divided by source of private funding, out-of-pocket represents 20 cents; private health insurance accounts for 33 cents; and other private sources, 5 cents. The rest, 42 cents, comes from public sources (Levit et al 1994). People who hold private health insurance policies usually work full time and receive their health plan as an employment benefit, paid for in whole or in part by their employer.

Although about 80% of the non-military population has some type of private health insurance, that insurance pays for only 20% to 32% of the national expenditures on personal health care (Knickman & Thorpe 1990). This gap occurs because covered services and liability (who-pays-for-what) vary widely. For example, many insurance policies pay physician and hospital charges if a person is hospitalized, but they do not pay physician charges if the person seeks preventive care or treatment as an outpatient. Most third-party payment systems, whether private or public, discriminate against mental health services as compared to other types of care (Gruenberg 1986).

There are various types of private health insurance plans, including managed fee for service, unmanaged fee for service, health maintenance organizations, and preferred provider organizations (Knickman & Thorpe 1990). "Managed" means any measure that seeks to reduce health care costs while maximizing value, such as controlling access to services and the quality of those services (Jonas 1992, pp. 43–44). Managed fee for service plans represent 43% of all private plans. The typical managed fee for service plan reduces the cost of reimbursement for care in a number of ways. The plan may require a second opinion before a surgical operation will be approved for payment, pre-admission authorization before a hospital stay may be ordered, and periodic reviews of the length of stay in the hospital. Thus, a managed service sets limits on the traditional physician-patient relationship by controlling the physician's decisions about treatment. The advantage to the subscriber, individual or employer, is the lower cost of coverage.

Managed fee for service plans are offered by various commercial insurance companies such as Blue Cross Blue Shield. Blue Cross Blue

Shield is the oldest type of health insurance, originating in a hospital prepayment plan for school teachers in Dallas, Texas in 1929. These plans are run by nonprofit organizations, usually controlled by hospitals and physicians. Commercial insurance companies entered the health care market in the 1940s. They are for-profit businesses that sell many types of insurance, including managed and unmanaged fee for service plans (Fein 1986).

Unmanaged fee for service plans represent 28% of private insurance plans. The plan specifies the services to be covered, but the subscriber has free choice of licensed physicians and hospitals. In general, there is no interference by the plan in the decisions made by the physician for the subscriber's treatment. However, the plan covers only part of the total cost. The subscriber must meet a deductible or co-insurance payment.

Independent plans include both profit and nonprofit organizations and may or may not have managed care features. Under the Employee Retirement Income Security Act of 1974, companies may self-insure for health benefits by establishing a self-funded, nonprofit health plan. Thus, they escape the taxes and regulations of state insurance laws.

Health maintenance organizations (HMOs) are another type of independent insurance. HMOs contract with an enrolled population to provide comprehensive health care on a prepaid basis as either for-profit or nonprofit agencies. HMOs may hire their own staffs or contract with a group practice, network of practices, or independent provider associations. They emphasize prevention and provide both inpatient and outpatient care. Services are guaranteed and prepaid, usually by employers or by employees through payroll deductions. Choice of providers is limited to those working for the plan. Since 1974, HMOs have become increasingly popular, currently enrolling about 18% of privately insured people. With the soaring cost of health care, many HMOs have raised premiums, limited benefits, and increased restrictions. Another version of this model is the *preferred provider organization,* which restricts the choice of physicians to those who agree to a reduced fee schedule. These plans enroll about 11% of the privately insured.

Contributions to philanthropic organizations support a wide variety of health-related services. Some philanthropies, such as the United Way, give funds to direct care agencies. Others provide direct services themselves, such as community hospitals and women's clinics.

Without these philanthropies, many people would have no health care at all.

Workers' compensation insurance provides health care and income replacement for workers who suffer work-related injury, disability, or death. Employers are liable for the cost of this insurance and must purchase a policy from a state-operated insurance fund, offer proof of self-insurance, or contract with a commercial insurance provider. Compensation and amounts awarded to workers are related to the degree and permanence of injuries and number of dependents. Recipients usually receive less than the wages they earned before their injury.

Employee health services began in 1887, when the Homestake Mining Company provided the first industrial medical department in the United States. In 1895, Ada Stewart was hired by the Vermont Marble Company as the first occupational health nurse. About that time Dr. Alice Hamilton began her work, becoming the foremost proponent of occupational safety and health of her day. The labor movement gained strength, and the Department of Labor was formed. In 1911, New Jersey passed the first workers' compensation act upheld by the courts. By 1948, all states had similar laws. In 1970, the Occupational Safety and Health Act made the health of workers a public concern. By 1990, employee health services offered education, direct services, referral, rehabilitation, counseling, and environmental surveillance.

Publicly Funded Programs

Voluntary health insurance does not help people who are unemployed or otherwise unable to purchase insurance. In the free-market system of the United States, the government has been unable and unwilling to provide a national health insurance plan for all its citizens or a tax-supported system of health care (Fein 1986). In spite of this, the government pays 42% of all health-care expenditures (Levit et al 1994). It provides comprehensive health care for Native Americans, members of the armed forces and their dependents, veterans, members of Congress, merchant marines, various groups of federal employees and their dependents, victims of Hansen's disease, and Medicare recipients. Federal grants enable states to provide health care for medically indigent persons through Medicaid. Other federal programs fund services for children with special needs, immunizations, injury control, and food assistance.

Medicare Medicare is a compulsory federal program providing health insurance for eligible persons 65 and older and for certain disabled individuals. It was created by 1965 amendments to the Social Security Act. Medicare is paid for by currently employed people through payroll deductions under the Federal Insurance Contributions Act. It is administered by the Bureau of Health Insurance within the Social Security Administration. Medicare has two parts: A and B.

Medicare Part A covers inpatient hospital services for 90 days per illness episode. Each year patients pay deductible costs equal to about one hospital day and a copayment of 25% of the cost of care for days 61 through 90. Other covered expenses include outpatient diagnostic services and 100 post-hospital days of skilled nursing services. The Omnibus Budget Reconciliation Act of 1981 added home health nursing and hospice services.

Medicare Part B covers physician's fees and other services such as diagnostic tests, rental of medical equipment for home use, and physical therapy in and out of the hospital. Medicare recipients pay monthly premiums, an annual deductible amount, 20% of an approved fee, and any amount above that fee. General tax revenues pay 80% of the approved fee (Levit et al 1994). Providers who agree not to charge more than the approved fee are said to "accept assignment." Those who do not accept assignment charge patients their normal fees, and patients must pay the difference or find other physicians. "Intermediaries," such as Blue Cross, process the claims. About 95% of the elderly are enrolled in Medicare as well as some younger persons who are disabled or have end-stage renal disease.

The cost of Medicare has increased about 18% per year since 1970. A major effort to control this cost is now underway in the form of a *prospective payment system*. This system is based on the average cost of care for a person of a given age with given medical diagnosis, belonging to a *diagnosis-related group (DRG)*. Hospitals are reimbursed according to DRGs. This reimbursement is based on the hospital's location (urban or rural) and the wage rate for the area. Additional payment is allowed if the hospital has a graduate medical education program (Prospective Payment Assessment Commission 1994). Provision is made for transfer of patients between hospitals and for a limited number of extended hospital days. The Health Care Financing Administration controls quality of care by sampling volume of admissions, case mix, and discharge status. *Peer review organizations* validate diagnoses and monitor quality of care and appropriateness of admissions. Regardless of length of stay or complications, hospitals must agree to accept a set fee as full payment. Thus, prospective payment is an incentive to discharge patients as soon as possible and has led to the growth of home care services.

Medicare legislation increased access to home care for the elderly by providing reimbursement for acute convalescent needs. However, this reform has not met the need for long-term care; less than 2% of public expenditures are reimbursed (Harrington 1994a). Medicare-certified home health agencies grew by 98% between 1981 and 1987. The rapid growth in this service has made it extremely difficult for federal and state governments to ensure basic safety and some measure of quality of care for a vulnerable group of patients (Harrington 1994b). Mundinger (1983) demonstrated the vital role nurses play in defining client profiles and outcome measures of health and functional status.

Medicaid Medicaid is a health assistance program providing medical services for the poor. Both federal and state funds pay for Medicaid, with the ratio of federal funding varying from 50% to 83%. Medicaid differs from Medicare in that the federal government does not entitle all poor persons to receive Medicaid as it entitles all persons over age 65 to receive Medicare. Instead, it gives money to the states. This allows considerable flexibility in the total scope of the program, including who will be eligible (Levit et al 1994). Some groups of people are eligible for Medicaid by mandate of the federal government. These include: (1) people who receive Supplemental Security Income for the aged, blind, and disabled; (2) families qualifying for Aid to Families with Dependent Children; and (3) people above the poverty level but within 130% to 200% of that level who belong to one of these groups: pregnant women, children under 6 years, Medicare enrollees, and recipients of foster care and adoption assistance under Social Security Title IV-E. The states may include other medically needy groups in the Medicaid program. In 1988, state income eligibility for the medically needy ranged from a low of 14.6% of the federal poverty level to 85.8%, with an average of 48.8%. Therefore Medicaid covers about 40% of persons defined as living in poverty.

The federal government defines minimum services for Medicaid-eligible persons, such as inpatient and outpatient hospital services, laboratory and X-ray services, and nursing home and home health care. States may provide additional benefits if they wish, such as inpatient psychiatric care, home health visits, eyeglasses, dental care, and drugs. Medicaid coverage is not a guarantee of access to care. Physicians may refuse to treat persons covered by Medicaid, citing low levels of reimbursement, burdensome record keeping, and delays in reimbursement from the state. Paying for Medicaid is becoming more difficult for states, which finance 43% of the cost (Laham 1993). Medicaid recipients will find that they must join state selected HMOs or PPOs as states introduce cost-control measures similar to those in the managed care plans of the private insurance companies.

In 1972, the Early Periodic Screening Diagnosis and Treatment Program was added to Medicaid services. It provides health screening and follow-up diagnostic services for infants, children, and adolescents who are classified as medically indigent or medically needy. The program provides outreach, health screening, and referral services, linking poor children with permanent sources of medical care.

Medicaid, not Medicare, is the chief source of funds for long-term care of the elderly. Medicare requires that covered long-term services be related to an acute illness. Medicare does not cover long-term care needed because of chronic disabilities. Personal resources must be used. When patients have used up all their resources, in a process called *spending down*, they may be eligible for Medicaid. Such forced impoverishment puts a critical hardship on the living spouse. It requires that a spouse either divorce the disabled spouse or become indigent by giving property away or allowing it to be debt-ridden in order to qualify for medical assistance.

Special Programs   Although Medicare and Medicaid are the most expensive and best known of federal and state programs, tax revenues support many others. These programs are of special interest because of the populations they serve and the impact they have on the health and quality of life of recipients. Family planning services are provided by both federal and state governments. Federal funds come from Title X of the Public Health Service Act, Title XIX (Medicaid) of the Social Security Act, and maternal and child health and social services block grants. Among patients served, 80% are below or slightly above the poverty level (Children's Defense Fund 1988). Food assistance is provided through federal food stamp, school food, and Women, Infant, and Children (WIC) programs. About 19 million persons participate in the food stamps program. Eligible families are given or purchase food stamps at a fraction of their value, using them to buy food in grocery stores. School food programs provide free or low-cost meals for poor children. The WIC food-supplement program provides nutrition counseling and food supplements such as milk for pregnant women and mothers with children up to 5 years of age.

Immunization grants from the federal government help states purchase vaccines to immunize their citizens. These federal-state programs, along with improved environmental conditions, have achieved a 99% reduction in diphtheria, pertussis, rubella, and polio. As a result of an internationally coordinated program by the World Health Organization, smallpox has been eradicated from the Western World. Two major concerns about immunization to children persist: costs and liability for adverse reactions to vaccines. Costs continue to rise as new vaccines are developed. In 1994, the estimated cost of vaccines to immunize a child against all vaccine-preventable diseases was $250, not including the price of program administration or provider fees for service. Fear of liability for reactions to vaccines has been reduced since many states now protect providers. Nurses in primary care and pediatrics have an obligation to stay informed of new vaccines, administration schedules, and contraindications. Providers are now liable for missed opportunities to vaccinate children. The American Academy of Pediatrics and the Advisory Committee on Immunization Practice of the Centers for Disease Control serve as a source of current information on immunizations.

Injury control is a serious concern throughout the world. Intentional injuries (homicides, suicides, and nonfatal assaults) and unintentional injuries (automobile crashes, falls, fires, and drowning) are the leading causes of death in people ages 1 to 44 years. The term *accident* is no longer used to describe these events because the word implies that little can be done to control the problem. Epidemiologic studies reveal that many injuries are preventable. The Centers for Disease Control; National Center for Environmental Health and Injury Control; the National Highway Traffic Safety Administration; and the National Institute for Occupational Safety and Health support a number of injury-control activities in the areas of surveillance, education, and research (Department of Health & Human Services 1992). The Children's Safety Network (1994) reports that $215 millions are being distributed through these agencies for injury-related research.

The Program for Children with Special Health Care Needs (CSHCN), formerly the Crippled Children's Service, was begun by

Title V of the Social Security Act of 1935 and retained in all subsequent Title V legislation. Federal funds, together with state matching funds, pay for treatment and rehabilitation for certain categories of disabilities. The states decide what they will cover and the amount of money they will spend. Many states overmatch federal funds. CSHCN has been notable in providing specialized medical care for children not otherwise assisted. It is supported by the private health sector, recruits qualified specialists, and promotes the treatment team concept, including nursing, social work, and other therapies. Case managers control expenditures, act as advocates for families, obtain appropriate specialty care, and conserve funds by developing interagency agreements with programs such as Medicaid. Unfortunately, CSHCN offers only specialty care, not overall health supervision (primary care). As a result, basic health needs such as immunizations, treatment of minor illness, and vision and hearing testing are not covered services. The policy to limit CSHCN to specialty care was made to avoid the appearance of government interference in the business relationship of primary care physicians with their patients.

Persons with acquired immune deficiency syndrome (AIDS) benefit from federal funding for research and treatment and also from the Ryan White Comprehensive AIDS Resources Emergency Act of 1990, the largest dollar investment made by the federal government to date ($348.1 millions in 1993) for the provision of services for people with human immunodeficiency virus (HIV) infection. This legislation enables metropolitan areas with large numbers of reported cases to meet emergency service needs. States can apply for funds to develop systems of care that combine out-of-hospital, community-based support services with in-hospital treatment in order to increase access to care, coordinate services, and reduce hospital admissions (Department of Health & Human Services 1993).

◇ Health Care Reform

The cost of health care in 1994 was estimated to be 13.2% of national income and is expected to soar (Starr 1994). As a consequence, efforts to reform the system have received national attention. In a free-market economy, ensuring access to health care and reducing costs is not easy because of the competing interests of consumers, providers, government, employers, and the insurance industry.

Consumers want access to the best possible health care from a provider of their choice. To achieve this, they need an affordable insurance plan that cannot be canceled if they become unemployed or acquire a long-term illness or disability. Providers, primarily physicians, want freedom from bureaucratic encroachment on their treatment decisions, relief from the high cost of malpractice insurance, protection from loss of earning power, and freedom to choose their area of practice. Employers, who are the primary payers of employee health insurance, want to control the costs of health care so that their businesses will prosper. Federal and state governments, who share responsibility for publicly funded health care coverage, want to contain costs because tax dollars are limited. The insurance industry wants to remain profitable, but its earnings are threatened under a system that insures everyone, regardless of risk. Obviously, in the interest of providing insurance at an affordable cost, each of these groups must compromise.

The Major Problems

There are two major problems: financial barriers to health insurance and the high cost of care. It is estimated that in the United States today, 37 million people are without health care insurance. Although most are employed, they cannot afford insurance premiums, yet they are not poor enough to qualify for public assistance. These people may receive some care, but they may not receive preventive care or treatment for illness to prevent complications. Furthermore, large numbers of people are vulnerable to losing their health insurance because they are at risk of being laid off or having their working hours reduced. Employers can save the cost of health insurance benefits by reducing workers to part-time status. It is estimated that over the course of the year, 1 in 4 Americans will be uninsured for part of the year.

The cost of care is enormous. The United States spends more on health care than any other industrialized nation, yet a significant portion of the population is excluded from the benefits of that care.

Some Solutions

One approach to health care reform is the *single-payer plan* (Himmelstein & Woolhandler 1994, Starr 1994). This plan creates a universal public system of health insurance, with comprehensive benefits financed by payroll taxes. All Americans would be covered in the same way that Medicare covers all elderly persons. The single-payer plan would replace Medicare and Medicaid. Costs would be controlled through administrative simplification and government-regulated payment for health care providers. Objections to single-payer plans, whether at the state or federal level, are that competition is blocked, choice of providers may be limited, and cost controls may be achieved by reducing services.

Managed competition is another approach to health care reform. It uses market forces to control costs and improve performance (Starr 1994). This approach characterizes several reform proposals. One plan sets up a system of competing regional purchasing groups to collect and distribute health care premiums, certify health plans, and offer them to consumers. The purchasing groups ensure that premiums grow no faster than federally set limits allow and contain costs by setting caps on fees. Consumers would be offered choices among HMOs and private providers who agreed to join the system. Some managed-competition plans are funded by employer mandates to pay for all their employees, regardless of the number of hours worked or pre-existing illness. Taxes would pay the premiums for nonworkers.

Some proponents of managed competition place the responsibility for obtaining health care coverage on the individual rather than the employer or the government. Every person would be required to have insurance either through their employer or by purchasing coverage in the private health insurance market. The government would subsidize premium costs for low-income individuals. Costs would be controlled by promoting consumer consciousness about costs of care, greater use of managed care plans, and greater competition among health plans. These methods of cost controls are features of *Nursing's Agenda for Health Care Reform*, the plan proposed by the American Nurses Association (1993). Other plans have neither an employer or individual mandate for insurance coverage but would reform private health insurance plans to ensure coverage regardless of pre-existing medical conditions. There would be subsidies for low-income people and assistance for small companies to purchase insurance for their employees.

Interim Reforms

While the American public awaits decisions from Congress on a comprehensive health care system, incremental reforms are occurring. In the private sector cost-saving measures include: (1) offering new forms and conditions for insurance such as PPOs, coinsurance, and deductibles, (2) requiring second opinions before surgery, (3) instituting a case-management system to limit the choice of providers to those charging the most reasonable fees, (4) offering incentives for less expensive services such as outpatient care, and (5) educating the public about healthful lifestyles.

In the public sector, with the number of people over age 65 growing, measures to reduce Medicare costs are urgently needed. These measures include limiting hospital payments by using a prospective payment system and shifting more of the cost to recipients. Proposals to reduce Medicaid costs include: (1) negotiating prospective payment contracts with hospitals, (2) limiting the choice of hospitals and providers through managed care plans, (3) permitting insurance companies to negotiate preferred provider agreements, (4) reducing the scope of coverage, (5) limiting the number of eligible people, and (6) returning the care of medically indigent adults from the states to the counties, which have their own tax base.

The present method of controlling health care costs leaves the poor with few choices. Social legislation of the 1930s and 1960s attempted to provide a system of health care for the poor that was equal to the private sector system. However, many forces have caused a return to the two-tiered system that prevailed when health care was paid out-of-pocket. Some of these forces include (1) inflation, (2) wasteful expansion of medical technology, (3) physician and insurance barriers to advanced practice by nonphysician health professionals, (4) failure of the health care system to respond to free-market forces, and (5) growth of for-profit health care corporations. Many believe that federally based comprehensive health insurance would achieve more equitable distribution of care. Much has been learned about responsible cost control since national health insurance was first proposed. Perhaps these lessons will serve as the basis for a more complete, equitable health care system (Starr 1994).

◆ Health Care Policy

A health care system develops from health policy decisions. These decisions reflect the economic constraints, cultural beliefs, and political ideology of a nation. They are made on the basis of *policy research*, a process by which information pertinent to an area of concern is gathered, tested, and made available to policy makers.

Data Collection

Collection of appropriate data is essential to policy research. It is carried out by federal, state, and local agencies. Federal agencies that collect and disseminate data about health in United States are listed in Table 6-3. The National Center for Health Statistics (NCHS) is the primary data-collection agency. It uses census data collected every ten years by the Bureau of Census to formulate the total population at risk for various vital events. The NCHS also conducts special surveys and publishes a wide range of health information. Its data are available on computer discs for research purposes, and its publications are listed in the *Catalog of Publications*, US Department of Health and Human Services.

The National Health Interview Survey is especially important to health policy research. This household survey of a probability sample of the population is valuable because it represents the perceptions people hold of their health status and needs. Data are classified by age and sex and used to predict the incidence of acute illness, injury, disability, limitation of activity due to chronic illness, and use of health care services. A limitation of the federal data-collection process is that it may take up to 5 years to analyze and publish information. Such delays complicate health planning but point out the value of local data-collection efforts.

All states have an office of vital statistics that collects health information. Data from local communities are sent to the state office and on to federal agencies. This information is used for health planning and policy development at all levels of government. Vital events such as births and deaths are routinely collected and reported. Other data are collected periodically by health professionals who carry out small surveys in work settings and local communities.

Major Indicators of Health Status

Major indicators of health status are *vital events*, such as births, deaths (mortality), and sickness (morbidity). *Demographic data* describe the size, distribution, structure, and change of a population over time. Vital events and demographics are usually expressed as proportions, called *rates*, with the vital event or descriptive feature

TABLE 6-3

Sources of Data	Types of Data
United States Department of Health and Human Services	
National Center for Health Statistics	The only federal agency specifically established for collection and dissemination of health data.
National Vital Statistics System	Collects and publishes data on births, deaths, marriages, and divorces
National Survey of Family Growth	Provides national data on demographic and social factors associated with childbearing, adoption, and maternal and child health
National Health Interview Survey	A nationwide, continuing, sample survey; data collected by personal household interviews on personal and demographic characteristics, use of health resources, illnesses, chronic conditions, injuries, impairments
National Health and Nutrition Examination	A nationwide sample survey; data obtained by direct physical examination, clinical and laboratory tests in order to measure and monitor indicators of nutritional status
National Health Provider Inventory	A comprehensive file of inpatient health facilities such as hospitals and nursing homes
National Nursing Home Survey	A nationwide sample survey of all types of nursing homes
National Hospital Discharge Survey	A nationwide sample survey that collects data about discharges from short stay hospitals
National Ambulatory Medical Care Survey	A national probability sample of ambulatory medical encounters in the offices of non-federally-employed physicians
National Center for Infectious Diseases	
Acquired Immune Deficiency Syndrome (AIDS) Surveillance	Local health departments collective information without personal identifiers for epidemiologic studies by the Centers for Disease Control

TABLE 6-3 *(continued)*

Selected Sources of Data on Health

Sources of Data	Types of Data
National Notifiable Disease Surveillance	Weekly provisional information on disease occurrence and public health implications; published in Morbidity and Mortality Weekly Report
National Center for Chronic Disease Prevention and Health Promotion	
Abortion Surveillance	Abortion service statistics by states
National Institute for Occupational Safety and Health	
National Traumatic Occupational Fatalities Surveillance System	Information from death certificates collected from the states
Health Resources and Services Administration	
Physician Supply Projections and Nurse Supply Estimates	Evaluates current and future supply of health care personnel designating shortage areas
Substance Abuse and Mental Health Services Administration	
National Household Survey on Drug Abuse	Data on use of marijuana, alcohol, cigarettes, and cocaine among persons 12 and older
Drug Abuse Warning Network	Data on drug abuse from emergency rooms and medical examiner facilities
National Institutes of Health National Cancer Institute	
Surveillance, Epidemiology and End Results Program	Data on cancer from 11 population base registries
National Institute on Drug Abuse	
Monitoring the Future Study	Survey of drug use and attitudes among high school seniors

➤

TABLE 6-3 *(continued from page 177)*

Selected Sources of Data on Health

Sources of Data	Types of Data
Health Care Financing Administration	
Estimates of National Health Expenditures	Compiled annually by type of expenditure and source of funds from an array of sources
Medicare Statistical System	Data on program effectiveness and tracking eligibility of enrollers
Medicaid Data System	Count of recipients and expenditure data
Department of Commerce	
Bureau of Census	Beginning in 1790, the Bureau has taken a census of population every 10 years; conducts monthly current population survey
Department of Labor	
Bureau of Labor	Prepares a monthly *Consumer Price Statistics Index,* a measure of changes in the average prices of goods and services purchased by urban wage earners and their families, showing trends in medical care prices by using specific indicators of hospital, medical, dental, and drug prices
Environmental Protection Agency	Collects data on pollutants for which national ambient air quality standards have been set; maintains Airometric Data Bank
United Nations	
Statistical Office	Prepares *Demographic Yearbook,* a collection of comprehensive international demographic statistics

Source: National Center for Health Statistics. *Health, United States,* 1993. Public Health Service, 1994.

the numerator and a total population at risk the denominator. The rate is expressed in relation to a unit of time, usually a year. The *crude death rate* is an expression of all deaths for a given year as a proportion of the total population. The *neonatal mortality rate* (deaths of infants in the first 28 days of life) reflects unaddressed health problems of pregnant women, such as poor nutritional status and anemia. It also may demonstrate problems that exist in preventing infant infection or trauma during labor and delivery. The *postneonatal mortality rate* (deaths of infants from age 29 days to 1 year) reflects unsafe feeding techniques and unintentional home injuries such as burns and falls. It also reflects environmental health issues such as unsafe water, improper sewage disposal, and inadequate food distribution. These data are especially important in developing countries of the world, where enteric and respiratory infections are a leading cause of infant death.

The *perinatal mortality rate* (fetal deaths and deaths of infants under 28 days) is of special concern in the United States. It is a relatively accurate measure of the impact of (1) prenatal care on a mother's health and (2) technology in the management of labor and delivery and support of fragile neonates. The perinatal mortality rate in the United States reveals that technology is only reducing birth weight–specific neonatal mortality. Providers of health care are able to save more very small babies, but the system is failing to prevent births of low birth weight babies, particularly African-American ones. Low birth weight accounts for the greatest proportion of perinatal deaths.

Total fertility rate is based on the number of births per woman of childbearing age (15 to 49 years). It represents the average number of children that would be born alive to a woman during her lifetime if she were to pass through all her childbearing years conforming to age-specific fertility rates of a given year. In 1993, the total fertility rate for the United States was 2.0; that is, women in the United States, on average, were having approximately two children throughout their childbearing years. During the same year the total fertility rate for Kenya, East Africa was between 6.7 and 6.8. That is, women in Kenya, on average, could expect to have over 6 children throughout their childbearing years (Population Reference Bureau 1994). Given such a rapid growth in population, it is easy to understand why African countries, such as Kenya, might have different priorities for maternal and child health planning than the United States.

Health Policy Research

As with other types of research, the first step in policy research is to formulate goals. These are expressions of values held by health professional and citizen groups. For example, a value identified by these organizations might be to make prenatal care available to all pregnant women regardless of ability to pay. That value might then become a policy goal. The next step is to review the history of a setting or situation relative to the goal and develop a methodology, identifying research objectives, significant vital events, and affected people. The research is conducted, data collected and analyzed, and findings presented to policy makers.

◆ Future Trends

Many people wonder if comprehensive health care is possible in a free-market economy. Indeed, the future of the United States health care system depends on the political and economic climate. The growth of managed competition is a major structural reform that shows promise of providing some choice of health care plans for consumers while helping employers to afford health care plans for their employees. Managed care plans are also being introduced into publicly funded health care coverage, such as Medicaid (California Department of Health Services 1993). In the absence of true health care reform these are incremental ways to keep the cost of health care under control. However, these incremental changes leave certain basic issues unresolved. Employer-based health care insurance will continue to exclude the unemployed and underemployed. The states are still faced with increasing numbers of uninsured persons for whom they must provide some basic health services. A political consensus to enact a national health care system has not yet been achieved. Even so, when the people and the profit-making corporations see a benefit from a comprehensive health care system, they will exert political pressure and a system will be adopted.

◇ Summary

Health care systems reflect the political and economic philosophy of the country in which they exist. These systems consist of the resources, functions, controls, and organization necessary to deliver health care. The United States health care system reflects the philosophy of a free-market economy. Its source of funding is diverse and complicated, made up of both public and private monies. There is general agreement on the urgent need to reform the US health care system to provide universal access to affordable care, but there is little agreement on how to achieve these goals. Nursing practice will be greatly influenced by the resolution of the health care reform debate. The ANA is monitoring proposals that focus on cost controls. The ANA's goal is to ensure that health care reform provides universal access to care and a better balance between illness/cure and wellness/care. By making policy research findings available to policy makers, it is expected that some change can be effected.

Critical Thinking Questions

1. Evaluate the practice used in cooperative/socialist health care whereby graduates of state-approved educational programs begin their practice without a licensure examination. In your opinion, should the United States adopt this practice? If so, what safeguards should be put in place?

2. Construct an argument to support the entrepreneurial and permissive system of health care in the United States.

3. Many people find that they are pulled in different directions because they hold conflicting values about health and health care systems. Use evaluative thinking (refer to the box "Questions That Stimulate Effective Thinking" in Chapter 5) to identify conflicting values you hold in regard to the kind of health care system the United States ought to have.

1. In a small group discuss the extent to which the health care resources in your community are accessible and adequate to meet the health needs of the population.

2. Describe a local health department program that is designed to serve a particular population, such as battered women. What is the purpose? What data were used to show a need for it? Was the source of the data valid? Are the goals and objectives clearly stated? How does the health department plan to evaluate the outcomes of the program?

3. Interview a financial officer of a health facility, such as a hospital, that accepts Medicaid reimbursement for patient care. Ask the officer: Does the facility participate in managed-care reimbursement plans? What impact has managed care or other types of cost control had on access to care, length of hospital stay, and cost of care of Medicaid patients in this facility?

4. Interview a member of the Gray Panthers, an advocacy group for the elderly. Ask that person to discuss access to health care for the elderly in your community.

Annotated Reading List

Harrington C, Estes CL (eds). *Health Policy and Nursing: Crises and Reform in the Health Care Delivery System.* Jones & Bartlett, 1994.

An excellent source of information, this book provides information on how the health care delivery system is structured, how it works, how the professions of medicine and nursing fit in the scheme of the US health care system, and how health care is financed. The book reviews the major reform proposals.

Laham N. *Why the United States Lacks a National Health Insurance Program.* Greenwood Press, 1993.

The author asks the question, "Why is the United States the only advanced industrial democracy in the world without national health insurance?" He provides a historical review of the politics of national health insurance in the United States, explaining the various positions of organized lobbyists over the years, such as the American Medical Association, the American Hospital Association, and the health insurance industry.

McCloskey JC, Grace HK (eds). *Current Issues in Nursing*, 4th ed. Mosby, 1994.

This useful reference gives the viewpoint of nursing through a collection of provocative discussions on such issues as the measurement of quality in nursing care, standard setting, reimbursement under health care reform, and credentialing and certification in nursing.

Starr P. *The Logic of Health Care Reform*. Penguin Books, 1994.

This small but powerful book offers information about what is wrong with the US health care system and makes proposals for correcting its inequities. The author describes each proposal and gives potential consequences for each course of action. A distinguished writer in the field of politics, health care, and American society wrote this as a handbook to inform legislative advocates and policy researchers.

References

American Nurses Association. *Nursing's Agenda for Health Care Reform*. ANA, 1993.

American Nurses Association. *Standards of Practice for the Primary Health Care Nurse Practitioner*. ANA, 1987.

American Public Health Association. *Publications 1993–1994*. APHA, 1994.

Arnett RH, McKusick DR, Sonnefeld ST, Cowell CS. Projections of Health Care Spending to 1990. *Health Care Financing Review* 1986; 7:1–36.

Blum HC. *Planning for Health*. Human Sciences Press, 1981.

Bulechek GM, Maas ML. Nursing Certification. In McCloskey JC, Grace HK (eds). *Current Issues in Nursing*, 4th ed. Mosby, 1994, pp.19–25.

California Department of Health Services. *Expanding Medi-Cal Managed Care*. Department of Health Services, 1993.

Children's Defense Fund. *A Children's Defense Budget: FY 1988*. The Children's Defense Fund, 1988, p. 71.

Children's Safety Network. *Childhood Injury: Cost and Prevention Facts*. National Public Services Research Institute, Economics and Insurance Resources Center, 1994.

Department of Health and Human Services, Public Health Service, Health Resources and Services Administration. *The Registered Nurse Population. Findings from the National Sample Survey of Registered Nurses*. Bureau of Health Professions, Division of Nursing, 1994a.

Department of Health and Human Services. Annual Update of the HHS Poverty Guidelines. *Federal Register*. US Government Printing Office, February 10, 1994b.

Department of Health and Human Services, Public Health Service, Centers for Disease Control. *The Third National Injury Control Conference, 1991.* US Government Printing Office, 1992.

Department of Health and Human Services, Public Health Service. *The Ryan White Comprehensive AIDS Resources Emergency Act of 1990.* Health Resources and Services Administration, Bureau of Health Resources Development, August, 1993.

Fein R. *Medical Care, Medical Costs: The Search for a Health Insurance Policy.* Harvard University Press, 1986.

General Accounting Office, United States. *Maternal and Child Health Block Grant: Program Changes Emerging Under State Administration.* General Accounting Office, GAO/HRD 84-35, May 7, 1984.

Gruenberg EM. Mental Disorders. In Last JM (ed). *Maxcy-Rosenau Public Health and Preventive Medicine,* 12th ed. Appleton-Century-Croft, 1986, pp. 1341–1384.

Grumbach K, Lee PR. How Many Physicians Can We Afford? In Harrington C, Estes CL (eds). *Health Policy and Nursing.* Jones & Bartlett, 1994, pp. 284–293.

Harrington C. The Nursing Home Industry: A Structural Analysis. In Harrington C, Estes CL (eds). *Health Policy and Nursing.* Jones & Bartlett, 1994a, pp. 192–204.

Harrington C. The Nursing Home Industry: A Structural Analysis. In Harrington C, Estes CL (eds). *Health Policy and Nursing.* Jones & Bartlett 1994b, pp. 236–243.

Harris R. *A Sacred Trust.* New American Library, 1966.

Henderson V, Nite G (eds). *Principles and Practice of Nursing.* MacMillan, 1978.

Himmelstein DU, Woolhandler SA. National Health Program for the United States: A Physicians' Proposal. In Harrington C, Estes CL: *Health Policy and Nursing.* Jones & Bartlett, 1994, pp. 476–489.

Hull K, American Hospital Association. Hospital Trends. In Harrington C, Estes CL (eds). *Health Policy and Nursing.* Jones & Bartlett, 1994, pp. 150–168.

Jonas S. *An Introduction to the U. S. Health Care System.* 3rd ed. Springer, 1992, pp. 23–48.

Knickman JR, Thorpe KE. Financing Health Care. In Kovner AR (ed). *Health Care Delivery in the United States.* Springer, 1990, pp. 240–269.

Kovner AR. *Health Care Delivery in the United States,* 4th ed. Springer, 1990, pp. 247–250.

Laham N. *Why the United States Lacks a National Health Insurance Program.* Greenwood Press, 1993.

Levit KR, Lazenby HG, Cowan CA, Letsch SW. National Health Expenditures. In Harrington C, Estes CL (eds). *Health Policy and Nursing.* Jones & Bartlett, 1994, pp. 14–27.

Mitchell M. Debate: How Can We Assure Health Care Quality. In McCloskey JC, Grace HK (eds). *Current Issues in Nursing.* 4th ed. Mosby, 1994, pp. 287–294.

Mundinger MO. *Home Care Controversy.* Aspen Systems, 1983.

Myers BA. Social Policy and the Organization of Health Care. In Last JM (ed). *Maxcy-Rosenau Public Health and Preventive Medicine,* 12th ed. Appleton-Century-Crofts, 1986, pp. 1639–1667.

National Center for Health Statistics. *Health, United States, 1993.* Public Health Service, 1994.

National Commission on Acquired Immune Deficiency Syndrome. *America Living with AIDS.* National Commission on AIDS. 1991.

Office of the Federal Register, National Archives and Records Administration. *The United States Government Manual 1993/94.* US Government Printing Office, 1993.

Population Reference Bureau. *1993 World Population Data Sheet.* 1994.

Prospective Payment Assessment Commission. Medicare and the American Health Care System. In Harrington C, Estes CL (eds). *Health Policy and Nursing.* Jones & Bartlett, 1994, pp. 169–178.

Roemer MI. *National Health Systems of the World.* Vol. 1, *The Countries.* Vol. 2, *The Issues.* Oxford University Press, 1991.

Schultz DS, Rafferty MP. Soviet Health Care and Perestroika. *American Journal of Public Health* 1990; 80:193–195.

Shonick W. Health Planning. In Last JM (ed). *Maxcy-Rosenau Public Health and Preventive Medicine,* 12th ed. Appleton-Century-Crofts, 1986, pp. 1669–1688.

Stafford M, Appleyard J. Clinical Nurse Specialists and Nurse Practitioners. In McCloskey JC, Grace HK (eds). *Current Issues in Nursing,* 4th ed. Mosby, 1994, pp. 19–25.

Starr P. *The Logic of Health Care Reform.* Penguin Books, 1994.

Styles MM. *Credentialing in Nursing: U.S.A. within a World View.* ANA, 1986.

US Census Bureau. *Statistical Abstract of the United States,* 113th ed. 1993.

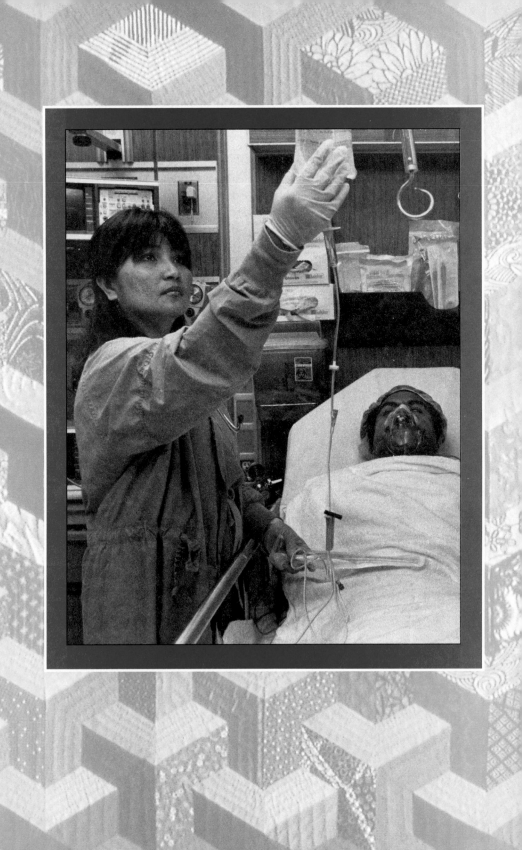

Ethical Concerns

7

◇ Learning Objectives

- Discuss the types, functions, acquisition, and importance of values.

- Apply values-clarification strategies to a nursing situation.

- Explain how belief systems develop and how they influence health care.

- Compare the stages of moral development according to Piaget, Kohlberg, and Gilligan.

- Compare deontological and teleological ethical theories.

- Formulate real-life examples of how deontological and teleological theories would affect ethical decisions.

- Discuss the difference between personal ethics and ethical codes.

- Compare the American Nurses Association and International Council of Nursing codes of ethics.

- Explain the ethical principles of respect for human life and dignity, beneficence, honesty, autonomy, and justice.

- Apply a decision-making process to an ethical dilemma in nursing practice, demonstrating how to resolve the dilemma.

Jamie was a beautiful 3-year-old. She was bright, well behaved, and much loved by her parents and 11-year-old brother. She delighted in going to the ocean, wading along the shore, and feeling the sand move under her toes as the waves rolled in and out on the beach. Her brother was permitted to go out to where the waves were high and the current swift because he knew how to swim. One afternoon, when her mother was distracted by a conversation, Jamie followed her brother out into the deeper water. A huge wave caught her and swept her under, but no one missed her for some time. When they did, it took nearly 30 minutes to find her. The EMTs finally got Jamie's heart started, connected her to a mechanical ventilator, started intravenous fluids and took her to the emergency room. Jamie never regained consciousness. Eventually, she was weaned from the ventilator. The intravenous lines were replaced by a feeding tube and she was transferred to a long-term care facility.

Now Jamie lies in a bed on the total care unit, unresponsive except to painful stimuli. Her care costs $1500/month. When she develops pneumonia, which is often, Jamie is taken to the acute hospital where the cost is $900/day. Her parents have exhausted their financial resources. Unable to "give up hope," they remain in a constant state of grief and guilt.

In the same community homeless children live in squalor, inadequately clothed and fed and chronically ill. Is Jamie's care an appropriate use of public money? Should her life be maintained at all costs? If not, how much cost? Who should decide?

◆

A few years ago, medical science knew no way to prolong life. The primary task of nurses and physicians was to support the sick until they healed or to comfort them until they died. There were no weighty decisions about who should live and who should die. Even when people desperately wanted to prolong life, no one had the knowledge or skill to do so.

Gradually at first, and now at an accelerated rate, scientific knowledge is expanding and health care providers have more and more control over life and death. Drugs and treatment can change the course of nature. Where once it was impossible to sustain life functions even for minutes, now it can be done for years. These advances have brought hope and joy, but they have raised profound questions. Is the presence of a heartbeat sufficient criterion to sustain it? Does the presence of a heartbeat mean the individual is "alive"? What about the person in whom that heart beats? What about the quality of life as opposed to its quantity (length)? Is it possible or reasonable to sustain everyone whose heart stops beating? If not, what criteria should be used to decide?

To help resolve these questions health professionals turn to *ethics*, that branch of philosophy that deals with the rightness or wrongness of human behavior. The result is a field of study called *bioethics*, the moral and social implications of medicine upon human life. Some of the concepts encompassed in bioethics are values, belief systems, and ethics.

◆ Values

Values are perceptions of worth that people place on objects, attitudes, ideas, and personal traits. They give direction and meaning to life and serve as general principles of conduct. People demonstrate their values every day by the choices they make and the actions they take. Values provide a frame of reference through which people integrate, explain, and judge ideas, events, and personal relationships.

A *value system* is a set of values arranged along a continuum of relative importance. For example, a father valued adherence to a religious doctrine. When his son left the faith, the father banished the son from the family even though doing so caused great sorrow. The father valued faith in a religious doctrine above the fellowship of his son.

Types of Values

People categorize values in many ways according to the way they view or use them. Steele and Harmon (1983) say that values relating to the maintenance of life, such as the value of food and water, are *intrinsic values* and that values originating outside the individual, such as the value of people, things, and concepts, are *extrinsic values* because they are not vital to life. *Personal values* are attributes that individuals hold dear, such as independence, artistic expression, and a sense of humor. *Professional values* are attributes prized by a professional group. For instance, artists and writers value creativity, and nurses value intelligence, empathy, and skill. *Cultural-societal-religious values* are attributes, including ethical principles, valued by a culture, society, or religion. For example, history reports that stoicism, the ability to bear pain without complaint, was a cultural value of the Stoics of ancient Greece. *Terminal values* are concerned with end states or goals, such as world peace and career success. *Instrumental values* are desirable modes of conduct, such as honesty and kindness.

The Functions and Importance of Values

Values serve many functions. They provide standards, reflect personal identity, furnish a basis on which to make decisions, give meaning to life, motivate behavior, and lead people to make "ought" and "should" demands on themselves and others. Values influence the choices people make and the way they use their time, spend their money, and expend their energy. Values affect their choice of friends, careers, and pleasurable pursuits. Even when people are not aware of values, their verbal and nonverbal behaviors reveal their values.

Acquisition of Values

Values are not inherited. They are taught by modeling and moralizing and caught by observation, reasoning, and experience. Children learn values as they are socialized into the family, school, and community. As they observe their parents and other role models and listen to what they say, children internalize their values and claim them as their own.

> *Olita's parents valued altruism and industry, modeled them in their lives, and taught them to their children. Olita incorporated these values into her value system and when her church established*

a homeless shelter, she was the first to volunteer. The values of altruism and industry were now her own.

Intellectual and emotional development influence values throughout the life span. Young children value concrete objects such as favorite toys and the physical closeness of parents. Older children value activities and the company of same-sex friends. Adolescents value peer approval more than family approval or even personal comfort. Young adults value achievement and intimate relationships. Middle-aged adults value personal and professional fulfillment. Older adults value health and association with family and friends.

Values Clarification

Because values influence us in so many ways, nurses need to know their own personal and professional values. The process of gaining this knowledge is called *values clarification.* The box on page 192 gives some strategies to help you identify your values.

The Valuing Process

In 1979, Raths, Harmin, and Simmons described the valuing process. It provides a means for people to sort out, analyze, and set priorities for their own values. The seven-step process is divided into three elements: choosing, prizing, and acting. See the box on page 193.

John had a secure position at the state hospital as a licensed psychiatric technician when he enrolled in an associate degree nursing program at the community college. He continued to work at the state hospital part-time. When John graduated, the hospital offered him a charge position. His family lives nearby, as does his girlfriend, and he values their support and closeness. However, since he has become an RN he has had many other career options. He uses the values-clarification process to make a choice about his career.

Choosing

1. John considers the many values he holds, including personal, financial, and professional security; being carefree; independence; challenge; adventure; and educational achievement. He realizes he cannot have all of these things at this time and must choose between them.

Values Clarification

Strategy: Voting

Indicate if you: (1) strongly agree, (2) agree, (3) don't care, (4) disagree, (5) strongly disagree

1. Women should have the right to have an abortion on demand.
2. Parents should have the right to discipline their children in any way they see fit.
3. Euthanasia is wrong in all circumstances.
4. Mentally retarded people should be sterilized.
5. People should have the right to purchase drugs without a prescription.
6. Life should be sustained at all cost, regardless of mental status.
7. The death penalty as a method of punishment is archaic and should be eliminated.

Strategy: Rank Ordering

Within each group of questions, rank each choice from 1 to 4, with 1 the highest priority and 4 the lowest priority.

1. With limited medical resources, which of the following clients should receive care?

    ___ Premature infants weighing less than 2 pounds at birth

    ___ Antepartal patients with complications of pregnancy

    ___ Men, ages 40–50, with acute myocardial infarcts

    ___ Women, ages 75–85, with crippling osteoarthritis

2. You are assigned to a client with cirrhosis of the liver. Rank the things you should do for her:

    ___ Explain the effects her drinking has had on her liver.

    ___ Make her as physically comfortable as you can.

    ___ Encourage her to talk about her feelings.

    ___ Allow her to make decisions about her care.

Strategy: Sentence Completion

1. If I had only six months to live I would . . .
2. If I won ten million dollars I would . . .
3. If I had a 12-month paid vacation I would . . .
4. If I were president of the United States I would . . .
5. If I wrote my epitaph it would say . . .

The Valuing Process

Choosing

1. Choosing freely

2. Selecting from alternatives

3. Choosing after consideration of the consequences of each alternative

Prizing

4. Being proud of and happy with the choice

5. Being willing to affirm the choice publicly

Acting

6. Making the choice part of one's behavior

7. Repeating the choice

2. John selects those values he holds highest from among the many. He decides that he most values independence, challenge, educational achievement, and financial and professional security.

3. John considers carefully the consequences of his choices. If he chooses security he will return to the state hospital where he will be professionally comfortable and financially secure. If he chooses challenge, adventure, and educational achievement he will go on for an advanced degree and become a nurse practitioner, but it will mean many years of hard work, financial sacrifice, moving to a large city away from his family and friends, and taking a part-time job in a new and unfamiliar hospital. John chooses challenge, adventure, and educational achievement.

Prizing

4. John is proud and happy about his choice. He feels elated about his decision.

5. John affirms his choice publicly by announcing his decision to his friends and his supervisor at the state hospital.

Acting

6. John makes the choice part of his behavior by sending for information about BSN and MSN nurse practitioner programs and by looking for a nursing position in the city.

7. John confirms his choice of action by applying for entrance into a BSN/MSN program; he goes for job interviews and looks for an apartment near his chosen university program.

Value Conflicts

Value conflicts occur when two or more values clash. When they are internalized values, the individual must prioritize them in order to resolve the conflict. When value conflicts occur between individuals, the people may agree to disagree, compromise, or expand the clash to open conflict.

◆ Belief Systems and Religions

Belief systems are organized patterns of thought regarding the origin, cause, purpose, and place of humans in the universe. These systems seek to explain the mysteries of life and death, good and evil, health and illness. Typically, belief systems include ethical codes that prescribe correct conduct. *Religions* are organized schemes of thought that include a belief system, organizational structures, and devotional rituals (Wach 1992), albeit, people do not need to subscribe to a religion to have a personal belief system, set of values, and ethical code of behavior.

Some sociologists believe that religions develop because humans feel the need to control the forces of nature and bring order (cosmos) out of disorder (chaos). Durkheim says that religion is an effort of humans to "pass science and complete it prematurely in an effort to keep the experience of chaos within limits that humans can sustain" (1915, p. 56). Religions often include ethical codes to govern social order, especially within families. These codes regulate sexual behavior, male and female roles, socialization of children, care of the sick and aged, ownership of property, and inheritance. Belief systems are no less important to people now than they were before the advent of the scientific method. They give meaning to life and provide a framework by which people order their lives. When people feel powerless and hopeless in the face of injustice and suffering, belief systems help them cope. They comfort the grief-stricken and give people identity and a feeling of importance. The ethical codes of belief systems give standards with which to measure right and wrong conduct.

Just as values and beliefs influence the way people respond to health status, so health status affects values and beliefs. A diagnosis of cancer may cause a young adult to value life as never before, a spinal cord injury may prompt the victim to appreciate mobility, and arthritis may cause the sufferer to value freedom from pain over life. Nurses help clients identify their values and beliefs in order to help them understand their reactions to injury and illness, integrate the experience of an injury or illness into their belief and value systems, and explore alternative plans when their goals are blocked. Nurses learn about client beliefs and values by reviewing health records for clues, talking with clients, and listening to the family and friends. They use this information to help clients plan actions that support their values and beliefs.

◇ Ethics

Ethics is the branch of philosophy that is concerned with the rightness or wrongness of human behavior and the goodness or badness of the motives behind it. Ethics implies that people can make choices about how they behave (Thiroux 1990, p. 2). Ethics is a subject that has fascinated people for centuries, one that has produced an enormous body of literature. Scholars divide these writings into three general categories: descriptive ethics, metaethics (analytical), and normative (prescriptive) ethics.

Descriptive ethics describes the moral choices of behavior that people make. *Metaethics* analyzes the language and words people use to discuss moral behavior. *Normative ethics* analyzes, evaluates, and develops norms or standards for dealing with moral problems. It raises questions about what is right, what is wrong, and how to decide. Normative ethics asserts that ethical decisions can be made from a way of reasoning represented by two ethical positions: teleological (consequentialist) and deontological (nonconsequentialist).

Teleological (consequentialist, utilitarian) theories are theories of end results or consequences (from the Greek *teleios,* meaning "end"). They affirm that the rightness or wrongness of an act is determined by its end results. To determine if an act is ethically right, one must compare the probable result of the act with the probable result of another act. The act that produces the greater good is chosen. The central issue of these theories is the principle of "greatest good." The utilitarian teachings of Jeremy Bentham (1962) and John Stuart Mill (1971) and the situation ethics of Joseph Fletcher (1966) maintain that end results and context are essential factors that must be considered.

Teleological theories foster morality by developing the capacity of humans to make better choices and by rejecting fixed moral rules of conduct and principles, such as "Thou shalt not steal" (Exodus 20:15). A mother in a war-ravaged land steals a bag of grain from the stores of a warlord to feed her starving children. According to teleological theories, her act was right and good because the end result (feeding her children) is a greater good than allowing them to starve.

Deontological (nonconsequentialist) theories are theories of duty or obligation to fixed laws. The term comes from the Greek *deontos,* meaning "duty to obey." The theorist most often identified with deontological approaches is Immanuel Kant. He maintains that some acts are inherently right or wrong, regardless of the end results; laws and rules are necessary (1972). Deontological theories foster morality by dictating behavior and controlling the right of people to make choices. There are no exceptions or mitigating circumstances. The mother who stole grain to feed her children was guilty of stealing. The law says stealing is wrong. According to deontological ethics, it is the duty of the mother to obey the law regardless of the end results.

Bioethics

Bioethics is the application of ethics to matters of life and death. Bioethics implies that a judgment should be made about the rightness or wrongness, goodness or badness, of a given medical or scientific practice. The term *bioethics* is used when life is involved. The term *ethics* is used when other areas, such as politics or economics are involved. Nurses are concerned about both bioethics and ethics.

Ethics, Morals, and Virtue

Although some authors use the word *ethics* to refer to standardized codes and *morals* to refer to common practices, both words mean habits or customs. Ethics comes from the Greek word *ethos*; morals, from the Latin word *mores*. Writers use the terms interchangeably to mean accepted standards of behavior, goodness, and virtue.

When someone asked Socrates how virtue was acquired, he is reported to have said, "You must think I am fortunate to know how virtue is acquired. The fact is that, far from knowing whether it can be taught, I have no idea what virtue is." His reply makes clear that the fundamental question is not how to become virtuous but what the nature of virtue or goodness might be. Philosophers and scholars have sought answers to this question for centuries.

Theorists

Sigmund Freud (1963) believes that the mechanism for right and wrong behavior within individuals is the superego, or conscience. He says that children absorb morals from their parents, especially from the one with whom they identify. He proposes that a son internalizes the moral standards and character of the father during resolution of the Oedipus complex, the time when a son identifies with his father and desires his mother, then hates his father as a rival. Freud hypothesizes that the id (the source of instinctive energy) is amoral and that the ego (the thinking, reacting mediator) is subject to the superego (the conscience).

Erik Erikson (1964), well known for his psychosocial developmental stages, proposes that moral development continues throughout life. He believes that if the conflicts of each psychosocial developmental stage are satisfactorily resolved, then an "ego-strength" or virtue emerges. His theory of moral development focuses on tasks to be achieved at various stages of life. The theory implies that love, fidelity, care, and wisdom are found only in adults.

Jean Piaget, through his studies of human intellectual development, sought to answer the question, "When and how do humans acquire morality?" He concludes that, because an understanding of what is "good" requires the intellect, then that understanding will change as the intellect develops. Piaget postulates two stages of moral development that must follow the initial stage of concrete action in young children. They are (1) rigid judgment based on edicts of external authority and (2) relativistic agreement to principles obtained from social contacts. The first is characterized by a mother saying, "You are a bad girl because you disobeyed me." The second stage is characterized by a child saying, "We don't like him because he is a tattletale" (1985).

Kohlberg's Stages of Moral Development

Level I: Preconventional
(Piaget's stage of preoperational thought in which a child begins to recognize relationships)

Person recognizes power of someone to enforce rules by physical force.

Stage 1: Punishment and obedience
What is right: Actions that avoid punishment. Obedience for its own sake.
Reason for doing right: To avoid punishment.
Social perspective: Egocentric viewpoint. Actions are considered in physical rather than psychologic terms. Confuses perspective of authority with the self.

Stage 2: Individualism; instrumental-relativism
What is right: Actions that satisfy one's needs and sometimes the needs of others. What is fair or agreed upon.
Reason for doing right: To serve one's needs in a world where one may have to recognize the needs of others.
Social perspective: Concrete individualistic. Aware that people have their own interests to pursue.

Level II: Conventional
(Piaget's stage of concrete operations in which a child begins to think logically, especially about concrete events)

Person maintains expectations of the self and the immediate group without regard for consequences. Conforms, and is loyal to, existing enforcers of social order.

Stage 3: Interpersonal conformity
What is right: Action that conforms to the society's expectations of the person's given role, showing loyalty, gratitude, and trust.
Reason for doing right: To be a good person in ones' own eyes and in the eyes of others.
Social perspective: Perspective of individual in relationship to others. Able to put the self in someone else's shoes, but not yet able to consider multiple relationships.

Stage 4: Social system and conscience; law and order
What is right: Actions that fulfill agreed-upon duties and keep the system

➤

Lawrence Kohlberg (1984) and his associates at Harvard University expanded on the work of Piaget. They focused their research on the questions: "Does personal morality change with intellectual development? If so, how?" They found a parallel between the stages of intellectual development described by Piaget and the stages of moral

going. Laws are to be obeyed except in extreme cases where they conflict with other fixed social duties.

Reason for doing right: To keep the institutions going. To avoid breaking down the system by not meeting obligations. The imperative of conscience.

Social perspective: Viewpoint of a system that defines rules and roles. Considers individual relations in terms of their place in the system.

Level III: Postconventional, Principled

(Piaget's stage of formal operations, in which child is able to think abstractly) Person tries to define moral values and principles apart from identity with the existing authority.

Stage 5: Utility and individual rights; social contract, legalistic

What is right: Being aware that people hold a variety of values and that these are relative. Usually upholds these relative rules in the interest of impartiality because they are a social contract. However, holds nonrelative values, such as life and liberty, regardless of majority opinion.

Reason for doing right: To fulfill one's obligation to law because of the societal contract to do so for the welfare of all people's rights. To provide the "greatest good for the greatest number."

Social perspective: Viewpoint of a rational individual aware of values and rights prior to social attachments and contracts. Considers moral and legal points of view and recognizes that they sometimes conflict. Finds it difficult to integrate them.

Stage 6: Universal ethical principles

What is right: Following self-chosen ethical principles that are based on universality and consistency. Principles are abstract rather than concrete and include justice, reciprocity, equality of human rights, and respect for the dignity of humans as individuals.

Reason for doing right: To fulfill one's personal commitment and belief in the validity of universal moral principles.

Social perspective: Viewpoint of a rational individual who recognizes that persons are ends in themselves and must be treated as such, that social arrangements derive from a moral perspective.

Adapted from Kohlberg L. Implications of Developmental Psychology for Education: Examples from Moral Development. *Educational Psychologist* 1973; 10:2–14.

development they identified. However, they discovered that some people attain much higher stages of moral development than Piaget described and that some people never move beyond the lowest ones. They identified six stages of moral development (see the accompanying box), which they grouped under Piaget's preoperational, concrete operations, and formal operations stages of intellectual development. People who reach the highest level of moral development base their conduct on abstract principles of right and wrong such as the Golden Rule rather than on concrete laws like the Ten Commandments.

Carol Gilligan found in her research that women consistently scored lower than men on Kohlberg's scale of moral development. She found that women see things from a *"care perspective* drawing attention to problems of detachment or abandonment and holding up an ideal of attention and response to needs."* Men, by contrast, see things from a *"justice perspective* drawing attention to problems of inequality and oppression and holding up an ideal of reciprocity and equal respect"* (Gilligan & Attanucci 1988, p. 73).

Gilligan describes three stages of developing an "ethic of care." Each stage ends with a transitional period when the person becomes uncomfortable with the present behavior and tries a new approach. Stage 1 is caring for oneself. The individual cares only for the self and feels isolated and disconnected from others. Stage 2 is caring for others. The individual recognizes the need for caring relationships and now defines good behavior as "caring for others." Such selflessness ignores personal needs and creates feelings of responsibility and resentment. Stage 3 is caring for oneself and others. The individual then sees a need to balance caring for others and for the self. Nonetheless, care remains the criteria by which one judges right and wrong behavior (Gilligan 1982, p. 74).

Ethical Principles

Ethical principles are fundamental concepts by which people judge behavior. These principles help people make decisions because they serve as criteria by which to measure actions. Laws flow from ethical principles, but they are limited to exact circumstances. Laws are rules made by an authority with power to enforce them. Ethical principles, by contrast, are on a higher plane than laws. They are not detailed rules about specific cases. Ethical principles speak to the "spirit" of a law, rather than its "letter."

Many philosophers recognize but one ethical principle. Jesus and Confucius teach versions of the Golden Rule: *Do unto others what you would they do unto you. Do not do unto others what you would not want them to do to you.* Kant (1964) holds that *duty* is the central issue; Mill (1971), *the interest of all;* Fletcher (1966), *love;* Scriven (1966), *equal rights*; Thiroux (1990), *human dignity*; Nodding (1984), *care*; Gilligan (1988), *care* and *justice*. A single, global principle for ethical behavior is an attractive concept, but when nurses face real-life issues, they need more specific guidance. Five such principles are: respect for human life and dignity, beneficence, autonomy, honesty, and justice.

Human Life and Dignity

Respect for human life and dignity is the most basic of all ethical principles. It requires that "individuals be treated as unique and equal to every other individual, and that special justification is required for interference with an individual's own purposes, privacy, or behavior" (Rawls 1971, p. 130). This principle calls for respect for the life, freedom, and privacy of all humans. Thiroux says that this principle is necessary for any moral system, because "there can be no human being, moral or immoral, if there is no human life" (1990, p. 88). He maintains that survival of the species requires respect for human life and dignity. Davis and Aroscar point out that the principle of human dignity recognizes that an individual is a member of a human community and that most of the decisions people make affect others. Therefore, respecting a person as an individual and a community member requires "consideration of duties and obligations to others as well as one's self in making decisions" (1991, p. 44). Gilligan's care perspective concerns the ethics of response and care in which moral problems are issues of relationships, resolved through the activity of care (Lyon 1988, p. 33).

Human Life and Dignity in Nursing Practice

Respect for human life and dignity requires that nurses

- Strive to save and sustain human life
- Respect decisions others make for themselves and their family members
- Respect the person and privacy of others, including colleagues
- Hold in confidence personal information they learn about others
- Discuss only professional issues that affect nursing care
- Respect the lifestyle and belief systems of others
- Support the basic needs of others, including the need for connectedness

A mother decides to bottle-feed rather than breast-feed her infant. Applying the principle of respect for human life and dignity, the nurse accepts the mother's decision and helps her bottle-feed her infant.

A man decides he does not want radical surgery that may halt the cancer growing in his larynx. After the nurse ascertains that his decision is made with full understanding of the possible results of his decision, the nurse helps him cope with the consequences of his decision.

A nurse seems overwhelmed by the demands of a new position for which she had no orientation. Applying the principles of respect for human dignity, a nursing colleague takes time to give information and encourage the new staff member.

Tanya, a 17-year-old high school junior, was admitted to the hospital with a diagnosis of pelvic inflammatory disease caused by a resistant gonorrheal infection. Lois, her nurse, started the prescribed intravenous infusion containing antibiotics and did what she could to make the girl comfortable. The mother stayed at the bedside, tearfully watching as her child's temperature soared and her condition worsened. Lois was especially moved because her own daughter was the same age as Tanya. When Lois went home she described the sad scene to her husband, omitting the girl's name, "because of confidentiality." At his office during coffee break the next day the husband bemoaned the "lack of morals of teens today." He illustrated his point by telling about a teenage girl who was near death in the hospital because "she played around and got clap." His friend told the story to his friend and soon the personal tragedy of Tanya became public knowledge. Although the infection finally subsided and her health returned, Tanya's reputation in the community had been seriously damaged. By disclosing confidential information, even though she did not mention the girl's name, the nurse violated the ethical principle of respect for human life and dignity.

Beneficence (Nonmaleficence)

Beneficence means doing good to benefit others. Nonmaleficence means refraining from doing harm. Davis and Aroskar said that "beneficence can be viewed on a continuum extending from noninfliction of harm (nonmaleficence) to benefiting others (positive beneficence)" (1991, p. 45). Beneficence dictates more than technical competence; it involves acting in ways that demonstrate caring: listening, empathizing, supporting, and nurturing. Beneficence is the motivating force behind caring. Nodding says, "To care is to act, not by fixed rule, but by affection and regard" (1984, p. 24).

According to Frankena, the principle of beneficence includes four things: (1) one ought not to inflict evil or harm, (2) one ought to prevent evil or harm, (3) one ought to remove evil or harm, and (4) one ought to do and promote good (1973, p. 47). Responsible citizens practice beneficence in their daily lives. They do not inflict harm. They prevent harm when possible, remove it from the neighborhood, and promote good.

Beneficence in Nursing Practice

Nurses continually practice the four "oughts" of Frankena. For example, they take special precautions to administer drugs accurately to do no harm. They use protective measures such as siderails to prevent harm. They report dangerous or unprofessional behavior of colleagues to remove harm. They provide empathic nursing care and continually update their nursing knowledge to promote the welfare of clients.

Beneficence does not mean doing for clients or coworkers in order to manipulate and control their lives. It means making the welfare of others the overriding goal of nursing actions. Beneficence means giving that extra nurturance that makes the difference, such as providing emotional support to the family of a comatose child. It means exercising patience while an amputee painstakingly ambulates with a new prosthesis, or a person with a colostomy changes the bag for the first time. Beneficence means showing "tough love" by insisting an adolescent take responsibility for destructive behavior. It means spending extra time listening to a distraught parent or holding the hand of a dying patient.

> José Sanchez was hospitalized and isolated because of a staphylococcal infection in a leg wound. He spoke little English, seldom looked at television, and had no visitors. Penny noticed how lonely he seemed as he silently gazed out the window day after day. She asked a Spanish-speaking nurse to explain the reason for his isolation and treatment. She ordered a portable radio from the maintenance department so that José could listen to a Hispanic station. By doing these things Penny went beyond technical competency. She demonstrated Frankena's fourth point of beneficence: "to do and promote good."

Beneficence may require nurses to take unpopular action to safeguard the welfare of others or themselves. They may have to stand up to administrators and insist on better staffing or safer protocols. They may have to report unprofessional conduct of coworkers.

Maria and Howard work nights in the intensive care unit. On several occasions in the last 2 months the narcotic count had been short. Maria notices that clients often complain of pain after Howard medicates them. She does not want to think that Howard might be taking the narcotics meant for people in pain, but she decides to watch him. Sure enough, Howard signs out a tubex of Demerol, but instead of giving it he slips it into his pocket. Maria reports her observation to the supervisor and together they confront Howard. He admits his narcotic dependency and subsequently enters a drug rehabilitation program.

Howard violated the first part of the principle of beneficence. He inflicted harm on his clients by not administering pain-relieving medication and then stealing the drug. Maria could have remained silent, but by taking action she demonstrated Frankena's second and third part of beneficence: to prevent harm and to remove harm.

Autonomy

Autonomy is the right of self-determination, independence, and freedom. Sandra J. Smith says that autonomy is the "ability to absorb information, comprehend it, make a choice, and carry out that choice" (1985, p. 10). The ethical principle of autonomy demands respect for the right of people to make decisions about themselves. Nurses implement this principle by providing information to clients and assisting them to understand it. They accept the client's decision because nurses respect the autonomy of the individual.

Autonomy, when expressed as respect for the unconditional worth of a person, is consonant with the thinking of Immanuel Kant. He viewed individuals as rational beings capable of making choices according to moral principles. He maintained that because of this capacity people ought to be treated as ends in themselves, not as means to an end (1964). When expressed as respect for the thoughts and actions of a person, autonomy is consonant with the philosophy of John Stuart Mill. A utilitarian, Mill believed that autonomous thoughts and actions are beneficial, both to individuals and to the state. He said that people should not interfere with this right as long as their actions do not limit the freedom of others or harm others (1971).

Mill held that it is in the public interest to allow people to make individual choices so that they can develop their full potential and be a tribute to the state. He maintained that one of the roles of government is to "foster social conditions that encourage the development of personal character so that citizens will base their choices on self-determined plans. The development of such character is fundamental to the moral order of the state and the concept of government" (1971).

The views of both Kant and Mill are reflected in the current definition of autonomy. According to Beauchamp and Childress, "the autonomous person determines his or her course of action in accordance with a chosen plan" (1989, p. 111). Such a person is able to understand the principles of conduct suggested by Kant and to follow a plan of action in harmony with the principles proposed by Mill. People with reduced autonomy are not able to act according to a chosen plan of action. Combining the views of Kant and Mill, we respect autonomy when we treat people as ends and respect their decisions. When we reject their plan or restrict their freedom to act on their plan, we disrespect their autonomy. Health professionals question a client's autonomy only when they view an action as harmful or when they question the capacity of an individual to make an autonomous choice. In that instance the duty to prevent harm outweighs the obligation to respect autonomy.

Thiroux observes that "autonomy resolves the problem of instilling flexibility within a moral system—a flexibility it needs because of very real diversity that exists among human beings" (1990, p. 167). By respecting autonomy, we take into account individual differences, permitting people to live out their lives in ways they choose. In authoritarian systems, autonomy is limited by laws, rules, and regulations. In democratic societies, individual freedom is valued and restricted only by the "common good" and the rights of others. Thus, the autonomy of one person ends where the rights of the next person begin.

Autonomy in Nursing Practice

In health care settings, the principle of autonomy requires that nurses respect the choices of clients even when they disagree with them. Nurses may interfere only when they believe a person does not have sufficient information or capacity to understand, or is being coerced. Once nurses determine that a client's decision is informed and freely made, they must not interfere. Even so, nurses have no duty to assist people to carry out damaging decisions, nor do they have a duty to assist people to harm themselves.

Mrs. Chan, an 88-year-old widow, listened intently to the treatment options the physician described for her stage II carcinoma of the breast: a lumpectomy followed by radiation and chemotherapy. The day before the scheduled surgery, Mrs. Chan phoned the office nurse to say that she had decided to cancel the surgery, the radiation, and the chemotherapy. The nurse was dismayed and expressed genuine concern. The nurse explained the reason for the proposed therapies and the likely outcome if they were not carried out. Mrs. Chan listened intently, then replied, "I understand, but I have decided that I do not want all that misery and expense. I have lived a good life and I am ready to die." The nurse must determine first, that Mrs. Chan understands the consequences of her choice of action and second, that she is making her choice freely, without coercion. According to the ethical principle of autonomy, the nurse then must respect the client's decision even though the nurse does not agree with it.

Honesty

The ethical principle of honesty requires truthfulness in word and deed. The principle is based on mutual trust and respect for human dignity. Without honesty, meaningful relationships break down. Thiroux said "all morality depends on agreements between human beings.... How can agreements be made or maintained without some assurance that people are entering into them honestly and truthfully?" (1990, p. 164). Honesty requires that people communicate truth, neither deceiving nor misleading one another. Deception is a purposeful effort to mislead, either by witholding vital information or by giving out false information. Cheating is deception by trickery, dishonesty, and fraud.

Honesty in Nursing Practice

Honesty and veracity are complicated for health care professionals because the truth may be painful and potentially harmful to those who receive it, and telling the truth may violate the principles of beneficence and respect for human dignity. The diagnosis of a disease for which there is no cure is a distressing truth to tell a client. Nurses do not want to be cruel, impersonal, or uncaring. Yet on occasion they must convey truth that is shocking and painful. When they must give such information, they can do so with empathy, warmth, and genuine concern. On rare occasions, when health professions believe the truth will cause harm, they may decide to use "benevolent deception." This is a strategy of delay or concealment until a client or family member is able to cope with the truth. Benevolent deception is not undertaken lightly. Nurses use it sparingly, balancing the principle of beneficence with that of honesty.

> Jeremy, age 9, was hospitalized for observation of a concussion following an auto accident in which both of his parents were killed. He repeatedly asked for his mother and father. The nurses did not know what to tell him. If they told him that both his parents were dead, they risk emotion-induced increased intracranial pressure. If they made up a story to explain why his parents did not come, they would violate the ethical principle of honesty and truthfulness. At a staff meeting they decided the immediate benefits of deception outweighed the potential for long-term harm. Therefore, on the basis of a "benevolent deception" they told Jeremy that his mother and father were in another unit and could not come to see him now. When Jeremy had recovered sufficiently, they brought his grandparents to the bedside and told him the sad truth.

On some occasions nurses must balance the principle of honesty (veracity) with that of human dignity (confidentiality).

> Susan, a nurse on the medical unit, was preparing to discharge a young man hospitalized with Pneumocystis carinii pneumonia, an opportunistic disease common in persons with AIDS. His girl friend drew Susan aside and bluntly asked, "Does Hal have AIDS?" Susan must protect the confidentiality of Hal's diagnosis. Yet Susan knows that AIDS is a deadly disease and that the woman might be infected if she has unprotected intercourse with Hal. Susan decided to avoid a direct answer, respecting the principle of confidentiality, and tell a general truth, respecting the principle of beneficence. She said, "I cannot tell you Hal's diagnosis, only he can do that. I can tell you that the virus that causes AIDS is passed from person to person in semen, blood, and other body fluids. To be absolutely safe, everyone should protect against infection."

Justice

The ethical principle of justice demands the impartial treatment of others, regardless of personal traits or circumstances. It implies fairness and equality. Like other ethical principles, justice is rooted in respect for human dignity. The historic image of justice is a blindfolded woman with a scale, weighing an issue on the basis of objective evidence and judicial precepts. The image suggests that absolute knowledge and clear legal guidelines are possible and available. Unfortunately, in nursing practice, such absolute knowledge is rarely possible. Even so, the ethical principle of justice demands that nurses strive for fairness and equality.

Theorists look at justice in many ways. Rawls sees justice as fairness, requiring a "veil of ignorance" like the blindfold on the woman with the scales. He describes this concept in two tenets: "each person is to have an equal right to the most extensive system of liberty for all, and social and economic inequalities are to be arranged so that they are to the greatest benefit of the least fortunate." He stresses that, of the two, liberty for all takes priority and "inequalities are allowed only to improve the condition of the least fortunate, such as children, the elderly, the poor" (1971, p. 302). Vaux says that the concept of fairness means "invoking the Golden Rule in such a way that one is truly committed to the well-being of another" (1974, p. 42). Davis and Aroskar discuss the issue of the "distribution of burdens and benefits in any society in which resources are limited." They conclude that "one needs to consider the morally relevant differences between individuals that justify differential treatment" (1991, p. 47). According to Rawls, the principle of justice has to do with distribution of what he calls "primary goods: income, wealth, liberty, opportunity, and the bases of self respect ... in which people come together to negotiate the principles of justice by which all are bound to live" (1971, p. 136–147). Gilligan and Attanucci say that "a justice perspective draws attention to problems of inequity and oppression and holds up an ideal of reciprocity and equal respect" (1988, p. 73).

Justice in Nursing Practice

The principle of justice is especially important to managers of nursing services. Justice demands the uniform application of performance standards, rewards, and penalties. It insists on fair and equal work assignments, vacation time, and opportunity for advancement.

Injustice, or its perception, undermines trust, destroys loyalty, and begets hostility.

> Greg had been a medic in a field hospital in Vietnam. He had worked at the community hospital for 11 years, first as an orderly, an interim permittee, and then a staff nurse on the medical unit. He received high performance evaluations and his pleasant nature won him friends throughout the hospital. Because perioperative nursing was his first love, Greg spoke to the OR supervisor about possible openings. She told him a new position would open soon and encouraged him to apply. When the position was posted, Greg immediately applied. He met all the published criteria. Two weeks later Greg found out that Candy, a new graduate and the daughter of a hospital trustee, got the job. Greg was furious. He had served the hospital for many years and had put in his time on a medical unit. He was well qualified for the perioperative position. Greg resigned and took a position in another hospital. Nursing management violated the ethical principle of justice and lost an excellent nurse.

The principle of justice is as important for clients and families as it is for employees. People expect hospitals to apply regulations equally to all clients, regardless of personal characteristics. To avoid frustration and anger hospitals need to publish their policies widely, state them clearly, and explain the rationale when possible.

> All the beds in the intensive care unit (ICU) were full. The emergency room called to report that a severely injured man was on his way to surgery and would be admitted to ICU afterward. Johanna, the supervisor, had to make room for the new client. After consulting her staff about the status of each client, she decided to move Mr. Lucas, a stabilized cardiac client, to the step-down unit. She told his wife of the impending move. Mrs. Lucas protested loudly. It was not right. Her husband had given generously to the building fund to expand ICU. She wanted him to stay in ICU for at least 2 more days. Johanna explained that beds in ICU were allotted according to acuity. Mr. Lucas was the only person stable enough to move. Reluctantly, the wife agreed. Both Johanna and Mrs. Lucas based their arguments on the ethical principle of justice. However, they were using different criteria. Johanna used client acuity; Mrs. Lucas used contributions. To avoid misunderstanding and support the ethical principle of justice, the hospital needs to let the public know the criteria used for clinical assignment.

Codes of Ethics

A code of ethics is a formal statement that sets standards of ethical behavior for a group of people. One of the hallmarks of a profession is that it has a code of ethics spelling out the ethical behavior of its members (see Chapter 1). For example, the code of ethics for judges emphasizes the ethical principle of justice. The code of ethics for nurses emphasizes the principle of respect for the life and dignity of clients.

Codes of ethics are not static documents but ever-evolving statements of values, reflecting social and professional change. The history of the ethical codes of nursing bears this out. Although not static, codes of ethics are not altered by every ebb and flow of thought. They are relatively constant. On this point Fowler writes, "Though it is not easy, ethical decision-making is not adrift in a rolling sea; it is anchored to the distinguished, distinctive, and definite moral and ethical tradition of the profession" (1992, p. 52). These changes are evident in the codes of physicians, nurses, and other health care providers.

An early effort to define ethical behavior among those who care for the sick is the Hippocratic Oath (470–360 BC). The American Medical Association adopted its first code of ethics in 1847. Since then, it has updated the code six times, most recently in 1980.

The first generally accepted code of ethics for modern nurses was written in 1893 by Lystra Gretter, Superintendent of the Farrand Training School, Detroit, Michigan. She patterned the code after the Hippocratic Oath and named it the Florence Nightingale Pledge. This pledge, or one of its many modified versions, is still recited at some nursing school graduation ceremonies. See the accompanying box.

The Florence Nightingale Pledge by Lystra Gretter, 1893

I solemnly pledge myself before God and in the presence of this assembly to pass my life in purity and to practice my profession faithfully.

I will abstain from whatever is deleterious and mischievous and will not take or knowingly administer any harmful drug.

I will do all in my power to maintain and elevate the standard of my profession and will hold in confidence all personal matters committed to my keeping and family affairs coming to my knowledge in the practice of my calling. With loyalty will I endeavor to aid the physician in his work, and devote myself to the welfare of those committed to my care.

American Nurses Association

In 1926, the American Nurses Association (ANA) tentatively adopted and published a code of ethics entitled "A Suggested Code" in the *American Journal of Nursing*, but the code was no. ratified by the membership. In 1940, the suggested code of 1926 was replaced by "A Tentative Code," reformulated in 1949 and adopted in 1950. It consists of a preamble and 17 provisions. The first major revision of the 1950 code was ratified in 1960. In 1968, the term *professional* was omitted from the title to indicate it applied to both technical and professional nurses, the preamble was dropped, and the number of provisions was reduced to 10. The 1968 version omitted reference to the moral character of nurses and focused on professional ethics. The 1976 revision updated the wording but maintained the same ethical principles of earlier codes. While the 1940 code disavowed discrimination on the basis of creed, nationality, or race, the 1976 version extends nondiscrimination to all personal attributes, socioeconomic status, and nature of health problems (Fowler 1992. pp. 149–151).

The most recent revision of the ANA code, entitled *Code for Nurses with Interpretive Statements*, was adopted in 1985. It revises and updates language but does not change any of the ethical principles of the prior version. The ANA describes the code as "more a collective expression of nursing conscience and philosophy than a set of external rules" (1985). See the box on page 212.

International Council of Nurses

In 1933, the International Council of Nurses (ICN) formed an Ethics of Nursing Committee. In 1953, the ICN adopted its first *International Code of Nursing Ethics*. In 1965, the council made minor revisions and changed the title to *Code of Ethics as Applied to Nursing*. In 1973, a new code was approved, beginning with a statement of the needs, responsibilities, and services rendered by nurses (1985). See the box on page 213.

Ethics Committees

Because nurses, physicians, and other health care providers must make bioethical decisions nearly every day, many hospitals appoint ethics committees to share the responsibility. These committees are made up of health professionals, ethicists, clergy, and public members. Some local, state, and federal regulations give these commit-

American Nurses Association Code for Nurses with Interpretive Statements

1. The nurse provides services with respect for human dignity and the uniqueness of the client unrestricted by considerations of social or economic status, personal attributes, or nature of health problems.

2. The nurse safeguards the client's right to privacy by judiciously protecting information of a confidential nature.

3. The nurse acts to safeguard the client and the public when health care and safety are affected by the incompetent, unethical, or illegal practice of any person.

4. The nurse assumes responsibility and accountability for individual nursing judgments and actions.

5. The nurse maintains competence in nursing.

6. The nurse exercises informed judgment and uses individual competence and qualifications as criteria in seeking consultation, accepting responsibilities, and delegating nursing activities to others.

7. The nurse participates in activities that contribute to the ongoing development of the profession's body of knowledge.

8. The nurse participates in the profession's efforts to implement and improve standards of nursing.

9. The nurse participates in the profession's efforts to establish and maintain conditions of employment conducive to high quality nursing care.

10. The nurse participates in the profession's efforts to protect the public from misinformation and misrepresentation and to maintain the integrity of nursing.

11. The nurse collaborates with members of the health professions and other citizens in promoting community and national efforts to meet the health needs of the public.

Reprinted by permission from *Code for Nurses with Interpretive Statements*. Kansas City MO, 1985.

tees a quasi-official role in making life-and-death decisions. Ethics committees also provide education for health professionals on ethical issues and offer nonbinding consultation to families. Because life-and-death decisions are so difficult, a committee approach helps share the responsibility and gives assurance to the hospital, family, and legal representatives that the best decision has been made.

Ethical Concepts Applied to Nursing, International Council of Nurses

The fundamental responsibility of the nurse is fourfold: to promote health, to prevent illness, to restore health, and to alleviate suffering.

The need for nursing is universal. Inherent in nursing is respect for life, dignity, and the rights of man. It is unrestricted by consideration of nationality, race, creed, color, age, sex, politics, or social status.

Nurses render health services to the individual, the family, and the community, and coordinate their services with those of related groups.

Nurses and People

The nurse's primary responsibility is to those people who require nursing care.

The nurse, in providing care, promotes an environment in which the values, customs, and spiritual beliefs of the individual are respected.

The nurse holds in confidence personal information and uses judgement in sharing this information.

Nurses and Practice

The nurse carries personal responsibility for nursing practice and for maintaining competence by continual learning.

The nurse maintains the highest standards of nursing care possible within the reality of specific situation.

The nurse uses judgement in relation to individual competence when accepting and delegating responsibilities.

The nurse when acting in a professional capacity should at all times maintain standards of personal conduct which reflect credit upon the profession.

Nurses and Society

The nurse sustains a cooperative relationship with co-workers in nursing and other fields.

The nurse takes appropriate action to safeguard the individual when his care is endangered by a co-worker or any other person.

Nurses and the Profession

The nurse plays the major role in determining and implementing desirable standards of nursing practice and nursing education.

The nurse is active in developing a core of professional knowledge.

The nurse, acting through the professional organization, participates in establishing and maintaining equitable social and economic working conditions in nursing.

Reprinted by permission of the International Council of Nurses, 1985.

Ethical Dilemmas

A *dilemma* is a perplexing problem that places a person in the position of choosing between equal but conflicting alternatives. An *ethical dilemma* is a moral problem that requires a choice between two or more conflicting actions, each based on a valid ethical principle. Each alternative has credibility, yet none will satisfy all of the ethical principles that apply. To complicate matters further, strong emotions such as grief and fear often accompany ethical dilemmas.

For example, if a long-comatose client is allowed to die during one of many bouts of pneumonia, the cost of care will end and the family will be free to complete their grieving and go on with their lives. This course of action is beneficent. However, to honor the principle of beneficence, the caregivers must violate the principle of respect for human life and dignity, because the action entails ending efforts to keep the person alive. Whatever action is taken, it will be charged with powerful emotions.

Resolving Ethical Dilemmas

Ideally, resolution of an ethical dilemma requires clear, rational thought and knowledge of ethical principles and law. It is also vital to know the ethical position of the decision makers, whether they follow a teleological (end-results, situational) tradition or a deontological (duty to obey, absolutist) tradition. Although ethical dilemmas may be more emotional than nursing problems, they require the same decision-making process nurses use every day.

Decision-Making Models

A number of decision-making models have been proposed to help nurses make ethical decisions. Purtilo (1993) suggests a five-step process: (1) gather relevant information, (2) identify the type of ethical problem, (3) determine the ethics approach to be used, (4) explore the practical alternatives, and (5) complete the action.

Thompson and Thompson (1985) suggested a ten-step process: (1) review the situation to determine health problems, decisions needed, ethical components, and key individuals; (2) gather additional information to clarify the situation; (3) identify the ethical issues in the situation; (4) define personal and professional moral issues; (5) identify moral positions of the key people; (6) identify value conflicts, if any; (7) determine who can make the decision; (8) identify the range of actions with anticipated outcomes; (9) decide on a course of action and carry it out; and (10) review the results of actions.

We suggest a decision-making process similar to a crisis-intervention model that takes legal issues into account. The process has seven steps:

1. Gather the facts: who the decision-makers are and whether they subscribe to teleological or deontological ethics.

2. State the problem.

3. List alternative solutions.

4. For each solution, state applicable ethical principles, laws, consequences, advantages, and disadvantages from the viewpoint of the decision maker.

5. Help the decision makers choose a solution based on their ethical position; if the solution is illegal, help them decide if they are willing to accept the consequences of breaking the law.

6. Provide emotional support for all affected persons.

7. Evaluate the decision-making process and its results in order to provide anticipatory guidance for the future.

Case Studies

Ethical dilemmas occur in every area of human experience. Although each situation is different, decisions about death, reproduction, scarce resources, behavior control, and professional relationships frequently raise ethical issues. Cases in each of these areas follow, with the decision-making model applied to the first dilemma.

Death *Quadriplegic woman.* A 28-year-old quadriplegic woman with severe cerebral palsy had herself admitted to a hospital. She asked to be kept comfortable with medications and physical care but allowed to die by starvation because her life was unbearable. Instead, the hospital force-fed her until the ethics committee could help them decide what to do.

1. Gather the facts: The woman is essentially alone, and the state pays for her care. She has no religious or moral problems with voluntary euthanasia, but cannot end her own life because of her helpless condition. The woman is mentally competent and states that she wants to die. The hospital is asked to take some action (administer pain-relieving drugs and provide care but refrain

from feeding her), so the hospital becomes the decision maker. The board of trustees of the hospital is committed to deontological (duty-to-obey) ethics.

2. State the problem: Should the hospital cooperate with the woman by allowing her to starve to death in their facility?

3. List alternative solutions:

   a. Give humane care but allow the woman to starve to death, per her request.

   b. Discharge the woman to her home with an attendant.

   c. Force-feed the woman until she can be placed in another facility.

4. State applicable ethical principles, laws, and consequences; list advantages and disadvantages for each possible solution:

   a. Give humane care but allow the woman to die.

   Ethical principles: Violates the principle of respect for human life and dignity (from the viewpoint of the hospital); supports the principle of autonomy (from the viewpoint of the woman).

   Legal issues: Possible criminal charges against the hospital for negligent homicide.

   Consequences: The "unbearable state" of the woman would end; the hospital might be charged with breaking laws; the deontological position of the hospital would be violated.

   Advantages: The misery of the woman would end.

   Disadvantages: The hospital might face civil and criminal legal action; the hospital would violate its ethical position.

   b. Discharge the woman to her home with an attendant.

   Ethical principles: Supports the principle of respect for human life and dignity (from the viewpoint of the hospital); violates the principle of autonomy (from the viewpoint of the woman).

   Legal issues: Possible charges of civil negligence by the woman.

   Consequences: The misery of the woman continues; the hospital avoids criminal charges, and the deontological position of the hospital is followed.

   Advantages: The hospital avoids legal charges and conflict with its ethical position.

Disadvantages: The woman does not have her wish fulfilled; there might be negative publicity for the hospital.

c. Force-feed woman until she is transferred elsewhere.

Ethical principles: Supports the principle of respect for human life and dignity (from the viewpoint of the hospital) because the woman is being kept alive; violates the principle of autonomy (from the viewpoint of the woman).

Legal issues: Possible legal action against the hospital (charges of battery, touching someone without his or her consent).

Consequences: The misery of the woman continues; she does not die from starvation in the hospital or at home; the hospital avoids criminal charges of negligent homicide but may be sued by the woman for battery.

Advantages: The ethical position of the hospital is upheld; legal action by the woman is unlikely.

Disadvantages: Possibly some negative publicity for the hospital.

5. Assist the decision maker to choose an action based on an ethical position: The decision maker is the hospital, whose ethics committee follows the deontological position. They decide to discharge the woman to her home with an attendant. In another hospital, the decision might be different, depending on its ethical position, its interpretation of the ethical principle of respect for human life and dignity, and the importance it assigns to the principle of autonomy.

6. Provide emotional support for those affected by the decision. In this case, the woman must continue to live in a condition she describes as "unbearable." She should be referred for counseling and emotional support.

7. Evaluate the decision-making process; provide anticipatory guidance for the future. Ethics committees learn from each decision they make. They may recommend that the hospital screen future admissions and that they publish the ethical position of the hospital so that physicians and prospective clients know what to expect in the future.

Osteosarcoma in a boy. A 12-year-old boy has just been diagnosed as having osteosarcoma of the femur. The only hope of a cure is radiation, chemotherapy, and amputation of the leg; however, a suspicious area in his lung suggests a possible metastasis. Without treatment, he will surely die. Even with treatment, his prognosis is poor. The treatment is painful, mutilating, and traumatic. The parent must decide.

Reproduction *Pregnant janitor.* A 28-year-old part-time janitor has just found out that she is pregnant for the fourth time. She has had three induced abortions and has decided to leave the man with whom she lives because he beats her. She is a recent convert to a religion that strongly opposes abortion and stresses the dominance of men over women. Her job pays too little to support her and a baby, and she opposes "going on welfare." Her support system consists of a widowed mother who lives nearby. How might the clinic nurse help her decide what to do?

Older mother. A 42-year-old woman is pregnant for the first time. Her physician recommends that she have an amniocentesis to find out if the baby has a birth defect such as Down syndrome. Her church opposes this procedure and teaches that a woman is to obey her husband. Her husband wants the amniocentesis done. She has told the office nurse of her quandary. How might the nurse help her decide?

Scarce Resources *Multiple birth defects.* A baby is born with multiple defects, and the mother is not able to care for the infant. He is placed in a state hospital, and a legal guardian is assigned. The medical staff outlines a proposed treatment plan that involves numerous operations over a period of several years at enormous expense to the state. The guardian and the medical staff have asked the hospital ethics committee to give them advice. What might that advice be?

Cardiac arrest in two men. Two men in the same hospital unit have a cardiac arrest within moments of one another. The first is a contentious 80-year-old man with many health problems. The other is the 42-year-old editor of the local newspaper, a husband and father of four children. There is only one cardiopulmonary resuscitation cart. A nurse heads the code team and must decide who to resuscitate first. How might the nurse decide?

Behavior Control *Electroconvulsive therapy.* A severely depressed woman is admitted as an involuntary client to a psychiatric facility. When antidepressants fail to help, the physician asks the client to sign a permit for electroconvulsive therapy (ECT). She refuses. Under state laws if three mental health professionals agree, ECT can be administered. How might the nurse decide?

Five-point restraints. A 7-year-old child is admitted to the psychiatric unit with a history of stabbing her sister to death with scissors. The child is incredibly strong and has frequent violent episodes when she attacks other clients and staff members. During these episodes staff members place her in five-point restraint in a seclusion room. The alternative to physical restraint is administration of large doses of sedatives. Members of the ethics committee are invited to a treatment team conference to help decide what to do. How might they decide?

Professional Relations *Assignment of holiday time.* The nursing supervisor is making holiday assignments. It is customary for the staff to rotate Thanksgiving, Christmas, and New Year's Day off. A nurse comes to the supervisor and asks for Christmas Day even though she had it last year. She explains that it is the last day before her brother is to enter the penitentiary to serve a 20-year sentence for child molestation. None of the staff know of her brother's criminal record. How might the supervisor decide what to do?

Medication error. Two clients on the unit have the same last name and are in adjacent rooms. Seconal is prescribed for one, Nembutal for the other. The evening nurse switches the medications. She realizes her error after the second client swallows the capsule and remarks that he had a orange capsule the night before. The nurse made two other medication errors last month and was warned that if she made another she would be dismissed. She is the sole support of three children and needs to work. How should she decide what to do?

◆ Summary

Because advances in medicine have raised ethical issues unknown in times past, modern nurses need to understand values, belief systems, and ethics. Values provide a frame of reference by which people integrate their lives. Values clarification helps people identify their values. Belief systems help explain the mystery of life and comfort believers; they may be a part of a religion or may exist independently. Ethics is concerned with judging the rightness or wrongness of actions. Such judgment may be based on teleological theories that say end results determine rightness or deontological theories that say obedience to

duty determines rightness. Respect for human life and dignity, beneficence, honesty, autonomy, and justice are ethical principles of special
concern to nurses. Codes of ethics are formal statements of the ethical behavior of professional groups. Ethical dilemmas occur when a
choice must be made between conflicting actions based on one or
more ethical principles.

Critical Thinking Questions

1. Which of your personal values might come into play if you were
   caring for a terminally ill AIDS client? How might values clarification assist a nurse who is caring for the client?

2. Describe how you feel about people who subscribe to deontological theories as a basis for deciding right and wrong. Is their view
   the same as or different from your own?

3. When trying to find a solution for an ethical dilemma, what do
   you feel is the most important thing to consider? What would
   you say to someone who does not agree that this consideration is
   the most important? What personal biases might have influenced
   your ideas about what is most important?

Learning Activities

1. Take the tests found in the Values Clarification box on page 192.
   What did you discover about your values? Do they differ from
   those of your classmates and parents?

2. Discuss what Durkheim meant when he said religion was "an
   effort of humans to pass science and complete it prematurely."

3. Write a paper explaining the ethical position you hold and why.

4. In small groups, discuss the moral development of Lucy of *Peanuts*
   and Scrooge of *The Christmas Carol* using the stages of Piaget,
   Kohlberg, and Gilligan.

5. Write a paper comparing the ICN *Codes for Nurses: Ethical Concepts Applied to Nursing* and the ANA *Code for Nurses with Interpretive Statements.*

6. In a small group discussion, resolve the ethical dilemma described in the vignette.

Annotated Reading List

Fletcher J. *Situation Ethics: The New Morality.* Westminster Press, 1966.

A classic, this book clearly and simply presents the concept of "agape," or God-like love. Its thesis is that our modern world would be a better place to live in if the law of love that considers circumstances replaced the rigid laws of right and wrong.

White GB, ed. *Ethical Dilemmas in Contemporary Nursing Practice.* American Nurse Publishing, 1992.

This book is a collection of ethical dilemmas, written by nurses working in various clinical settings across the United States. The 10 case studies were selected from 94 responses to a call for papers by *The American Nurse.* The cases reflect "a shift in the discipline of ethics from a focus on rights-based universalizable principles to a concern with individual stories embedded in particular communities" (p. xiii).

References

American Nurses Association. *Code for Nurses with Interpretive Statements.* ANA, 1985.

Aristotle. *Nicomachaen Ethics.* Trans. by Martin Ostwald. Bobbs-Merrill, 1962.

Beauchamp TL, Childress JF. *Principle of Biomedical Ethics,* 3rd ed. Oxford University Press, 1989.

Bentham J. *The Works of Jeremy Bentham.* Bowring J, ed. Russell & Russell, 1962.

Davis AJ, Aroskar MA. *Ethical Dilemmas and Nursing Practice,* 3d ed. Appleton & Lange, 1991.

Durkheim E. *The Elementary Forms of the Religious Life.* Harvard Press, 1915.

Erikson EH. *Insights and Responsibility: Lectures on the Ethical Implications of Psychoanalytic Insight.* W. W. Norton, 1964.

Fletcher J. *Situation Ethics*. Westminister Press, 1966.

Fowler MD. A Chronicle of the Evolution of the Code for Nurses. In White GB, ed. *Ethical Dilemmas in Contemporary Nursing Practice*. CNA, 1992.

Frankena WK. *Ethics*. Prentice-Hall, 1973.

Freud S. *The Ego and The Id and Other Works*, vol. 19. Trans. by James Strachney. Hogarth Press and Institute of Psychoanalysis, 1961.

Gilligan C, Attanucci J. Two Moral Orientations. In Gilligan C et al, eds. *Mapping the Moral Domain*. Harvard University Press, 1988.

Gilligan C. *In a Different Voice: Psychological Theory and Women's Development*. Harvard University Press, 1982.

International Council of Nurses. *Code for Nurses: Ethical Concepts Applied to Nursing*. ICN, 1985.

Kant I. *Groundwork for the Metaphysics of Morals*. Trans. by HJ Patton. Harper & Row, 1964.

Kohlberg L. Implications of Developmental Psychology for Education: Examples from Moral Development. *Educational Psychologist* 1973;10:2–14.

Kohlberg L. *The Psychology of Moral Development: Essays on Moral Development*, 2nd ed. Harper & Row, 1984.

Lyon NP. Two Perspectives: On Self Relationships and Morality. In Gilligan C et al eds. *Mapping the Moral Domain*. Harvard University Press, 1988.

Mill JS. *Utilitarianism: With Critical Essays*. Gorowitz S, ed. Bobbs-Merrill, 1971.

Nodding N. *Caring*. University of California Press, 1984.

Piaget J. *The Moral Judgment of the Child*. Free Press, 1985.

Purtilo RB. *Ethical Dimensions in the Health Professions*, 2nd ed. Saunders, 1993.

Raths LE, Harmin M, Simmons SB. *Values and Teaching*, 2nd ed. Charles E. Merrill, 1979.

Rawls J. *A Theory of Justice*. Harvard University Press, 1971.

Rokeach M. *The Nature of Human Values*. Free Press, 1973.

Scriven M. *Primary Philosophy*. McGraw Hill, 1966.

Smith SJ. The Principle of Autonomy. In *Ethics: Principles and Issues*. CNA, 1985.

Steele SM, Harmon V. *Values Clarification in Nursing*, 2nd ed. Appleton-Century-Crofts, 1983.

Thiroux JP. *Ethics, Theory and Practice*, 4th ed. Macmillan Publishing, 1990.

Thompson J, Thompson H. *Bioethical Decision-Making for Nurses*. Appleton-Century-Crofts, 1985.

Vaux K. *Biomedical Ethics: Morality for the New Medicine*. Harper & Row, 1974.

Wach J. *Sociology of Religion*. University of Chicago Press, 1992.

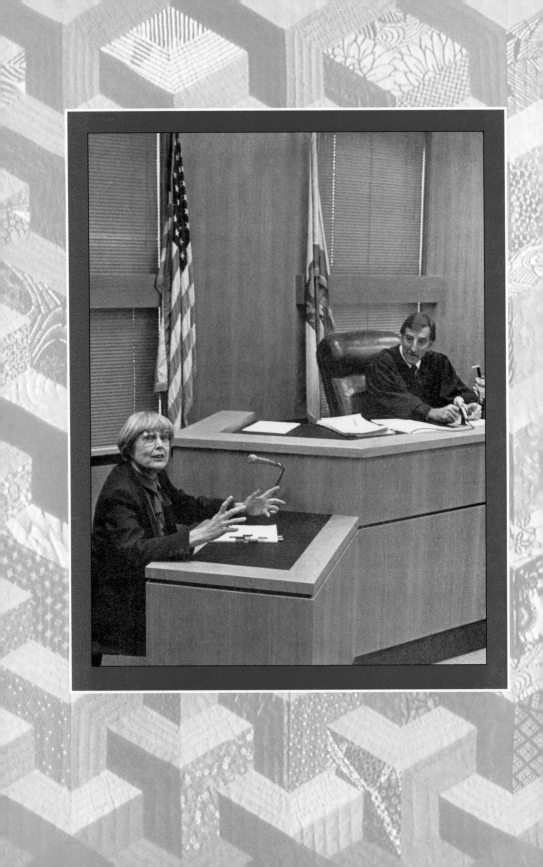

Legal Issues

8

◇ Learning Objectives

- Discuss the origin of constitutional, administrative, statutory, and case (common) law.

- Describe the judicial system and its functions.

- Compare civil law and the civil trial process with criminal law and the criminal trial process.

- Discuss four roles nurses play in trials.

- Describe various tort actions in which nurses may be involved.

- Discuss negligence, including the essential elements that must be established.

- Explain the concepts of individual responsibility, *res ipsa loquitur, respondeat superior,* and standard of care as they relate to professional negligence.

- Compare the Bill of Rights of the US Constitution and the American Hospital Association Patient's Bill of Rights.

- Discuss strategies nurses can use to prevent malpractice claims.

- Explain factors nurses need to consider in regard to professional liability insurance.

- Describe actions nurses can take to defend themselves if served with a summons and complaint.

Ina *stared at the official-looking envelope handed to her by the stranger. The return address said: Superior Court. Fear swept through her body as she tore open the envelope. She found two documents inside, one entitled "Summons," the other "Complaint." The documents named her, Ina Jaffe, as a defendant. It also named the Community Hospital and Simon Anslow, MD, an emergency department physician.*

Shocked and confused, Ina shut the door and walked to a chair. She felt numb. She tried to read the documents but the language was strange, its implications unclear. Only vaguely could she remember an incident that might have prompted the allegations. What did this mean? What should she do? To whom should she turn? Should she call an attorney? Her supervisor? The regional office of her state nurses association?

Ina started to call the hospital, then she remembered that she had paid premiums for professional liability insurance. Fearful that her policy might have expired, Ina rushed to her file and found the insurance folder. Yes, she was covered, and there were instructions about what to do and what not to do if she ever had a problem. There was also an 800-number.

Ina picked up the phone and dialed the number. As she waited for it to ring, Ina realized how vulnerable she was and how little she knew about the legal system.

◆

Although aware of some legal regulations in nursing practice, few nurses have a working knowledge of the judicial system. Fewer still are prepared for the crisis a subpoena might bring. To protect themselves, nurses need to understand the basis of law in the United States, the structure and function of the legal system, and the difference between civil and criminal law. They need to know how the trial process and professional liability insurance work and how to defend themselves if they face a lawsuit.

◇ The Basis of Law in the United States

Law in the United States is based on the old English system where the monarch held supreme power over the land and the people. He acted according to his "divine right." As a consequence, his decisions became the law of the land, known as *common* or *case law*. Creighton noted that the "practice of building a system of rules and sanctions by the accumulation of case-to-case decisions [remains a]…unique characteristic of Anglo-American jurisprudence" (1986).

The Magna Carta, granted by King John in 1215, is considered the foundation of English constitutional liberty and a landmark in the struggle for human freedom. It effectively limited the power of the monarchy and protected individual rights and property. Thus, English law came to have two functions: to protect and enforce the rights and privileges of individuals and to provide an organized government with limited powers. Not surprisingly, the United States incorporated those same functions into its judicial system.

◇ The Legal System

In the United States, the Constitution is the supreme law of the land. It protects individual rights and balances the powers of government. The first ten amendments of the Constitution, called the Bill of Rights, and various of the other amendments place restrictions on the power of government and establish specific individual freedoms, such as the right to free speech, assembly, and equal protection under the law. When individuals believe they have been denied any of these

The Bill of Rights (US Constitution, Amendments 1–10, and 14, Section 1)

1. Congress shall make no law respecting an establishment of religion, or prohibiting the free exercise thereof; or abridging the freedom of speech, or of the press; or the right of the people peaceably to assemble, and to petition the Government for a redress of grievances.

2. A well-regulated Militia, being necessary to the security of a free State, the right of the people to keep and bear Arms, shall not be infringed.

3. No Soldier shall, in time of peace be quartered in any house, without the consent of the Owner, nor in time of war, but in a manner to be prescribed by law.

4. The right of the people to be secure in their persons, houses, papers, and effects, against unreasonable searches and seizures, shall not be violated, and no Warrants shall issue, but upon probable cause, supported by Oath or affirmation, and particularly describing the place to be searched, and the persons or things to be seized.

5. No person shall be held to answer for a capital, or otherwise infamous crime, unless on a presentment or indictment of a Grand Jury, except in cases arising in the land or naval forces, or in the Militia, when in actual service in time of War or public danger; nor shall any person be subject for the same offense to be twice put in jeopardy of life or limb; nor shall be compelled in any criminal case to be a witness against himself, nor be deprived of life, liberty, or property, without due process of law; nor shall private property be taken for public use, without just compensation.

rights, they can seek redress in federal courts. Similarly, state constitutions guarantee the individual rights of citizens. See the accompanying box.

The US Constitution establishes three separate branches of government within the federal system: executive, legislative, and judicial. The states follow that same pattern. This tripartite system authorizes specific powers and responsibilities for each branch so that no branch becomes more powerful than another. This system exemplifies the doctrine of separation and balance of powers. The US Constitution also provides for a balance of power within the judicial branch. The Constitution grants specific powers to the federal government, called *express powers*. All other powers are retained by the states under the Tenth Amendment (Creighton 1986).

6. In all criminal prosecutions, the accused shall enjoy the right to a speedy and public trial, by an impartial jury of the State and district wherein the crime shall have been committed, which district shall have been previously ascertained by law, and to be informed of the nature and cause of the accusation; to be confronted with the witnesses against him; to have compulsory process for obtaining witnesses in his favor, and to have the Assistance of counsel for his defence.

7. In Suits at common law, where the value in controversy shall exceed twenty dollars, the right of trial by jury shall be preserved, and no fact tried by a jury, shall be otherwise reexamined in any Court of the United States than according to the rules of the common law.

8. Excessive bail shall not be required, nor excessive fines imposed, nor cruel and unusual punishments inflicted.

9. The enumeration in the Constitution, of certain rights, shall not be construed to deny or disparage others retained by the people.

10. The powers not delegated to the United States by the Constitution, nor prohibited by it to the States, are reserved to the States respectively, or to the people.

14. Section 1. All persons born or naturalized in the United States, and subject to the jurisdiction thereof, are citizens of the United States and of the State wherein they reside. No State shall make or enforce any law which shall abridge the privileges or immunities of citizens of the United States; nor shall any State deprive any person of life, liberty, or property, without due process of law; nor deny to any person within its jurisdiction the equal protection of the laws.

The executive branch enforces the law. It delegates its duties to various departments that enforce laws and promote regulations within their jurisdiction. For example, at the federal level, the Department of Health and Human Services is established under the authority of the executive branch of the federal government. Boards of nursing are established under the executive branch of state governments. The chief executive officer in both federal and state governments is granted specific powers and required to administer and enforce the law. The legislative and judicial branches keep a close watch on the executive branch at both the federal and state level.

The legislative branch of the federal government enacts laws, but that ability is limited. Federal and state constitutions specify the areas in which laws may be enacted. At the federal level, Congress can, among other acts, coin money, provide for the general welfare, and amend the Constitution by a two-thirds vote. Other areas are delegated to the states.

The judicial branch of government interprets the law and adjudicates (decides) disputes in accordance with the law. Its purpose is to administer justice without partiality. To carry out this purpose, the judiciary resolves disputes, modifies behavior, allocates gains and losses, and makes policy. As an arbiter of disputes, the court may interpret administrative regulations, determine whether or not the civil rights of individuals have been violated, and resolve contract disputes between individuals. As a modifier of behavior, the court may impose sanctions on impermissible behavior such as indecent exposure. The court may reward acceptable behavior by action such as reducing a jail sentence for "good behavior." As an allocator of gains and losses, the court may be asked to decide which party will bear the cost of breaking an agreement. For instance, the court may be asked to decide if a hospital has broken a labor contract with its nurses. As a policy maker, the court may recognize new causes for action or may determine that individuals have a clear personal interest in suing (standing to sue) for injuries.

Sources and Types of Law

Table 8-1 describes four sources of law and two major divisions of law. It illustrates the differences among the various categories of law that guide the decisions of the federal and state court systems.

TABLE 8-1

Sources and Types of Law in the United States

Sources of Law

Constitutional Law
Source: United States Constitution, the supreme law of the land
Functions: Establish executive, legislative, judicial branches of government
Grant specific powers to federal and state governments
Protect substantive rights (specific freedoms) of individuals
Protect procedural rights (right to due process) of individuals

Statutory Law
Source: Laws passed by legislative bodies at federal, state, and local level
Functions: Protect and provide for the general welfare of society

TABLE 8-1 *(continued)*

Sources and Types of Law in the United States

Administrative Law

Source: Power of executive branch, as delegated by the legislative branch, to regulate at federal, state, and local levels

Function: Delegate authority to various agencies to carry out special duties

Examples: Federal administrative law: National Labor Relations Board makes rules to regulate collective bargaining State administrative law: Boards of nursing make rules to regulate nursing practice in the state

Common (Case) Law

Source: Precedents, customs, traditions, "court-made"

Based on: *Stare decisis:* to adhere to things decided (past decisions) to resolve present disputes

Res judicata: a matter settled by judgment; once decided and appeals exhausted, parties cannot take the case to court again

Functions: Avoid duplication and unnecessary expenditure of resources

Types of Law

Criminal Law

Function: To protect society from actions that directly threaten its orderly existence. Criminal acts, while aimed at individuals, are offenses against the state; perpetrators are punished (fined, imprisoned, etc.); victims usually are not compensated

Categories: *Felony:* most serious offense (homicide, evading income tax, violating a nurse practice act or its rules and regulations)

Misdemeanor: lesser offense (traffic violations, unlawful assembly)

Juvenile: crimes committed by minors (age varies with states and crime)

Proof: Beyond a reasonable doubt; unanimous jury decisions may or may not be required

Civil Law

Function: To redress wrongs and injuries suffered by individuals, usually in the form of monetary compensation

Categories: *Contract:* legally binding agreement between two or more parties

Tort: any civil wrong other than breach of contract (negligence, slander, malpractice, assault, battery, false imprisonment, and invasion of privacy)

Proof: By a preponderance of the evidence; jury decisions may not be unanimous

The Criminal Trial Process

Initiation of a Suit

Law enforcement officers present investigative data to either state or federal prosecutors. If government attorneys believe there is sufficient evidence, they prepare a *complaint of information (indictment)*. If the crime is a felony or a violation of federal law, a grand jury is convened to decide if there is *probable cause* to believe a crime was committed. If so, government attorneys file a *complaint*. Some states also use grand juries to decide probable cause.

Arraignment

If the accused is not already in custody, the court issues an *arrest warrant*. Police bring the defendant before a judge for an *arraignment* (bail hearing) to decide if the accused should be released on bail until the trial.

Pleas

At the arraignment, defendants must plead "nolo contendere," "guilty," or "not guilty" to the charges. If they plead "guilty," defendants waive their right to a trail.

Discovery

The process of gathering information includes: pre-sentence investigation; requests for disclosure or notices to produce specific documents. Criminal defendants have more protections than civil defendants, eg, prosecutors must give defense attorneys evidence concerning the guilt or innocence of a defendant. During the discovery period, defense attorneys may attempt to arrange a

➤

Federal Courts

The Constitution gives the Supreme Court exclusive jurisdiction when states are the litigants (parties) in a legal action and appellate jurisdiction (power to review and decide appeals) when cases from lower federal and state appeal courts involve federal law. United States district courts are the trial courts of the federal system. Circuit courts of appeal review cases decided by district courts. These courts are organized according to geographic areas that may include several states, such as the Seventh Circuit, made up of Illinois, Michigan, Indiana, and Wisconsin. Federal courts have exclusive jurisdiction over cases that involve constitutional disputes or other federal questions and those arising between citizens of different states when the amount of money in controversy exceeds $50,000 (28th USC: 1331, 1332 1994).

plea bargain agreement by which a defendant pleads "guilty" to a lesser charge in exchange for a more lenient sentence. If no plea bargain agreement is made, the case often goes to trial.

Trial

Jury selection: The judge and attorneys examine prospective jurors.

Opening statements: The prosecuting and defense attorneys state what they will prove.

Testimony: Prosecution witnesses testify, then defense witnesses. Unlike in civil trials, defendants do not have to disprove the government case. They can remain silent or can testify in their own behalf. Once both sides have presented their cases, the judge instructs the jury about its responsibility and applicable law.

Jury deliberation: The jury then retires to deliberate.

Verdict

If a decision is reached, the jury returns and delivers its verdict. If the jury cannot agree, it notifies the judge who then declares a *mistrial*. When the jury finds a defendant not guilty, the person goes free and cannot be tried again for the same offense. If found guilty, the defendant is sentenced to a punishment, such as imprisonment, a fine, or a special work assignment.

Appealing the Verdict

Defendants may appeal the verdict.

State Courts

The state court system is much like the federal system in organization. Each state has its own trial, appellate (appeals), and supreme court, although they may have different names. As with their federal counterparts, the constitution and laws of the states give state courts specific powers. Trial courts hear cases dealing with civil and criminal violations of state statutory and common laws. Many judicial systems establish divisions to handle special kinds of cases, such as traffic courts and municipal courts for minor disputes or infractions.

The Trial Process

By understanding the steps involved in criminal and civil trials, nurses can reduce confusion about a complex process. See the boxes on the trial process beginning on pages 232 and 234.

The Civil Trial Process

Initiation of a Suit
Individuals who believe they have been injured consult attorneys who advise them as to whether there is a credible *cause* (grounds) *of action.* If so, attorneys draft a *complaint* that includes counts (charges), alleging damaging actions they must prove. They also prepare a *summons* listing the names of the *plaintiffs* (persons making the charge) and the *defendants* (ones being charged).

Filing the Complaint
The attorneys take or send the complaint and summons to the courthouse where a clerk stamps it with a date and time and assigns a case number and an appearance date.

Service and Court Appearance
A deputy sheriff or service agent delivers the complaint and summons to the defendants, who usually obtain legal counsel. Defendants or their attorneys appear in court as stipulated by the summons.

Preparation of Answers to the Complaint
If grounds to dismiss the complaint are not available, the defendants and their attorneys write a response to each and every allegation in the complaint and file their answers with the court.

Counterclaims and Third Party Complaint
Defense attorneys may file a counterclaim against plaintiffs, but it must be about the same event as the original complaint. If other people had a part in

➤

Roles of Nurses in the Trial Process

Nurses may be involved in the legal process as plaintiffs, defendants, factual witnesses, or expert witnesses. As plaintiffs, nurses may be initiators of suits alleging harm from the actions of others. For example, nurses may believe that their professional competence has been maligned by untrue oral or written statements of other health professionals. As plaintiffs in such suits, they may seek compensation for damage to their reputation caused by slanderous (oral) or libelous (written) statements. As defendants, nurses may be charged with committing civil wrongs, such as professional negligence (malpractice), or criminal wrongs, such as violations of the nurse practice act of their state. In either case, nurses who are defendants need to protect their rights by obtaining competent legal advice. As factual wit-

the alleged injury, either attorneys for defendants or for plaintiffs may file a *third-party complaint*.

Discovery
The information gathering process includes: written interrogatories (questions); notices to produce documents; and depositions (oral statements). During the discovery period, defense attorneys may call for a *summary judgment* by the court and plaintiff attorneys may move for a *voluntary dismissal*.

Pretrial Hearings
A pretrial judge attempts to help parties resolve the dispute without going to trial. If the judge is not successful, a trial is scheduled. It may be a *bench trial* (judge only) or a *jury trial* (when either party files a jury demand).

The Trial Procedure
Jury selection: The judge and the attorneys examine prospective jurors.

Opening statements: The attorneys for both parties state what they will prove.

Testimony: Witnesses for plaintiffs testify, then witnesses for defendants. In malpractice cases expert witnesses often testify. Either side may ask the judge for a *directed verdict in their favor.* If denied, the case goes to the jury.

Jury deliberation: The jury retires to deliberate. A unanimous decision may not be required.

Verdict
The jury returns and delivers a verdict that may be quite complicated.

Appealing the Verdict
Either party may appeal the verdict.

nesses, nurses give testimony about what they saw or remember about incidents or circumstances. For instance, a colleague may witness an event that triggers a complaint and summons against another nurse. The colleague may be subpoenaed (summoned) to testify as to what she or he saw and heard relative to the event. Even before the trial, the witness probably would be subpoenaed to give a deposition (sworn pretrial testimony) about the incident.

As expert witnesses, nurses inform the jury about the standard of care in a particular situation. They must have a thorough knowledge of the nurse practice act of the state and the standard of care in the same field as the case at issue. Expert witnesses describe what an ordinary, reasonable, and prudent nurse in the same or similar circumstance in the same or similar community would have done. They may be asked to evaluate the behavior of the defendant and state whether or not the defendant upheld that standard. Many malpractice cases are won or lost as a result of such testimony. Serving as an expert witness is one of the rewarding and challenging roles nurses play in the legal process.

◆ Criminal Law and Nursing Practice

Criminal law is concerned with harm against society, that is, with actions that directly threaten the orderly existence of society. It deals with criminal statutes and their enforcement. Criminal acts, while aimed at individuals, are offenses against the state. Fenner explains, "To tolerate such actions would directly endanger the state's right to maintain an orderly social existence" (1980). Therefore, in criminal cases the government attorney, on behalf of the people, is the prosecutor. When a guilty verdict is returned, the victim usually does not receive redress (compensation). Instead the person who committed the crime is punished in some way, such as being sentenced to jail, fined, or placed on probation. Conviction of a crime requires proof beyond a reasonable doubt. Criminal acts of special concern to nurses are violation of nurse practice acts and narcotics laws.

Violations of Nurse Practice Acts

The purpose of nurse practice acts is to protect the public by setting and enforcing standards of nursing education and practice. As an extension of that purpose, regulatory boards make rules and regulations that affect many issues such as scope of practice. See Chapter 3. Violations of nurse practice acts are criminal offenses. When people believe that a nurse has violated a provision of a nurse practice act, they may complain to the board of nursing. The board investigates the allegations, and attorneys for the board file a complaint against the licensee if the board finds evidence that supports the allegations.

Although nurse practice acts vary from state to state, they contain similar grounds for complaints, including: (1) diverting controlled substances from health care agencies for personal use, (2) obtaining a nursing license by fraudulent means, (3) being convicted of a felony in any state, and (4) practicing nursing in a grossly incompetent or negligent manner.

Because a state license cannot be taken away without due process, licensees have the right to a hearing about alleged violations. They have the right to be represented by an attorney and the right to present witnesses on their behalf. The result of such a hearing may be that: (1) no action is taken against the nurse, (2) a reprimand is given, (3) the license is suspended or revoked, or (4) the nurse is placed on probation. See Chapter 3. Because conviction of violating a nurse practice act has such serious consequences, nurses facing such allegations should seek legal counsel.

> *Herniez, a nurse practitioner, examined and treated two patients without a physician's order. The Florida State Department of Professional Regulation suspended her license. On appeal, the court upheld the suspension because Herniez went outside the scope of practice of her license (Herniez v. Florida State Department of Professional Regulation, 1980).*

Violations of Narcotic Laws

Two federal laws govern the use of drugs in the United States: (1) the Comprehensive Drug Abuse Prevention and Control Act, which regulates drugs that are subject to abuse, and (2) the Food, Drug, and Cosmetic Act, which restricts interstate shipment of drugs not approved for human use and outlines the testing and approving of drugs. Nurses are responsible for a standard of care that includes accounting for and administering drugs safely. This means they use the "five rights" of drug administration: the right drug, the right patient, the right time, the right dosage, and the right route. Nurses must account for controlled drugs accurately and must not take the drugs of patients for their personal use.

◇ Civil Law and Nursing Practice

Civil law is concerned with harm against another individual, including breaches of contract and torts. It seeks to make right the wrongs and injuries suffered by individuals, usually in the form of monetary compensation. A *contract* is a legally binding agreement between two or more parties, such as exists between employers and employees (see Chapter 12). Breaking such an agreement is called a breach of contract. A *tort* is any civil wrong other than a breach of contract. Assault, battery, false imprisonment, invasion of privacy, and defamation of character are intentional torts. Negligence is an unintentional tort and malpractice (professional negligence) is usually brought as an unintentional tort.

Assault and Battery

Assault is saying or doing anything that makes people fear they will be touched without consent. *Battery* is touching people without their consent, whether or not they are harmed. The key element of assault is fear of being touched. "If you don't let me give you this injection, I'll put you in restraints" is an example of assault. For battery to occur, unconsented touching must take place. The key element of battery is lack of consent. Therefore, if a client bares her arm for an injection, she cannot later charge battery, saying that she did not give consent. If, however, she agreed to the injection because of a threat, the touching would be deemed battery, even if she benefited from the injection and it was properly prescribed. Clients have the right to refuse treatment except in rare circumstances. Other examples of assault and battery are (1) forcing clients to submit to treatments for which they have not consented orally, in writing, or by implication; (2) moving a protesting client from one place to another; (3) forcing a client to get out of bed to walk; and (4) in some states, performing blood alcohol or other tests without consent (*Nurse's Handbook* 1992).

Informed Consent

To prevent allegations of assault and battery and to comply with the law, nurses must obtain voluntary and informed consent from clients for all medical treatment. *Voluntary* means that no coercion is applied, and *informed* means grasping the full import of a proposed treatment. Clients must understand the relative value, alternatives, and risks of having and of not having a treatment. Informed consent may be either verbal or written; however, written consent is preferred because it provides a record. Consent forms must state the specific proposed treatment. Broad consent for "any necessary procedure" is not enough. Physicians are responsible for informing clients and obtaining their consent for medical treatment. Nurses, however, may present the form for clients to sign and may witness their signatures. If clients do not seem well informed, nurses should notify physicians so that they can give their clients more information. Nurses have an ethical obligation to both clients and to physicians to provide proper care, even though nurses are not legally liable for informed consent.

Right to Die

In a landmark case, *Cruzan v Director, Missouri Department of Health*, the parents of Nancy Cruzan petitioned to have their comatose daughter's tube feedings discontinued. In 1990, the US Supreme Court held that the state has the right to refuse to stop life-sustaining treatment unless "clear and convincing evidence" exists about the patient's wishes. Because this standard was not met, the Court did not allow the tube to be removed. It implied, however, that if clear and convincing evidence existed, the client's wishes would be respected. Two months later the Cruzans petitioned the local court with new evidence, and a judge granted them the right to remove Nancy's feeding tube. She died soon thereafter. The Cruzan case alerted the public to the need for providing medical directives.

Most states have *living will laws* (natural death or right to die) that recognize a client's right to die by refusing extraordinary measures when there is no hope of recovery. Some laws permit the next of kin to speak for the client. However, the best evidence is written, either a living will or a durable power of attorney. See the boxes beginning on pages 240 and 242 for samples of these documents.

In 1991, Congress passed the Patient Self-Determination Act requiring hospitals, nursing homes, health maintenance organizations, hospices, and home health care agencies that participate in Medicare and Medicaid to inform clients of their right under state law to refuse treatment if they become incapacitated. The law requires the health care agency to note in the medical record if the person has a written rejection of life support. Nurses should take care to follow this law.

Living Will*

Declaration made this_____ day of_____ 199__.

I,_____, being of sound mind, willfully and voluntarily make known my desire that my dying shall not be artificially prolonged under the circumstances set forth below, and do declare:

If at any time I should have an incurable injury, disease, or illness certified to be a terminal condition by two doctors who have personally examined me, one of whom shall be my attending doctor, and the doctors have determined that my death will occur whether or not life-sustaining procedures are utilized and where the application of life-sustaining procedures would serve only to artificially prolong the dying process, I direct that such procedures be withheld or withdrawn, and that I be permitted to die naturally with only the administration of medication or the performance of any medical procedure deemed necessary to provide me with comfort or care or to alleviate pain.

In the absence of my ability to give directions regarding the use of such life-sustaining procedures, it is my intention that this declaration shall be honored by my family and doctors as the final expression of my legal right to refuse medical or surgical treatment and accept the consequences from such refusal.

I understand the full import of this declaration and am emotionally and mentally competent to make this declaration.

Signed _____   Address _____

➤

False Imprisonment

False imprisonment is confining people against their will by physical or verbal means. Some examples of false imprisonment are (1) restraining a client without written consent by an authorized person, (2) restraining a mentally ill client who is not a danger to self or others, (3) detaining an unwilling client in the hospital if the person insists on leaving, and (4) detaining a person who is medically ready for discharge for an unreasonable period of time.

Obviously, restraining clients with leather straps or locking them in a room is false imprisonment. However, removing their clothing

I believe the declarant to be of sound mind. I did not sign the declarant's signature above, for or at the direction of the declarant. I am at least 18 years of age and am not related to the declarant by blood or marriage, entitled to any portion of the estate of the declarant according to the laws of interstate succession of the _____ or under any will of the declarant or codicil thereto, or directly financially responsible for the declarant's medical care. I am not the declarant's attending doctor, an employee of the attending doctor, or an employee of the health facility in which the declarant is a patient.

Witness _____   Witness _____

Before me, the undersigned authority, on this_____ day of_____,
199___, personally appeared _____, _____, and _____,
known to me to be the Declarant and the Witnesses, respectively, whose names are signed to the foregoing instrument, and who, in the presence of each other, did subscribe their names to the attached Declaration (Living Will) on this date, and that said Declarant at the time of execution of said Declaration was over the age of 18 years and of sound mind.

(Seal)
My commission expires:

_____

Notary Public

_____

*Check requirements of individual state statute.

This sample form is reprinted from *Modern Maturity* (June/July 1988), p.33, with permission of the American Association of Retired Persons (AARP). The form originally appeared in the AARP's *A Matter of Choice*, prepared for the US Senate Special Committee on Aging.

to prevent them from leaving or threatening them if they try to leave are also acts of false imprisonment. If, for safety, clients need to be restrained, nurses should try to gain their cooperation. If this attempt fails, the legal representative of the client must give permission. If these options are not available, nurses should document the need for restraints, consult with the admitting physician, and follow agency policies. Nurses can protect themselves from charges of false imprisonment by discussing safety needs with clients and families and by recording and reporting client behavior to supervisors and physicians.

Durable Power of Attorney for Health Care*

I, _____, hereby appoint: Name _____,
Home address _____, Home telephone number _____,
Work telephone number _____ as my agent to make health care
decisions for me if and when I am unable to make my own health care decisions. This gives my agent the power to consent to giving, withholding, or stop-
ping any health care, treatment, service, or diagnostic procedure. My agent
also has the authority to talk with health care personnel, get information, and
sign forms necessary to carry out those decisions.

If the person named as my agent is not available or is unable to act as my
agent, then I appoint the following persons to serve in the order listed below:

1. Name _____   Home address _____
   Home telephone number _____   Work telephone number _____
2. Name _____   Home address _____
   Home telephone number _____   Work telephone number _____

By this document I intend to create a power of attorney for health care which
shall take effect upon my incapacity to make my own health care decisions
and shall continue during that incapacity.

My agent shall make health care decisions as I direct below or as I make
known to him or her in some other way.
(a) Statement of desires concerning life-prolonging care, treatment, services,
and procedures:

_____

(b) Special provisions and limitations:

_____

By signing below I indicate that I understand the purpose and effect of this
document.

➤

By statute and case law, at both state and federal levels, psychiatric clients cannot be admitted to mental hospitals against their will
without due process of law. Once admitted, they cannot be placed in
restraints or seclusion unless there is demonstrable clinical need.
Even then, regulations define the circumstances, length of time, and
type of restraint that may be used. Clients who voluntarily seek
admission to a psychiatric unit cannot be restrained against their
wishes any more than clients in nonpsychiatric facilities can. Nurses
who work in psychiatric facilities need to know specific state and federal laws pertaining to patient rights.

I sign my name to this form on _____ (date).
My current home address: _____
Signature _____

Witnesses: I declare that the person who signed or acknowledged this document is personally known to me, that he or she signed or acknowledged this durable power of attorney in my presence, and that he or she appears to be of sound mind and under no duress, fraud, or undue influence. I am not the person appointed as agent by this document, nor am I the patient's health care provider or an employee of the patient's health care provider.

First witness:
Signature _____   Home address _____
Print name _____   Date _____
Second witness:
Signature _____   Home address _____
Print name _____   Date _____
(At least one of the above witnesses must also sign the following declaration.)

I further declare that I am not related to the patient by blood, marriage, or adoption, and to the best of my knowledge, I am not entitled to any part of his or her estate under a will now existing or by operation of law.

Signature _____

I further declare that I am not related to the patient by blood, marriage, or adoption, and to the best of my knowledge, I am not entitled to any part of his or her estate under a will now existing or by operation of law.

Signature _____

*Check requirements of individual state statute.
From *Modern Maturity* (June/July 1988) p 88. Reprinted with permission of the American Association of Retired Persons. The form originally appeared in the AARP's *A Matter of Choice*, prepared for the US Senate Special Committee on Aging.

Invasion of Privacy

Clients have a right to privacy with respect to their personal lives. This right derives from interpretation of the US Constitution and is expressly stated in some state laws. All information about a person belongs to that person. Nurses who divulge information without authorization from clients or from their legal guardians may be held liable. Without the express permission of the client, nurses may not release private information to a third party, allow them to read medical records, take pictures, or observe medical procedures. Only those professionals who are involved in the care of a client should have access to the medical record. Those who are not must have specific written authorization or a court order. The only exceptions to this rule are the mandatory reporting of certain communicable and new-born infant diseases to public health authorities and the reporting of child abuse, adult abuse, rape, and gunshot wounds to law enforcement officials.

Privileged Communication

Privileged communication is information that does not have to be revealed in a court of law. It is confidential information that clients disclose to certain trusted individuals, namely to physicians, clergy, attorneys, or spouses within the scope of the relationship. Not all states recognize the nurse-client relationship as privileged, and not all communication is considered privileged. If the court determines that certain communication is not privileged, the witness may be required to reveal it.

> *In a therapy session a week before her husband was shot to death, a woman told her nurse-therapist that she sometimes stayed awake at night thinking of ways to kill her abusive husband. The woman was charged with homicide. At her trial the nurse-therapist was required to give the court the dates of her therapy sessions with the woman. However, she was not required to reveal the client's incriminating statement because in that state the law designated the nurse-client relationship as privileged. The woman was acquitted. One of her husband's drinking buddies confessed to the killing.*

Defamation of Character

Defamation of character is communication to another that is damaging to a person's reputation. The communication need not be false or intentionally damaging. When the communication is oral, it is called *slander;* when it is written, it is called *libel.* If nurses write libelous statements in client records, such as, "The boy's mother rudely demanded a dinner tray," the woman may charge that the statement adversely affected the care of her child by prejudicing nurses against him. Prudent nurses record only objective data, documenting facts, and avoid giving opinions. When it is necessary to report inappropriate care or error, or to evaluate another employee, nurses should use the procedures specified by the institution and limit their remarks and written reports to objective evidence. Factual appraisal reported through appropriate channels is generally protected from legal action.

Negligence and Malpractice

Negligence is a failure to act as any reasonable, prudent person would, with consequent injury or damage to people and property. When negligence is alleged, the conduct of the accused is measured by what a reasonable, prudent individual would have done in the same or similar circumstances. This provision seeks to ensure that an objective standard is used to determine whether or not negligence was present. Negligence is an unintentional tort, a civil cause of legal action. When individuals sustain injuries or suffer damages, they seek redress, usually money, in negligence actions. Four elements must be proven for negligence actions to be successful:

1. There must be a duty, by law, that dictates expected behavior to avoid unreasonable and foreseeable risk of harm to another.

2. There must be a breach of that duty, or a failure to uphold that duty.

3. The breach must be the proximate (probable) cause of injury to the victim.

4. Actual damages recognized by law must be suffered (Creighton 1986).

Malpractice is professional negligence, the improper discharge of professional duties, or failure to meet standards of care, resulting in harm to another person. Some important principles affecting malpractice actions include individual responsibility, *respondeat superior, res ipsa loquitur,* and standard of care.

Individual Responsibility

An important concept in any negligence action is the principle that each person is responsible for his or her own actions. Even when other people or organizations are involved in a situation, it is difficult for any individual to remain free of all responsibility and shift all liability to others.

A patient, ambulating in the hall of a busy surgical unit, slipped on a water spill and broke her hip. In her suit she named every nurse who worked on the unit that day, alleging malpractice for not noticing the spill and wiping it up. The court agreed with the patient and held each nurse responsible.

Respondeat Superior

Respondeat superior literally means "let the master speak." This doctrine holds employers indirectly and vicariously liable for any negligence of their employees when employees act within the scope of their employment and when negligent acts occur during employment. This doctrine allows an injured party to sue both the employee and employer, to sue only the employee, or to sue only the employer for alleged injuries. Although each person is responsible for her or his own acts, nurse managers and faculty members are responsible for the acts of those they oversee (*Nurse's Handbook* 1992).

> *A first-year nursing student was assigned by an instructor to care for an elderly man. Using a hydraulic lift, the student put the man into in a tub of hot water, burning him badly. The man's family sued the physician, hospital, head nurse, student, faculty member, and school of nursing. The court held the student responsible to the standard of care of a RN because the student was performing RN functions. If the student was not able to function safely without supervision, she should not have been permitted to carry out those functions. The court held the hospital liable under* respondeat superior, *because hospitals are liable for student actions as if they are employees. The court held the head nurse liable because she was responsible for the care of all the clients in the unit. It found the instructor liable because she did not properly assign or adequately supervise the student. Applying the principle of* respondeat superior, *the court held the nursing school liable because the director used poor judgment in employing or assigning the faculty member to her teaching responsibilities.*

Res Ipsa Loquitur

Res ipsa loquitur literally means "the thing speaks for itself." It is a rule of evidence designed to equalize the positions of plaintiffs and defendants, when otherwise plaintiffs (those injured) could be at a disadvantage. The rule allows a plaintiff to prove negligence by circumstantial evidence when the defendant has the primary and sometimes only knowledge of what happened to cause the injury. Usually, plaintiffs must prove every element of a case against defendants. Until they do, the court presumes that the defendants met the applicable standard of care. When the court applies the *res ipsa loquitur* rule, the burden of proof for causation shifts from plaintiffs to defendants. Defendants must prove that the injury was caused by something other than their negligence. Plaintiffs can ask the court to invoke the *res ipsa loquitur* rule if three elements are present: (1) the act that caused an injury was in the exclusive control of the defendant; (2) the injury would not have happened in the absence of negligence by the defendant; and (3) no negligence on part of the plaintiff contributed to the injury (*Nurse's Handbook* 1992).

> *A laparotomy sponge was left in a patient's abdomen after surgery. Applying the principle of* res ipsa loquitur, *the court held the physician, the hospital, and the operating room nurses liable. The court did so because the sponge was in the exclusive control of the defendants; it would not have been left in the abdomen except for the negligent act; and the patient did not contribute to the injury.*

Standard of Care

Professional negligence (malpractice) deals with negligent acts of professionals such as nurses and physicians. All of the elements and principles that apply to negligence also apply to professional negligence, with one exception. The principle of standard of care is different for professionals than nonprofessionals. When alleged negligent behavior is judged, the conduct of nurses is measured by a standard of care that is "what any reasonable, prudent professional nurse would have done in the same or similar circumstances in the same or similar community" (*Nurse's Handbook* 1992). The words "same or similar community" might be construed to mean the standard of care found in the local community. This is not the case. The "community" of health care professionals is the national community, the entire United States. Thus, it is imperative that nurses know national standards of care for nursing practice. These standards are set forth by well-known experts and authors and by professional organizations such as the ANA and NLN. When health professionals represent themselves as specialists, they are held to a standard of care of specialists such as those identified by credentialing organizations. They must also meet state licensing requirements.

Good Samaritan Laws

Good Samaritan laws protect nurses and physicians from civil liability when they give emergency care. When nurses come to the aid of accident victims, two kinds of law protect them: common law and statutory law, often called good Samaritan laws. All states now have good Samaritan laws that cover nurses and physicians when they aid disaster and accident victims. Some states even have duty to rescue statutes, requiring all citizens to come to the aid of anyone they know is in grave danger. In all cases, nurses must observe professional standards of care. The following are guidelines to help nurses reduce the risk of a malpractice action when they come upon an accident:

- Give cardiopulmonary resuscitation as needed.

- Stop bleeding with pressure; avoid tourniquets if possible.

- Move victims only to protect them from further injury.

- Assess for consciousness, pain, and possible fractures.

- Keep victims warm.

- Avoid speculating about who or what caused the accident.

- Allow only skilled personnel to attend or treat the victim.

- Stay at the accident site until skilled personnel arrive to assume care of victims.

- Guard the personal property of victims, releasing the property only to the police or family. (*Nurse's Handbook* 1992, p. 188)

Selected Malpractice Cases

Wound Monitoring

John Daniel incurred a leg injury and was treated at Gladewater Municipal Hospital. Osteomyelitis developed in the injured leg. In his complaint Daniel alleged that the condition was caused by negligent care by the nurses and the physician, Dr. Marashi. Specifically, Daniel alleged that the nurses were negligent because they failed to change his bandages and did not inform the physician of drainage from the wound. He alleged that the physician failed to monitor the wound properly and sued the physician and the hospital, as the nurses' employer. At the trial, testimony showed that the plaintiff's bandage was changed only two times during his 39-day stay in the hospital. The first change occurred 13 days after surgery. Further testimony showed that the surgical site drained heavily during this time and the drainage was malodorous.

The plaintiff produced two expert witnesses: Dr. Jacobs, a physician, and Ms Dole, a nurse. Dr. Jacobs testified that the physician who cared for Daniel did not uphold the standard of care relative to monitoring the wound and changing the dressings. Ms Dole testified that the conduct of the nurses did not meet the standard of care of professional nurses because they failed to change the dressings and to notify the physician of drainage from the operative site. Based on testimony by the experts, the jury returned a $100,000 verdict in favor of Daniel, against the physician and the hospital (Gladewater Municipal Hospital v. Daniel 1985).

Patient Teaching

In another case, patient teaching became the focus of alleged negligence on the part of a nurse in an emergency room.

Mrs. Crawford's son was involved in a fight during which the son was stabbed in the shoulder and hit on the head with a baseball bat. The injured man was rushed to one hospital, then transferred to Earl Long Hospital, where he was seen in the emergency department. The attending physician asked the nurse to call the mother and ask her to come and take her son home. The nurse did so. The nurse testified that when Mrs. Crawford arrived at the hospital she gave the mother specific instructions about how to care for her son at home. She told the mother to awaken her son at regular intervals, question him to see if he was alert and knew who and where he was, and determine if his eye pupils were the same size. The mother seemed to understand the instructions and took her son home. The mother testified that on arriving at home she went to bed and that her son stayed up a while longer. When she awoke the next morning, Mrs. Crawford went to check her son and found that he was dead. She brought suit against the hospital as the employer of the nurse, alleging that the emergency room nurse was negligent because she failed to give home care instructions. The nurse testified that she gave instructions to the mother, albeit orally. She did not document her instruction giving in the record.

The court carefully evaluated the testimony of the nurse and concluded that she was truthful when she testified that she had given the required instructions to the mother. By expert testimony, the court determined the standard of care in 1975 was to give oral instructions to family members or other responsible persons for the care of individuals sent home with head injuries. The court gave great weight to the fact that the nurse insisted the mother come to the hospital to pick up her son rather than send him home in a taxi as the mother requested. The nurse's insistence, they concluded, was evidence that she intended to give home care instructions directly to the mother. The court entered a verdict in favor of the hospital. Although the verdict supported the nurse and hospital, the whole affair could have been avoided. The nurse should have given both oral and written instructions to the mother and documented her action in the record (Crawford v. Earl Long Memorial Hospital 1983).

Drug Reaction Monitoring

Four recovery room nurses and a cardiologist were sued for the death of a client due to negligent care following surgery. Torbert, the plaintiff, was undergoing surgery for closure of a colostomy. He developed premature ventricular contractions (PVC) of his heart shortly after the anesthesia was induced. Dr. Befeler, a cardiologist, was consulted. He ordered medication to suppress the abnormal heart contractions and then approved completion of the surgical procedure. In the recovery room the PVCs continued, and about 3 hours after surgery the patient suffered cardiac arrest. Although revived, the man sustained brain damage and died several weeks later.

The family brought suit against the nurses and physician, alleging professional negligence in not adequately monitoring the patient. Testimony at the trial revealed that the head nurse in the recovery room interpreted existing protocols at the time of the incident to mean that one-to-one monitoring of the client was to occur only until he stabilized. The team leader, also a defendant, testified that she gave Demerol about 45 minutes before the arrest but did not monitor the man to detect an adverse reaction to the medication. It was determined that a reaction to the medication caused the arrest. Finally, the nurse assigned to monitor the man testified that she was not monitoring him at the time of his cardiac arrest. As a *result, the client was not attended by a nurse for at least 10 minutes after the cardiac arrest.*

The jury returned a verdict against the nurses and the cardiologist, apportioning fault at 45% for the head nurse, 45% for the team leader, 5% for the nurse who did not monitor the patient, and 5% for the cardiologist. This case demonstrates that nurses are liable for their actions whether they give direct client care or supervise others giving such care. When nurses perform at a level below the standard of care, they are professionally negligent and responsible for the injury (Torbert v. Befeler 1985).

◈ Patient's Bill of Rights

Not long ago people accepted the notion that hospitals cared for clients with omniscient concern, like beneficent parents. People who entered the hospital relinquished their basic human rights. Although the National League for Nursing (NLN) published the first patient's bill of rights in 1959, few people challenged the system. If they did, they were intimidated by custom or left to file malpractice suits. In 1973, a federal commission attributed much of the malpractice crisis to violations of patient rights. That same year the American Hospital Association (AHA) approved a statement entitled "A Patient's Bill of Rights," Minnesota passed the first state patient rights law, and Congress passed the Rehabilitation Act guaranteeing the same rights to handicapped as to nonhandicapped people. In 1980, Congress enacted the Mental Health Systems Act, a comprehensive federal law on mental health services. Though much of the law was repealed, the Patient's Bill of Rights survived. In 1987, Congress passed the Omnibus Budget Reconciliation Act, imposing minimum standards to protect the rights of long-term clients. The law granted relatives and officials the right of access to investigate complaints (*Nurse's Handbook* 1992, p. 64). In 1992, the AHA revised its "Patient's Bill of Rights," removing sexist language and reflecting public awareness of patient rights (see the box on page 252). All these laws and standards flow from the ethical principles of autonomy and respect for human dignity.

The American Hospital Association Patient's Bill of Rights

1. The patient has the right to considerate and respectful care.

2. The patient has the right to and is encouraged to obtain from physicians and other direct caregivers relevant, current, and understandable information concerning diagnosis, treatment, and prognosis.

Except in emergencies when the patient lacks decision-making capacity and the need for treatment is urgent, the patient is entitled to the opportunity to discuss and request information related to the specific procedures and/or treatments, the risks involved, the possible length of recuperation, and the medically reasonable alternatives and their accompanying risks and benefits.

Patients have the right to know the identify of physicians, nurses, and others involved in their care, as well as when those involved are students, residents, or other trainees. The patient also has the right to know the immediate long-term financial implications of treatment choices, insofar as they are known.

3. The patient has the right to make decisions about the plan of care prior to and during the course of treatment and to refuse a recommended treatment or plan of care to the extent permitted by law and hospital policy and to be informed of the medical consequences of this action. In case of such refusal, the patient is entitled to other appropriate care and services that the hospital provides or transfer to another hospital. The hospital should notify patients of any policy that might affect patient choice with the institution.

4. The patient has the right to have an advance directive (such as a living will, health care proxy, or durable power of attorney for health care) concerning treatment or designating a surrogate decision maker with the expectation that the hospital will honor the intent of that directive to the extent permitted by law and hospital policy.

Health care institutions must advise patients of their rights under state law and hospital policy to make informed medical choices, ask if the patient has an advance directive, and include that information in patient records. The patient has the right to timely information about hospital policy that may limit its ability to implement fully a legally valid advance directive.

5. The patient has the right to every consideration of his privacy. Case discussion, consultation, examination, and treatment should be conducted so as to protect each patient's privacy.

6. The patient has the right to expect that all communications and records pertaining to his/her care will be treated as confidential by the hospital, except in cases such as suspected abuse and public health hazards when reporting is permitted or required by law. The patient has the right

to expect that the hospital will emphasize the confidentiality of this information when it releases it to any other parties entitled to review information in these records.

7. The patient has the right to review the records pertaining to his/her medical care and to have the information explained or interpreted as necessary, except when restricted by law.

8. The patient has the right to expect that, within its capacity and policies, a hospital will make reasonable response to the request of a patient for appropriate and medically indicated care and services. The hospital must provide evaluation, service, and/or referral as indicated by the urgency of the case. When medically appropriate and legally permissible, or when a patient has so requested, a patient may be transferred to another facility. The institution to which the patient is to be transferred must first have accepted the patient for transfer. The patient must also have the benefit of complete information and explanation concerning the need for, risks, benefits, and alternative to such a transfer.

9. The patient has the right to ask for and be informed of the existence of business relationships among the hospital, educational institutions, other health care providers, or payers that may influence the patient's treatment and care.

10. The patient has the right to consent to or decline to participate in proposed research studies or human experimentation affecting care and treatment or requiring direct patient involvement, and to have those studies fully explained prior to consent. A patient who declines to participate in research or experimentation is entitled to the most effective care that the hospital can otherwise provide.

11. The patient has the right to expect reasonable continuity of care when appropriate and to be informed by physicians and other caregivers of available and realistic patient care options when hospital care is no longer appropriate.

12. The patient has the right to be informed of hospital policies and practices that relate to patient care, treatment and responsibilities. The patient has the right to be informed of available resources for resolving disputes, grievances, and conflicts, such as ethics committees, patient representatives, or other mechanisms available in the institution. The patient has the right to be informed of the hospital's charges for services and available payment methods.

Reproduced by permission of the American Hospital Association. *A Patient's Bill of Rights* was first adopted in 1973. This revision was approved by the AHA Board of Trustees in 1992.

◆ Preventing Malpractice Claims

Without doubt, the trust the public once held for the medical profession has diminished. Today people know more, are more assertive, and are more involved in their personal health care. They question treatments and act when they believe care is inadequate. When people view the health care industry as predatory and impersonal, they are more apt to take legal action for perceived error. Hospitals, physicians, and especially nurses can do much to change that dynamic and prevent malpractice suits. Here are some suggestions:

- *Recognize suit-prone clients and intervene.* When people feel frightened and powerless, they are critical and demanding. By avoiding such clients or reacting defensively, nurses may confirm client fears. If, however, nurses listen actively, discuss treatment plans openly, and involve clients in decision making, they can foster trust and respect. As a consequence, clients will be less inclined to pursue legal action.

- *Develop self-awareness.* Nurses need to recognize their strengths and weaknesses and use continuing education to grow. They should not be afraid to admit lack of knowledge in some area and should refuse assignment to a specialty where they lack critical skills.

- *Delegate duties cautiously.* Supervisors are responsible for subordinates, equipment, and supplies on their units. If they assign a task that is beyond the ability or scope of practice of a caregiver and an error occurs, the supervisor is responsible. When an employee is incompetent, supervisors should follow accepted performance-evaluation procedures.

- *Follow agency policies and procedures.* These documents are designed to prevent errors. If a mistake occurs, such as a drug administration error, and legal action results, the court will want to know if the nurse followed accepted procedures. Even if the incorrect dose was dispensed by a pharmacist, the nurse could also be liable if the nurse did not follow the normal procedure designed to prevent errors.

- *Document actions accurately.* If a nurse does not document an action, it may be difficult to prove to the court that the nurse performed it. Nurses should write notes as if they will be read out loud in court. The notes should be accurate, objective, and without subjective judgments that could be construed as libelous. Accurate, detailed documentation is the best defense in court.

- *Write detailed incident reports.* However unpleasant they may find the task, nurses need to describe all errors, injuries, and accidents in incident reports. Do not record the fact that an incident report was written in a client's record. The risk manager receives these reports, analyzes them, and recommends policy and procedural changes to prevent future incidents. Because long periods of time may elapse between an incident and a court action, an incident report may be the only detailed account of what really happened.

- *Prevent accidents.* Nurses must be alert for hazards that cause accidents. Water spills, broken equipment, cluttered halls, protruding apparatus, blood-contaminated sharps, and exposed electric wires are accidents waiting to happen. When they do, and people suffer injuries, nurses may be held liable.

◆ Professional Liability Insurance

The likelihood of being sued is real. Lawsuits are costly and awards may reach millions of dollars. Even when a verdict is favorable, the price of defending oneself can be immense. Given these realities, nurses should become informed consumers of liability insurance. The box on page 256 lists some important features of professional liability insurance policies that nurses need to know.

◆ Defending Yourself

If you are served with a summons and complaint, you will need to act right away. If you do nothing and fail to answer the complaint, a default judgment could result. Here are some suggestions for what to do and what not to do:

Do (if personally insured):

- Immediately telephone the company that provides your liability insurance. Usually a toll-free number is provided on the cover

Important Features of Professional Liability Insurance

Definition

Professional liability insurance shifts the cost of a suit and its settlement from one person to others. It covers acts committed while functioning in a professional capacity.

Two types of coverage

1. Occurrence covers any incident that occurs during the time a policy is in effect, no matter when a claim is filed, even after the policy ends (more costly).
2. Claims-made covers only claims made during the time the policy is in effect. Tail-coverage may be purchased to effectively turn a claims-made policy into an occurrence policy.

Coverage limits

No policy is limitless. Some important limitations are:

1. The maximum dollar amount that will be paid in a settlement. Excess judgments, amounts over the amount covered by the policy, must be paid by the defendant from personal assets.
2. Whether the negligent acts of those the policy holder is supervising are covered.
3. Whether the following negligent acts of the policy holder are covered: misuse of equipment, errors in reporting or recording, failure to properly teach clients, errors in giving medication, and mistakes in giving emergency care outside the employment setting.
4. Whether the policy will provide protection if the employer sues the policy holder.

Individual or employer policies

An individual policy gives the named holder more power to control decisions than if the person is insured only under the policy of the employer. Employer

➤

letter that accompanies the policy. The company spokesperson will tell you how to proceed. If you do not contact the insurance company within the time specified by the policy, the insurance company may refuse to cover you.

policies cover nurses only when they are on the job, working for that employer, within the scope of the job description of the employer.

Exclusions

Many policies exclude coverage of criminal acts; intentional torts such as assault, battery, and false imprisonment; and disciplinary actions brought against nurses by licensing boards.

Right to decide about settlements

Nurses need to know if the insurance policy gives them the right to decide about the settlement of the case, or if the insurance company has that right alone.

Scope of practice

Advance practice nurses (APN) in independent practice need to know if an insurance policy covers them or only nurses employed by health care agencies. APNs may be able to purchase liability insurance from their professional organizations.

Duration of coverage

Liability insurance policies are contracts that are renewed or canceled each year. The policy usually states how it is to be canceled and how many days of notice must be given.

Cautions

A liability insurance policy is a legal contract between an insurance company and a policy holder. False information on the application may void the policy. Liability insurance does not cover acts outside the scope of practice or licensure, or intentional torts such as assault, battery, false imprisonment, invasion of privacy, and slander.

- Fill out the informational forms sent by your insurer as completely as possible.
- Follow all instructions the insurance carrier gives, such as telephoning a specific attorney in your area. Send lawsuit papers by certified mail, return receipt requested; save the receipt.

- Create your own legal file of all documents, receipts, and correspondence about the case.

- Contact the legal department of the institution where the incident occurred.

- Work closely with the attorney the insurer assigns to you.

- Take steps to protect your personal property; many states have *homestead laws* that permit you to protect property such as your home from judgments against you.

Do (if not personally insured):

- Contact the legal department of the institution where the incident occurred. Notify them that you have been served.

- Work closely with the attorney assigned to your case by the institution's insurance company.

- If it seems that your interests are not being protected, you may decide to retain your own legal counsel. Look for an attorney who is experienced in medical malpractice.

Do not (whether insured or not):

- Talk to anyone about the incident except the insurance carrier and your attorney, including personal and professional acquaintances and news media.

- Sign any papers or give any written statements to plaintiffs or their attorneys without legal counsel.

- Even think about trying to defend yourself against a lawsuit. Your opposition will have experienced attorneys who would make short work of your amateur defense.

◇ Summary

In United States there are four sources of law—constitutional, statutory, administrative, and common (case)—and two types of law—criminal and civil. Criminal law is concerned with harm against society and includes violations of nurse practice acts and narcotic laws. Civil law is concerned with harm against individuals and includes assault, battery, false imprisonment, invasion of privacy, defamation of character, and negligence. The trial process of both criminal and civil cases follows a step-by-step sequence. Professional negligence is decided by measuring nursing actions against the standard of what any reasonable, prudent nurse would do in the same or similar circumstances and community. Patient bills of rights codify basic human rights guaranteed by the US Constitution. Nurses need to know how to avoid lawsuits, how to choose liability insurance, and what to do if legal action is taken against them.

Critical Thinking Questions

1. What underlying pattern or principle do you see in the first ten amendments to the US Constitution?

2. What are the similarities between the civil and criminal trial processes? What are the differences? What changes would you make to improve either process?

3. Given the existence of the first ten amendments to the US Constitution, how do you explain the need for a Patient's Bill of Rights?

1. Observe a jury trial, preferably one involving professional negligence (malpractice).

2. Interview a nurse who has served as an expert witness; determine what made that person an expert and what kinds of questions were asked at the trial.

3. Imagine that you are a prosecuting attorney looking for evidence of negligence; evaluate the nurses notes you find in a client's chart for accuracy, objectivity, and completeness.

4. Review protocols in your health care agency for incident reports, telephone prescriptions, controlled substances, and permission for surgical procedures.

5. Read the vignette at the beginning of the chapter; in a group discussion, role-play explaining the trial process to Ina.

Annotated Reading List

Calfee BE. War Stories. The State License Hearing—Information for Empowerment. *Revolution, The Journal of Nurse Empowerment* Winter 1993; 69–71.

This valuable article describes the legal fact that nurses "answer to two masters," their clients and their licensing board. When nurses are found liable in malpractice suits, the fact is reported to the licensing board. The board has the responsibility to investigate. They may schedule a hearing to determine whether the nurse's license should be suspended or revoked. The article describes the process and lists five guidelines for nurses who may find themselves involved in a license dispute with their licensing board.

Meubauer MP. Careful Charting, Your Best Defense. *RN* Nov 1990; 77–80.

In this brief, fact-filled, useful article, the author asks, "How does your charting measure up against these examples?" She gives examples of sketchy charting that would leave a nurse little defense. Then she states clearly what to include and what to omit in what she calls "defensive" record keeping.

References

Crawford v. Earl Long Memorial Hospital. 431 So. 2d 40 (La. App.) 1983.

Creighton H. *Law Every Nurse Should Know.* 5th ed. Saunders, 1986.

Cruzan v. The Director, Missouri Deptartment of Health, 110 S Ct. 2841, 111 L. Ed 2d 224 1990.

Fenner KM. *Ethics and Law in Nursing, Professional Perspectives.* Van Nostrand, 1980.

Gladewater Municipal Hospital v. Daniel, 694 S.W. 2d 619 (Tx. App.) 1985.

Herniez v. Florida State Department of Professional Registration, 390 So. 2d 194 (Dist. Ct. App.) 1980.

Nurse's Handbook of Law and Ethics. Springhouse, 1992.

Torbert v. Befeler, No. L-17463-81, Union City Superior Court, April 25, 1985, *Atlanta Law Reporter* (December) 1985.

28th USC 1331,1332. 1994.

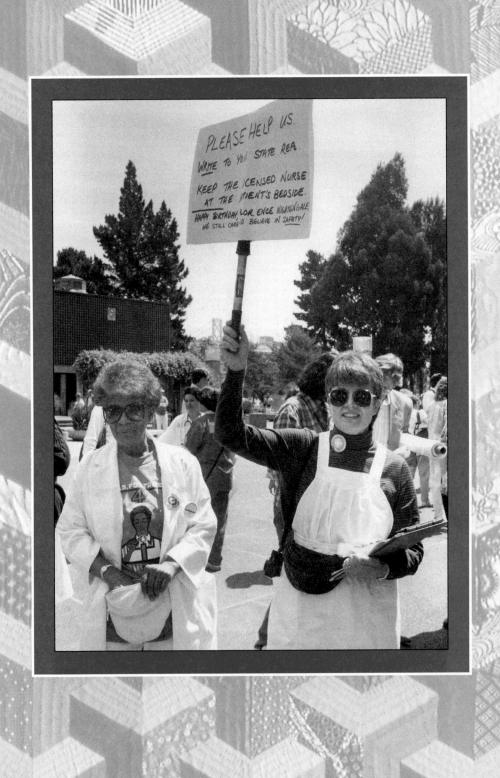

Change, Power, and Politics

9

◈ Learning Objectives

- Discuss the characteristics and types of change.

- Compare rational, paradoxical, normative, and coercive models of planned change.

- Identify the criteria for choosing each model of planned change.

- Define and describe the characteristics and types of power.

- Discuss the sources of power, giving examples of each source.

- Explain how nurses can use power with themselves and others to bring about change.

- State the do's and don'ts of writing to elected representatives.

- Describe political actions nurses can take relative to the government, professional organizations, workplace, and community.

- Discuss the socialization of women relative to power and politics.

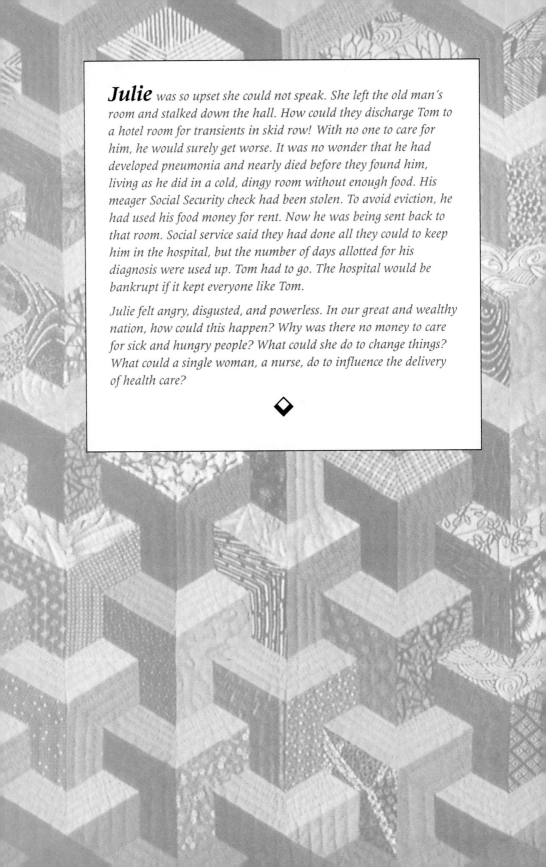

Julie was so upset she could not speak. She left the old man's room and stalked down the hall. How could they discharge Tom to a hotel room for transients in skid row! With no one to care for him, he would surely get worse. It was no wonder that he had developed pneumonia and nearly died before they found him, living as he did in a cold, dingy room without enough food. His meager Social Security check had been stolen. To avoid eviction, he had used his food money for rent. Now he was being sent back to that room. Social service said they had done all they could to keep him in the hospital, but the number of days allotted for his diagnosis were used up. Tom had to go. The hospital would be bankrupt if it kept everyone like Tom.

Julie felt angry, disgusted, and powerless. In our great and wealthy nation, how could this happen? Why was there no money to care for sick and hungry people? What could she do to change things? What could a single woman, a nurse, do to influence the delivery of health care?

◆

The realities of contemporary health care often conflict with the humanistic ideals of nursing. Yet for decades nurses have accepted these realities as inevitable. Women dominated the profession, but the passive role they learned as women kept them from challenging the status quo and acting to bring about change. However, in recent years, women have begun to assert themselves, to confront the rigid gender roles that restricted them, and to assert themselves as copartners in society. With strong leadership and changing attitudes, the nursing profession has begun to make its voice heard. To continue this progress, all nurses need to understand the concepts of change, power, and politics and put that knowledge to work in their daily lives.

◆ Change

The primary reason for nurses to learn about power and politics is to produce change. But what is change? *Change* is action, movement, alteration, and transformation. It is conversion from one state to another. Brooten and colleagues defined change as "the process which leads to alteration in individual or institutional patterns of behavior" (1988). Change is the process by which alterations occur in the function and structure of society. Planned change is a deliberate, collaborative effort to improve the operation of a human system. It is a goal-directed process that includes a change agent and a client system. The system may be an individual, a group, or a social institution.

Change agents are the ones who initiate change or who assist others to make modifications in a system. Change agents rely on a systematic body of knowledge about change to guide the change process. They plan and implement change in what are called target systems. Nurses act as change agents when they apply the nursing process to client problems: assessing needs, planning strategies, implementing, and evaluating the effectiveness of those strategies to bring about change. Change agents may be formally or informally designated by institutions. They may come as external change agents from outside an institution or as internal change agents from inside an institution. Because they work with human systems, these agents must assume a leadership role. As such, they accurately assess situations, build trust and hope in those with whom they work, communicate effectively, and commit themselves to the process of change.

Characteristics of Change

Change is inevitable. In open, living systems, change goes on continually. Sometimes it occurs slowly and subtly, and sometimes quickly and dramatically. Regardless of its speed, change in any part affects the whole system. By continually adapting to change, systems have a tendency to maintain a uniform, steady state within and between their parts. Thus, to produce stability, a system must constantly adapt.

Change is neither good nor bad. It is the use of change that decides its rightness or wrongness. Change for the sake of change is of no value and may even cause damage. However, positive change produces growth, relieves boredom, heightens self-esteem, increases productivity, and invigorates participants.

Resistance to change is affected by self-interest and group norms. In the broadest sense, all behavior is caused and is motivated by self-interest. As a result, people resist change that threatens their beliefs, values, status, personal security, or the norms of their group. Sometimes change penalizes people in terms of time, money, and effort. Sometimes it creates suspicion because people fear its effects. The stages of resistance to change are:

1. Undifferentiated resistance,

2. Lining up of sides for and against change and development of positions,

3. Direct conflict between the two sides, with resistance gradually reduced or overcome,

4. The assumption of power by the people for the change,

5. The beginning of aceptance by those against the change,

6. Repression of the memory of opposition to change by all but a few (Stevens 1975).

Acceptance of change is a predictable process. The six stages of acceptance of change are (1) gradual awareness of new idea, system, or practice, (2) search for more information, (3) evaluation of information as it relates to the situation, (4) mental imaging of the proposed change, (5) tentative use of change, (6) adoption of the change and integration of the system (Stevens 1975).

Emotional Phases of Change

Perlman and Takacs (1990) identify ten emotional phases people experience as they experience change, beginning with equilibrium and ending with reemergence. They are

1. Equilibrium, characterized by emotional and intellectual balance, high energy, and harmony of personal and professional goals

2. Denial, in which the individual denies the reality of the change and experiences various degrees of physical, cognitive, and emotional malfunction

3. Anger, manifested by rage, envy, and resentment

4. Bargaining, an attempt to eliminate the change

5. Chaos, characterized by diffused energy and feelings of powerlessness, insecurity, and loss of identity

6. Depression, with ineffective defense mechanisms, self-pity, and little energy for productivity

7. Resignation, when the change is passively accepted

8. Openness, when there is some renewal of energy to implement new roles or assignments that result from the change

9. Physical and emotional reunification, in which there is willful expenditure of energy to explore new events

10. Reemergence, when the person again feels empowered and begins to initiate new projects and ideas.

Types of Change

Change has been categorized in various ways by different theorists. In one of their early writings, Bennis et al (1976) identify eight types of change: indoctrination, interactional, socializing, coercive, technocratic, natural, emulative, and planned. Sampson (1971) suggests three types: developmental, spontaneous, and planned change, and Duncan (1978) says there are only two types: haphazard and planned change. Notice that each theorist identifies planned change. Planned change involves problem solving and decision making as well as interpersonal competence. It is deliberate and carried out consciously to influence the condition of oneself or another organism or situation.

Models of Planned Change

Theorists have explained change by the use of models that describe several kinds of change, including rational, paradoxical, natural, and coercive change. These models are classified by the amount of resistance they predict can be overcome. Before choosing a model to use, change agents must assess the degree of resistance they expect to encounter. The *rational model* is useful when the least amount of power is needed to overcome resistance, the *paradoxical model* is somewhat more useful when more power is needed, the *natural (normative) model* is more useful when even more power is needed, and the *coercive model* is best in situations requiring the most power. Each model has appropriate uses.

Rational Model

The rational model for planned change is based on the belief that people would change if they knew a better way to accomplish a goal. Therefore, this model includes no strategy to overcome resistance. Instead, the model focuses on the proposed change. One of the best-known rational approaches is called *diffusion of innovation* (Rogers & Shoemaker 1971). The diffusion of innovation model has three steps: (1) invention of the change; (2) diffusion (communication) of information, with success depending on compatibility with existing values, complexity in using or understanding, trialability (use on a trial basis), and observability of positive results; and (3) consequences, that is, adoption or rejection of change.

Application of the Rational Model

The rational model works well when an individual or group is motivated and simply needs guidance to make a change. The rational model may take the form of a public information campaign such as the "Just say NO!" slogan initiated to reduce the incidence of substance abuse. The effectiveness of this approach depends on the motivation of the target system and their acceptance of the proposed method of producing results.

> The staff of a busy same-day-stay unit found the admitting procedures cumbersome and time-consuming. They asked the nurse manager to help them devise a more efficient system. She formed a committee that surveyed the literature, met with various department heads, and devised a new procedure. With the approval of all con-

cerned, the staff instituted the new system for a 9-week trial. Throughout the trial, the staff evaluated the new procedure, suggesting minor adjustments. At its conclusion they voted to endorse the revised procedure and sent it to administration for approval, implementing a rational model of planned change.

Paradoxical Model

A paradox is a contradictory, illogical event. This model grew out of the study of human communication by Watzlawick, et al (1974). These researchers are remembered for their description of double-bind communication and for paradoxical psychotherapy in which therapists prescribe the symptom. They propose that change occurs at two levels: logical, first-order change and illogical, second-order change. *First-order change* involves rearranging existing elements of a system in a logical fashion. Such change may appear to fix a problem for a while, but in time it may create greater frustration because people become discouraged and the problem remains.

Second-order change requires an innovative approach. It asks change agents to look at a problem creatively from a different perspective, called reframing. The process of second-order change is as follows: (1) define the problem in concrete terms, (2) list the solutions attempted so far, (3) define a realistic change, and (4) create and implement an innovative solution for the problem. The unique thing about second-order change is innovation. Second-order change is not a mere rearrangement or improvement of old methods. It is a fundamental change, a novel approach requiring a thorough assessment of the goals to be achieved.

Application of the Paradoxical Model

A long-term care unit regularly used more clean linen than was budgeted. The administrators decided to mount a campaign aimed at reducing laundry costs using the rational model of change. The nurse manager, the change agent, set up meetings with staff nurses to publicize the high cost of clean linen, asked staff to reduce linen use, and finally, issued a quota of linen per client per day. The nurses tried to comply, but they were unable to reduce linen use. After a 3-month trial, linen use was just as high as it had been before the campaign. First-order change did not solve the problem. The nurse manager, working with the staff, decided to implement a paradoxical model.

1. They defined the problem: *Even though bowel and bladder training is ongoing, clients require frequent bed baths, linen changes, and large amounts of clean linen.*

2. They listed possible solutions:
   a. *Place clients in paper diapers, use paper towels to clean up after incontinence, and change bed linen but once a week.*
   b. *Install a washing machine and dryer on the unit and ask the staff to wash the linen if it becomes soiled.*
   c. *Give fewer baths and only minimum cleansing after incontinence.*
   d. *Place client in bath chairs and wash them thoroughly in the shower.*

3. They defined realistic change: *Linen usage will drop 10%.*

4. They created an innovative solution: *Remodel the bathroom into a shower room with a hand-held spray unit, purchase shower chairs with wheels, and give inservice education to staff on how to use the new equipment.*

The nurse manager presented the idea to the hospital administrator, who convinced the board of trustees to authorize the construction project.

Three months after the new system was instituted, there was a 15% reduction in laundry use, fewer decubitus ulcers, greater mobility of clients, and higher staff morale. Although the solution required the initial expense of remodeling the bathroom and purchasing shower chairs, the cost was soon recovered in savings. Client welfare and staff morale improved markedly.

Normative (Natural) Models

Normative models of planned change are more holistic than rational ones. They take into account the nature of the change, the change agent, and the target system. They recognize the effects of feelings, needs, attitudes, and values on the people who are to change. Two classic normative models are those of Lewin and Havelock-Lippitt.

Lewin Model Lewin (1951) identifies three phases that occur in all change: unfreezing, changing, and refreezing. He recommends that the process of planned change begin with a thorough analysis of the target system and its environment to identify forces for and against

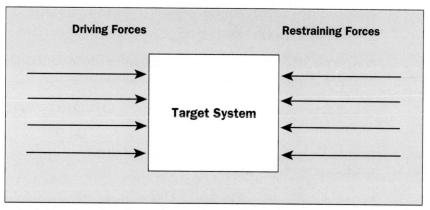

Figure 9-1 Force field analysis: forces for and against change in a target system.

change. Those that push the system toward change he calls driving forces; those that pull the system away from change he calls restraining forces. See Figure 9-1.

Unfreezing. Once the driving and restraining forces are known, Lewin recommends three tactics to unfreeze, or destabilize the system to get it moving in the direction of change. He describes these tactics as disconfirmation, inducing guilt and anxiety, and providing psychologic safety. Disconfirmation is confronting the target system with conflicting evidence so that people will feel uncomfortable or dissatisfied with its present condition and will want to change. Disconfirmation may consist of information or experience that challenges the present condition. Inducing guilt and anxiety is accomplished by showing that important goals or values are not being met or upheld. This is done to upset the balance between driving and restraining forces and raise the level of tension within the system. Psychologic safety is given to help people feel comfortable enough to reduce their defensiveness and attempt to change.

Changing. Once the system is unfrozen and moving toward change, the change agent begins putting the planned change into effect. At this point in the process, Tappen (1989) suggests that the change agent:

1. Introduce information needed to implement changed behavior,

2. Encourage new behavior and allow practice and experimentation with changed behavior,

3. Continue supportive climate to reduce defensive behavior and resistance,

4. Provide opportunities to ventilate feelings of frustration and anxiety regarding the change,

5. Provide feedback on progress and clarify goals to reinforce change and keep up momentum,

6. Encourage trust, keep communication open, and support the driving forces,

7. Continue to use disconfirmation, guilt, and anxiety to overcome resistance,

8. Be enthusiastic, keeping interest high and the change process moving forward.

Refreezing. The purpose of refreezing is to stabilize the system and integrate the change so that it becomes a part of the regular functioning of the system. During this phase the change agent continues to guide the process, acts as an energizer to continue the process, and delegates an increasing amount of responsibility to others in the system.

Application of the Lewin Model

Administrators of a state psychiatric hospital were smarting from media criticism. Client violence had caused many serious injuries to staff nurses and other clients. Administration appointed a panel of experts to study the problem. The panel recommended that clients be assigned to nursing units on the basis of aggressive behavior, diagnosis, and age. These assignment criteria would replace the regional ones that had been in place for 20 years whereby clients were assigned to hospital units according to their home geographic area. Administrators decided to make the change.

Unfreezing. *Unfreezing began by analyzing the system to identify driving forces that would facilitate the change and restraining forces that would work against change as shown in Figure 9-2. To unfreeze the system the change agents (administrators) used disconfirmation by citing comparative safety records of other psychiatric hospitals, guilt and anxiety by citing recent deaths and serious injury to clients and staff members, and psychologic safety by encouraging staff participation. Administration announced the plan for reassignment of clients. It was to be implemented gradually. To begin the process staff members were asked to sort clients by 12 categories, including age, aggressive behavior, and level of functioning.*

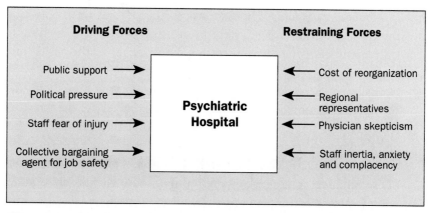

Figure 9-2 Forces for and against change in a psychiatric hospital.

Changing. *The change took more than 2 years. Before, during, and after, the administrators and staff exchanged information by written memos and group discussions. During these meetings staff had the opportunity to voice their concerns. Administrators clarified goals and kept the momentum going. To reduce anxiety, a calendar for each move was published in advance so that clients and staff members knew when and where they were going. Administrators visited the nursing units to encourage and keep the process moving.*

Refreezing. *Refreezing took many months. After the initial large-scale moves of clients and staff, administrators delegated more and more of the process to unit managers. They instituted an impartial priority system for transfer of personnel from unit to unit. The system gradually stabilized as it integrated the change into its regular operations. Although resistance to change was substantial at first, with time the staff saw the benefits of the change, adjusted to their new assignments, and accepted the change. The incidence of staff and client injury dropped significantly.*

Havelock-Lippitt Model The change process described by Havelock (1973) and Lippitt (1973) focuses on how the leader brings about change using a democratic style of leadership. In fact, the term *change agent* came from this model. It assumes a good working relationship between the leader and target system. The six steps in this model are (1) build a relationship, (2) diagnose the problem, (3) assess resources, (4) set goals and select strategies, (5) implement the change, and (6) stabilize, consolidate, and reinforce the change.

Build a relationship. The first task of the change agent is to gain the respect of the target system by relating personally, listening to staff members, and demonstrating knowledge, enthusiasm, and leadership.

Diagnose the problem. The next step is to identify a problem that the target system considers important and needing change. The change agent acts as an energizer, promoting trust and encouraging and guiding movement toward a consensus about the problem.

Assess resources. The third step is to assess available resources. These include motivation, commitment, knowledge, skill, time, energy, power for implementation, financial backing, social norms, roles, and values that support the change.

Set goals and select strategies. After diagnosing the problem and assessing available resources, the group sets goals and specific objectives. Group members in the target system are actively involved just as they were in the second and third steps. The leader acts as guide, supporter, resource person, and energizer.

Implement planned change. Implementation of planned change is greatly facilitated by beginning at a *leverage point,* which is a person or group that is most likely to be receptive to change. Instituting the change at the leverage point minimizes resistance, making change more likely.

Stabilize, consolidate, and reinforce. In the final step, the change agent works to stabilize the system, consolidate, and reinforce the changes. The leader continues to give participants feedback and to support the change.

Application of the Havelock-Lippitt Model

A new nurse administrator was hired by the trustees of a 35-bed hospital in a small town. She had excellent credentials and a reputation for effective leadership, but the staff was skeptical. Soon after arriving, the new administrator set up individual and group meetings with the nurses to learn about their problems. Her openness, honesty, evident knowledge, and concern gained their confidence. However, she found so many problems that she had to decide where to begin. A poll of the staff indicated that the most vexing problem was the haphazard performance-evaluation process for determining salaries and promotion.

The next step was to assess available resources. The nursing administrator gained the support of the hospital administrator. She gathered samples of evaluation methods from other hospitals and the American Nurses Association. Staff members offered their time and effort. The nurse administrator identified the shift lead nurses as the leverage point, because they were the ones most dissatisfied with the old process. Therefore, she asked these nurses to serve on a coordinating committee. At their first meeting, the committee defined its goal and strategies. The goal was to develop performance-evaluation criteria for each staff position and a fair, comprehensive process for retention and promotions. When completed, the process would be presented to the trustees for approval and then implemented. The nurse administrator gave ongoing encouragement and support. When the project was completed and approved, the nurse administrator implemented the new evaluation process.

Coercive Model

The coercive model is an authoritarian approach to change that assumes resistance will be substantial. It is used when more democratic, participatory approaches have failed or are expected to fail. This model recognizes human needs, values, feelings, and attitudes but does not bow to them. Those who use this approach enter a win-lose situation in which they must have enough power to overcome all resistance. The change agent assesses the target system, decides on the change to be made, plans the sequence of steps for its implementation, and selects strategies for overcoming resistance.

Application of the Coercive Model

Several nurses complained to the nurse administrator that many of their peers arrived late to work and took many breaks and long lunch periods. The concerned nurses said such behavior placed an unfair burden on those who were punctual. Furthermore, they said such behavior was unethical and violated their employment contract. The administrator checked the employment contract. Indeed, such behavior was a clear violation of the nurses' contract. She decided to monitor the situation for a week and see if the complaints were true. She found they were.

The nurse administrator decided to use a coercive approach to change. She sent a notice to all units reminding nurses that they had agreed to report to work on time and to take two 10-minute breaks and one 30-minute lunch period. If consistent tardiness or excessive break-taking continued, a time-clock would be installed, pay would be docked for missed time, and attendance records would become an item in performance evaluations.

Change occurred immediately. The nurses began arriving for work on time and limiting the number and length of breaks in accordance with their contractual agreement. The hospital had the ethical responsibility and legal power to overcome resistance and to enforce the change.

◆ Power

Power is an uncomfortable concepts for nurses, perhaps because they see power as the opposite of caring, or because they view themselves as powerless. Nonetheless, if nurses are going to influence the delivery of health care and advance their role as health care providers, they must learn the meaning, characteristics, types, and uses of power and must understand its role in effecting change.

Definitions of Power

Power is defined as the ability to influence behavior. Morrison defines power as the "force or energy required to accomplish a task, meet a goal, promote changes, or influence others" (1993, p. 104). She believes that nurses must clearly understand and value power before they can exert their collective efforts toward acquiring and increasing power, both individually and as a group. Hendricks (1992) says "power is a positive force for creative change and is a central issue in nursing's struggle to define itself," and Stevens (1979) says that "power is the capacity to modify the conduct of others in a desired manner, while avoiding having one's own conduct modified in undesired ways."

Characteristics of Power

Power, like change, is a neutral concept, neither good nor bad in itself. When it is used constructively to reach a useful, productive, and benevolent goal, we think of it as good. When it is used to enslave, destroy, or harm others, we think of it as bad. Lord Action's famous remark, "Power tends to corrupt, and absolute power corrupts absolutely" speaks to the misuse of power associated with authoritarian control and dictatorial rule. When people take control of their lives and assume responsibility for their destiny, we say they are "empowered." Empowerment is an important goal for nurses, individually and collectively. Wynd (1985) believes that "the effective use of power is associated with a high degree of responsibility, accountability, the ability to form alliances and procure resources, and the courage to take action, often in a competitive mode, in the face of obstacles and outside power." Schlomann (1993) says that "empowerment strategies, rather than stress-reduction exercises, are more appropriate for dealing constructively with burnout/exploitation."

Power is reciprocal. When one person assumes control, another gives it up. Power cannot be taken without the permission or coercion of the one who surrenders it. People relinquish power to meet a basic need or to follow a strong belief. In 1993, in Waco Texas, more than 75 people relinquished control of their lives to a religious leader named David Koresh and died with him in a fire that consumed their communal fortress. It is important to remember that the possession of power is fleeting, never permanent, always subject to challenge by those who want to seize it for themselves.

Types of Power

Power has been typified as personal, shared, political, and collective. Personal power is defined as "the drive within a person to overcome both internal and external resistance to reaching one's goals...not a desire to exercise control over others, but to have control within oneself.... [It is] the energy and means to use what is needed to reach the 'pot of gold,' a way of living, not a way of responding" (Hamilton & Kiefer 1986). Personal power develops as a result of life experiences, values, and how people view their place in the world.

Shared power has been described as team power. As applied to leadership, Kelly (1992) says that shared power places an emphasis on interdependence in relationships and human interaction as a source of power and differs from the personal power seen in a male style of leadership, which is direct, aggressive, and competitive. Research indicates that women tend to prefer shared power more than personal power (Gorman & Clark 1986). This preference may occur because women are socialized to be more concerned than men about human connectedness (Gilligan & Attanucci 1988).

Political power is associated with governmental control of people, using the prestige of office and the coercive power of the state. In a broad sense, political power is a type of shared power. In a democracy the citizens have some control over the laws that govern them. Even so, they often feel powerless because changing laws and influencing those who interpret them is difficult and expensive.

Collective power is the power of numbers, uniting their collective energy to achieve a goal. When a professional group exercises such power, it is called *professional power*. Hamilton & Kiefer (1986) say that nurses' professional power is "the ability of nurses to reach goals with patients, function autonomously, and effect change within a work setting, such as knowing how to work within the system...to reach goals." Nurses exercise professional power in many ways, by demonstrating expert skill and knowledge, participating in quality-assurance activities, and working through official nursing organizations to advance the profession.

Sources of Power

The ability to exercise power by influencing the behavior of others is derived from a number of sources. Some are more available and ethically acceptable to nurses than others. Recognizing these sources is the first step toward developing power strategies. They include informational, legitimate, associative, reward, coercive, collective, and charismatic.

Informational power (expert knowledge) comes from a perception of an ability to access, withhold, or possess key information, exceptional talent, skill, or expertise. Such people as researchers, clinical specialists, and "old hands" (experienced nurses) possess informational power.

Legitimate power (positional) derives from a formal position or title in an organization that gives the holder authority to make decisions. It is possessed by such persons as nursing administrators, faculty members, and nursing school deans.

Associative power arises from a perception that people connected with powerful or renowned people also have power. Those with associative power include alumni of great universities and friends, relatives, and employees of the rich and famous.

Reward power comes from a perception of an ability to bestow rewards or favors on others such as promotions, grades, money, and days off. It is possessed by such persons as instructors, scheduling clerks, and performance evaluators.

Coercive power (legal, physical, financial) arises from a perception of an ability to punish, threaten, or withhold rewards. It is possessed by such persons as nursing instructors, officers of the law, and nurse administrators.

Collective power arises from the sheer weight of numbers of people, as found in groups such as the American Medical Association and American Nurses Association.

Charismatic power (referent, personal) arises from a personal sense of self and an ability to communicate personal attributes so that others admire, identify with, and are motivated to follow the person. "Natural" leaders, respected teachers, and role models often possess charismatic power.

Uses of Power

Power is a neutral concept of control, neither good nor bad in itself. It is the use of power that is constructive or destructive. Nurses use power in relation to the self, and their peers, subordinates, and superiors.

With the Self

To use power for yourself you must take control of your life. The first step is to become self-aware, "to know thyself," as Socrates advised. You need to assess your physical, emotional, and intellectual capacities, values, beliefs, talents, limitations, prejudices, aspirations, and needs. With such knowledge you can then identify your large general goals. Then, for each of the goals, list specific, attainable objectives to achieve in a given period of time. Here are some strategies to help you achieve your objectives:

- "Package" yourself to fit your objectives. If you want to be considered for promotion to an administrative position, dress with impeccable care; look like an executive. If you want to be a university professor, earn higher academic degrees. If you want more friends, be friendly.

- Be adaptable and flexible, temporarily altering your course, if necessary, to reach long-range goals. As a new graduate you may have to work in a skilled nursing facility before you can work in home health care.

- Practice assertive communication. With courtesy and sincerity, (1) say what you see, objectively; (2) say how you feel, honestly; (3) listen to the other person, attentively; (4) say what you want, clearly. Such behavior is healthy and empowering.

With Peers

To use power with peers you must demonstrate respect, collegiality, kindness, accountability, and professionalism. Too often interpersonal power is destructive rather than constructive. It is mean-spirited and seeks to destroy rather than build. When nurses feel powerless, they are more likely to be critical, competitive, and cruel. If a colleague makes an error they quickly rush to report it, magnify the significance of the error, and dissociate themselves from the one who made it. Such lack of charity often arises in institutions where a top-down leadership prevails. The classic research of Lewin et al (1939) on styles of leadership shows that in authoritarian-led groups, members are more competitive and hostile and less creative than in democratic-led groups. Nurses do not need to remain victims of such systems. Using interpersonal power they can behave differently. Using shared power they can change the work environment to one that fosters collegiality.

With Subordinates

The constructive use of power with subordinates involves accepting responsibility, communicating clearly, and encouraging feedback. It includes assessing subordinates accurately, matching assignments with abilities, delegating duties appropriately and fairly, giving compliments and reproofs sincerely and without favoritism, and explaining rationales for decisions. In short, the constructive use of power with subordinates means treating others as you would like to be treated yourself.

With Superiors

You can use power with superiors by demonstrating professional competence, using assertive communication, and being flexible and willing to compromise. Even when nurses behave in these ways, problems may arise. If so, nurses need to remember that a group is more powerful than an individual. Professional organizations offer expert advice on the use of collective power to effect change.

With the Public

The media has not been kind to nursing. It has portrayed nurses as sex-craved, incompetent servants with time to gossip and flirt. Too often sensational stories of rare criminal acts by nurses get front-page coverage while autonomous, noble acts are ignored. Nurses can change this state of affairs and use power with the public. They can (1) support health and human welfare legislation; (2) submit stories of courage, achievement, and independence to the media; (3) communicate their objections to demeaning roles in media productions and argue for roles that portray nurse as independent professionals with moral principles and rewarding personal lives; (4) maintain high standards of professional competence; (5) deliver sensitive nursing care to clients.

◇ Politics

Politics is the science or art of government. It is the business of conducting the affairs of state, setting public policy, and implementing laws that affect the lives of citizens. In a democratic system of government, every citizen has political responsibilities because the government is of and by the people.

Political Action

Political action means getting involved in the process of change. Such involvement is most effective when nurses use what Vance (1985) calls the three C's of political action:

- *Communication* that is assertive, clear, and concise

- *Collectivity,* a source of power and the foundation for networking, coalition-building, and collaboration

- *Collegiality,* a sense of community, sisterhood, and camaraderie, the foundation for building esteem and trust and supporting and nurturing associates

Nurses can use communication, collectivity, and collegiality to take political action. To do so they must become informed, vote, communicate with elected representatives, and contribute time, money, and effort.

Become Informed

Listen to daily news and in-depth reports of public radio and television stations. Read news magazines and news sections of professional journals. Seek out special reports of such nonpartisan groups as the League

How a Bill Becomes a Law

Formation of idea	By the President, members of Congress, or citizen group for a new law.
Writing the idea into legal form	By legislative attorneys.
Sponsorship by members of House or Senate	Up to 25 Representatives and any number of Senators may cosponsor a bill; taxation bills originate in the House.
Introduction of bill; assignment of number; first reading	Sponsor introduces bill by handing it to the clerk or placing it in a box called a hopper; clerk gives bill a number and reads title into the *Congressional Record*, called the *first reading*.
Assignment to committee for study	Speaker of House and Vice-President of Senate assign the bill to appropriate committee.
Study by committee	Committee hears testimony from experts and interested persons; they can revise, pass, report out, or table the bill.
Placement on calendar	In House, the Rules Committee can delay action, limit debate, limit and prohibit amendments; in Senate, bills are usually scheduled in order; leader of majority party may push bills ahead.
Consideration by full House	In House, at *second reading*, entire bill is read; *third reading* is by title only after amendments have been added and before final vote; most bills pass by simple majority (one more than half the number of votes); then bill goes to Senate.

➤

of Women Voters and Common Cause, or partisan groups such as the Republican and Democratic Party. As a member of American Nurses Association (ANA), subscribe to *Capital Update,* a legislative newsletter published by the ANA. Learn the names and addresses of your elected representatives by calling a public library or local newspaper. Learn how a bill becomes law (see the accompanying box). Obtain copies of proposed state laws by asking for them by number from state printing offices. Obtain proposed federal laws from US Senate Documents

Consideration by full Senate	In Senate, debate can last indefinitely unless there is an agreement to limit debate; when the debate ends, vote is taken; most bills require a simple majority to pass; if bill passes it goes to Conference Committee.
Conferencing	Conference Committee is made up of members of both houses. They work out differences between House and Senate versions of the bill; revised bill is sent back to both houses for final vote.
Printing of bill	Bill is printed by Government Printing Office, a process called *enrolling*.
Signing of bill	Speaker of House and Vice-President sign enrolled bill, now called an *Act of Congress*.
Consideration by President	President can sign or veto an act, or by waiting 10 days, excluding Sunday, can allow act to become law without signature; if Congress adjourns before 10 days are up, act dies; this is called a *pocket veto*.
Reconsideration by Congress of vetoed bill	A two-thirds majority vote of both houses of Congress *overrides* a presidential veto; act, also called bill, becomes law.
Becoming a law	When an act becomes a law it is given a number, indicating the number of the Congress that passed it; a new Congress forms every 2 years after the election; for example, a law enacted by the 96th Congress might be designated 96-146.

Office, Washington, DC 20510 or Doorkeeper of the House of Representatives, US Capitol, Washington, DC 20515.

Vote

The most fundamental political action citizens can take is to vote. Nurses may feel they are too poor to contribute money, too busy to work for candidates, or too involved to serve on boards and committees. However, nurses everywhere can be informed and vote.

Communicate with Representatives

Elected officials represent the people of their district or state. They seek input from, pay attention to, and vote in accordance with the wishes of their constituents. The people who make their opinions known influence the outcome of issues. Address your letters to:

US Representatives: Honorable _____,
House Office Building, Washington, DC 20515.

US Senators: Senator _____,
Senate Office Building, Washington, DC 20510.

When you write to elected officials, *do*:

- Identify the issue or the bill by number.

- Time your letter or telegram to arrive before a vote.

- Be brief and to the point. "Please vote no on Bill # _____."

- Give your reasons; state how the bill affects people. "Because…"

- Be constructive; offer an alternative approach if you can.

- Give praise when it is due.

- State your own views, in your own words, on your own stationery. (Form letters and petitions are less effective.)

When you write to elected officials, *do not*:

- Threaten, berate, or demean.

- Send long, rambling essays.

Contribute Time, Money, and Effort

Political action takes time, money, and effort. Besides telephoning, writing letters, and sending telegrams, nurses can work on the campaigns of candidates and referendums, testify at public hearings, contribute money, serve on voluntary boards and commissions, seek appointment to positions of authority that will influence health policy and practice, and run for public office. By doing so, nurses provide pertinent facts, represent the viewpoint of nursing, and increase its prestige and viability.

Political Focus

In the Community

Nurses can become politically active in their communities in count-less ways, from serving on school lunch committees to becoming mayors of cities. Because they are articulate, intelligent, highly moti-vated, and energetic people, nurses are natural leaders. They can pur-sue their interests and make a difference in every area of life: in health care facilities and prisons; in the area of infant and aged care, highway safety, and air quality; in self-help groups and food distribu-tion centers. Wherever there are people, nurses can apply their knowledge of power and politics and work for a more humane and healthful society.

In Professional Organizations

Professional nursing organizations are devoted to advancing the pro-fession and influencing health care. They exercise collective power by presenting a united voice for nursing. Individual nurses can partic-ipate in the activities of these groups in numerous ways at many lev-els. Professional organizations influence the delivery of health care by serving in advisory capacities to governmental agencies and by sup-porting public and private initiatives. Political action committees (PACs) are agencies devoted to advancing the interests of groups. Because not-for-profit organizations such as the ANA are prohibited by law from engaging in political action, they use PACs to carry out their agendas.

In the Workplace

Nursing is hard work. It requires enormous amounts of energy. Not much is left over for political action in the workplace. However, if nurses leave decisions about client care to others, others will make the decisions. If nurses are to exert power, they must become involved. By applying the interpersonal skills of political action (com-munication, collectivity, collegiality), nurses can effect change in the workplace. Here are some specific strategies:

- Volunteer to be a member of standing committees that make pol-icy recommendations.

- Use both the formal and informal information network of your agency to influence others. Many health care providers have an in-house newsletter or official communication system. All agencies have an informal communication network. Remember, people who control information hold power.

- Use employee representatives if the agency has a collective-bargaining organization.

- Pursue endeavors that earn respect and recognition, such as research and nursing excellence.

- Seek positions of authority. By serving in administrative positions, nurses gain the power to make decisions and to access others who hold power.

Political Strategies

While *politics* is the art or science of government, *political strategies* are tactics people use to influence governmental decisions. With energy and commitment, nurses can effect change by using the strategies listed in the box on page 287.

Restrictions on Political Activities

In an effort to prevent unfair political influence, the US Congress passed the Hatch Act in the 1930s. It prohibits employees of tax-supported agencies from engaging in activities on the behalf of a political party or in support of legislation that could be construed as support from a government agency. The act does not interfere with the right of private citizens to support parties, candidates, or ballot measures. However, employees must be careful to speak and act *only* as private citizens, *not* as agency representatives. Because many states have their own versions of the Hatch Act, nurses should learn about restrictions in their state.

Women, Power, and Politics

In our culture, power and politics are associated with masculinity. Until recently, women have been socialized to be noncompetitive, meek, compliant, passive, and subservient and to shun power. In this view, authority and power are the birthright of men; compliance, the lot of women. In fact, in most world cultures today, men are the rulers and spiritual leaders. In general, women take over the reins of government only when family inheritance outweighs sexual bias, and efforts to produce a male heir fail. Small changes are being made,

Eighteen Strategies For Political Action

1. Develop a sense of self and the ability to communicate effectively.

2. Seek positions that give you authority to grant rewards and mete out punishment.

3. Become an expert in an area of interest, earn degrees, and gain special skills.

4. Form coalitions with powerful persons of like mind.

5. Avoid people with sullied reputations.

6. Control information, either by giving or withholding it.

7. Do your homework; learn all you can about an issue you wish to change.

8. Be ready to move on issues; "strike while the iron is hot."

9. Compromise, if necessary; "half a loaf is better than none."

10. Display confidence; "nothing ventured, nothing gained."

11. Be prepared to give something in return, "qid pro quo."

12. Be patient; "Rome was not built in a day."

13. Watch for any change or weakening of position; "get your foot in the door."

14. Become sensitive to hidden agendas; "read between the lines."

15. Refrain from commitments that limit maneuverability or influence.

16. Try to understand another position; "walk a mile in the other person's moccasins."

17. Don't be discouraged by setbacks; "look at the big picture."

18. Gain collective power by joining the American Nurses Association and other nursing groups.

but women have a long way to go before they gain a significant share of the positions of power.

Because 88% of nurses in the United States are women (NLN DataSource 1993), it is no surprise that nurses have difficulty assuming power or using power in the political arena. Many women nurses feel angry and sad but powerless to change the system. Many nurses still think of power as antifeminine, inappropriate, and unprofessional. They view powerful nurses with suspicion and fear. This point of view is self-defeating and demeaning. Nurses have superior intellects and organizational abilities. Moreover, they are nurturers and caregivers, committed to high ethical standards. What better group is there to lead the nation in areas of public policy and action? Nurses need not shun power but embrace it. They need to apply their knowledge of power and politics to their personal, professional, and public lives to bring about constructive change.

◆ Summary

A working knowledge of the concepts of change, power, and politics can help nurses make a difference in government, the community, their professional organizations, workplaces, and personal lives. Change is a process for altering a system. It can be haphazard or planned. To institute planned change, change agents use rational, paradoxical, normative, and coercive models. Power is the ability to influence behavior. Neither good nor bad, power may be personal, shared, political, or professional. Its sources are informational, legitimate, associative, reward, coercive, collective, and referent power. Power can be used with the self, peers, subordinates, superiors, and the public to bring about change. To do so, nurses must use political action and apply political strategies in every area of their lives.

Critical Thinking Questions

1. What evidence can you give to support the claim that "change is neither good nor bad?"

2. Evaluate this argument: "Because 88% of nurses are women, it is not surprising that nurses have difficulty assuming political power."

   A. What is the factual information in the argument? What sources could you use to check the accuracy of the facts?

B. What is an unstated assumption in the argument?

C. Is the argument adequately supported by facts of evidence? If not, what other evidence would you need to make that claim with confidence?

3. Some people believe that nurses should focus less on acquiring autonomy and power, and more on caring and collaboration. What do you think? Why?

Learning Activities

1. Identify a specific change that is needed in your nursing school. Select a model for planned change that you believe will be effective. Outline a plan for change, including a timeline.

2. Explain the steps of the Lewin and Havelock-Lippitt models for planned change to a group of nurses; give an example of each model.

3. Write a brief sketch of someone who possesses each of the following sources of power: informational, legitimate, associative, reward, coercive, and referent power.

4. Give a 5-minute talk entitled, "Women, Power, and Politics."

5. Assign one or more political strategies to each of a group of students. Ask each group to state when the strategy might be appropriate, giving an example.

6. Attend a community health planning meeting; assess the political strategies being used.

7. Write to the US House or Senate printing office for a specific health-related bill.

8. Write a draft letter to a member of Congress about a current concern. Critique the letter for clarity, brevity, and appropriateness.

Annotated Reading List

Costello-Nickitas DM. Legislative Update, Making a Case for Nursing: Earning a Seat at the Policy Table. *Revolution: The Journal of Nurse Empowerment.* Winter 1993, p. 58.

This powerful article tells how nurses can make sure nursing is present at the policy table as decisions about health care are made. The author says it is time for "action-packed politics" and discusses six specific actions nurses can take to have their voices heard, to take "the system back by getting involved in policy change and development."

Wheeler CE, Chinn PL. *Peace and Power: A Handbook of Feminist Process,* 3d ed. National League for Nursing, 1991.

This book, selected by the *American Journal of Nursing* as book of the year, focuses on a consensus-building approach to group interactions. It integrates the essence of feminist theory with practical suggestions to help individuals and groups develop principles of unity, share leadership skills, encourage participation, and transform conflicts into growth-enhancing experiences.

References

Bennis WG, Benne KD, Chin R, Corey KE. *The Planning of Change,* 3rd ed. Holt, Rinehart, and Winston, 1976.

Brooten DA, Hayman L, Naylor M. *Leadership for Change: A Guide for the Frustrated Nurse.* Lippincott, 1988.

Duncan WJ. *Essentials of Management,* 2nd ed. Dryden Press, 1978.

Gilligan C, Attanucci J. Two Moral Orientations. In Gilligan C, Ward JV, Taylor JM, eds.: *Mapping the Moral Domain.* Harvard University Press, 1988.

Gorman S, Clark N. Power and Effective Nursing Practice. *Nursing Outlook* May/June 1986, p 129.

Hamilton JM, Kiefer ME. *Survival Skills for the New Nurse.* Lippincott, 1986.

Havelock RG. *The Change Agent's Guide to Innovation in Education.* Educational Technology Publications, 1973.

Hendricks D. The Power Problem. *Nursing Management* Oct 1992.

Kelly LY. *The Nursing Experience: Trends, Challenges, and Transitions.* Macmillan, 1992.

Lewin K. *Field Theory in Social Science: Selected Theoretical Papers.* Harper and Row, 1951.

Lewin K, Lippitt R, White RK. Patterns of aggressive behavior in experimentally created "social climates." *Journal of Social Psychology* 1939; 10:271–299.

Lippitt GL. *Visualizing Change: Model Building and the Change Process.* La Jolla, CA: University Associates, 1973.

Morrison M. *Professional Skills for Leadership: Foundations of a Successful Career.* Mosby, 1993.

NLN Nursing DataSource, Publ. #19-2526. National League for Nursing, 1993.

Perlman D, Takacs GJ. The Ten Stages of Change. *Nursing Management* 1990; 21(4):33–38.

Rogers EM, Shoemaker FF. *Communication of Innovation,* 2nd ed. Free Press, 1971.

Sampson E. *Social Psychology and Contemporary Society.* Wiley, 1971.

Schlomann P. Burnout or Exploitation. *Revolution: The Journal of Nurse Empowerment.* Winter 1993.

Stevens B. Effecting Change. *Journal of Nursing Administration.* 1975; 5:23–25.

Stevens B. Power and Politics for the Nurse Executive. *Nursing Health Care* Nov 1979; 1:208.

Tappen RM. *Nursing Leadership and Management: Concepts and Practice,* 2nd ed. Davis, 1989.

Vance C. Political Influence: Building Effective Interpersonal Skills. In Mason DJ, Talbott SW, eds.: *Political Action Handbook for Nurses.* Addison-Wesley, 1985.

Watzlawick P, Weakland J, Fisch R. *Change: Principles of Problem Formation and Problem Resolution.* Norton, 1974.

Wynd C. Packing a Punch: Female Nurses and the Effective Use of Power. *Nursing Success Today* Sept 1985; 2:15–20.

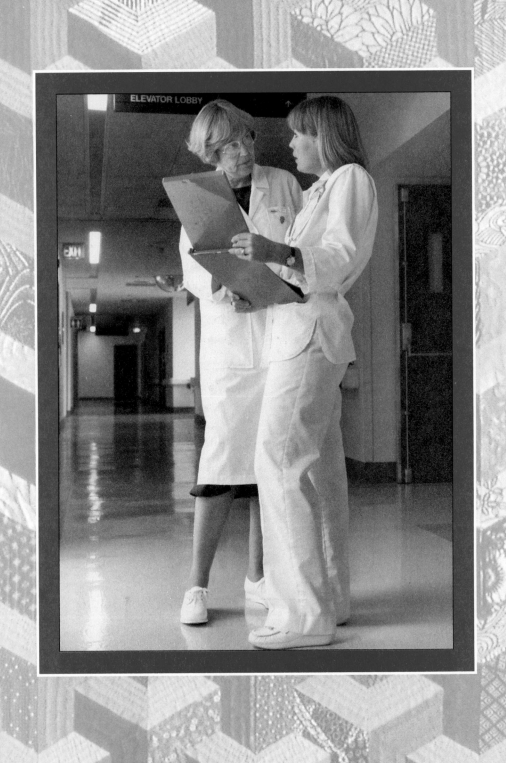

Managing Nursing Care

10

◆ Learning Objectives

- Apply general systems theory to a health care agency.

- Compare a manager to a leader.

- Describe the steps of the management process.

- Describe the four phases of the budgetary process.

- Identify measures to manage time effectively.

- Compare bureaucratic structures with adaptive structures.

- Describe the staffing process, from analysis of the work to scheduling people to do it.

- Discuss communication, teaching, motivation, conflict resolution, and morale building relative to nurse management.

- Explain how accountability relates to the components of controlling.

- Compare risk management with quality assurance.

- Discuss the purposes and process of performance evaluations.

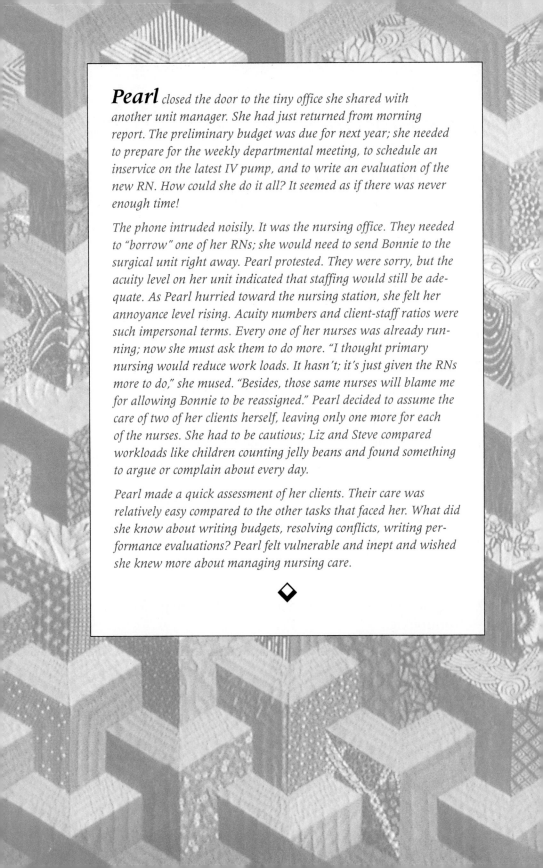

Pearl closed the door to the tiny office she shared with another unit manager. She had just returned from morning report. The preliminary budget was due for next year; she needed to prepare for the weekly departmental meeting, to schedule an inservice on the latest IV pump, and to write an evaluation of the new RN. How could she do it all? It seemed as if there was never enough time!

The phone intruded noisily. It was the nursing office. They needed to "borrow" one of her RNs; she would need to send Bonnie to the surgical unit right away. Pearl protested. They were sorry, but the acuity level on her unit indicated that staffing would still be adequate. As Pearl hurried toward the nursing station, she felt her annoyance level rising. Acuity numbers and client-staff ratios were such impersonal terms. Every one of her nurses was already running; now she must ask them to do more. "I thought primary nursing would reduce work loads. It hasn't; it's just given the RNs more to do," she mused. "Besides, those same nurses will blame me for allowing Bonnie to be reassigned." Pearl decided to assume the care of two of her clients herself, leaving only one more for each of the nurses. She had to be cautious; Liz and Steve compared workloads like children counting jelly beans and found something to argue or complain about every day.

Pearl made a quick assessment of her clients. Their care was relatively easy compared to the other tasks that faced her. What did she know about writing budgets, resolving conflicts, writing performance evaluations? Pearl felt vulnerable and inept and wished she knew more about managing nursing care.

◆

Although nurses use management skills from the first day they care for clients, they also need to understand the management process as well as some important management concepts. These concepts include systems theory, management theories, leadership, decision making, problem solving, and technological competence.

◇ Management Concepts

Systems Theory

Systems thinking is especially useful for nurse managers. A general systems view of the world was proposed by von Bertalanffy (1968) as a way of viewing various entities, including social structures. Von Bertalanffy defines a *system* as an organized whole unit that produces an effect or a product whose interdependent component parts interact with the environment. Systems are classified according to their relationship to the environment (open or closed), position in relation to other systems (suprasystems, focal systems, or subsystems), and the nature of their component parts (animal, vegetable, mineral).

Closed systems are those in which there is no input or output of energy, therefore, no change in component parts, no renewal, and no life. A closed system represents the end result of a process where the components reach an inactive steady state. *Open systems* are those in which there is an exchange of energy, materials, and information with the environment. They are characterized by

- Uniqueness formed when separate parts come together
- Internal organization with boundaries between the system and environment
- Input of energy into the system
- Throughput during which the system processes, changes, and reorganizes imported energy
- Output of energy into the environment in the form of goods, services, and intellectual products
- Feedback by which a part of the output returns to the system, creating change (positive) or maintaining a steady state (negative)
- Interrelatedness of component parts, so that a change in any part affects the whole

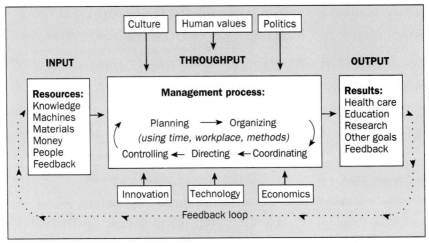

Figure 10-1 The management process within a system.

- Dynamic equilibrium, as in homeostasis

- Continual renewal

- A cyclical pattern with continual input, throughput, output, and feedback.

When we view a health care agency as a system, with *input* (people, knowledge, equipment, money, and feedback) and *output* (health care, education, research, and feedback), we see that *throughput* is the working core of the system, the place where the management process takes place. See Figure 10-1.

Management

Management is the process of coordinating input resources of a system to achieve goals and generate services and products. The *management process* transforms the goals of an organization into tangible objectives, using materials and human resources. It does this within ethical, physical, cultural, and legal constraints in accordance with the philosophy and policies of the agency. The process is divided into five functions or operations: planning, organizing, coordinating, directing, and controlling.

Planning includes these steps: (1) identifying the goals and objectives of the organization in accordance with its purpose and philosophy, (2) selecting work that will accomplish the goals and objectives, (3) creating policies and procedures, (4) formulating an operating budget of time and materials, (5) solving problems, and (6) modifying the plan in response to evaluation (control) results.

Organizing includes these steps: (1) creating an organizational and work-unit structure, (2) clarifying the values and norms of this structure, (3) writing the policies and procedures in accordance with the values and norms of the institution, (4) writing job descriptions for those who will assume responsibility, and (5) adjusting the structure in response to control results.

Coordinating (staffing) includes the following: (1) recruiting, interviewing, hiring, and scheduling staff, (2) communicating with, developing, and involving staff in problem-solving, and (3) praising, reprimanding, and resolving individual conflicts as necessary.

Directing includes these functions: (1) providing a motivating climate, (2) setting up channels of communication, (3) managing competition and facilitating collaboration, and (4) mediating differences.

Controlling (evaluating) includes: (1) comparing results with plans; (2) identifying ideal behaviors; (3) evaluating processes, product, and workers; (3) acting within legal and ethical boundaries; and (4) taking corrective action as indicated.

Levels of Management

To accomplish its work, many organizations use a hierarchy of top-, middle-, and first-level managers. Top-level managers oversee the total operation of an organization. They establish goals, policies, and strategies; make business arrangements with outside firms; and represent the agency to the community. They report to the owner, board of directors, or electorate, and have titles like chief executive officer, president, vice-president, and administrator. Middle-level managers are responsible for coordinating several units within an organization. They convert broad policies and strategies into specific objectives and programs. Middle managers report to top managers, serve as links between first-level managers and top managers, and have titles such as supervisor, line manager, director, and coordinator. First-level managers are directly responsible for service and the implementation of specific objectives. They report to middle managers, serve as links between staff and middle management, and function as unit managers, case managers, and primary care nurses. In recent years, less hierarchical, "flatter" models of management have emerged that allow for greater autonomy, particularly in organizations with large numbers of professional employees.

Management Theories X, Y, and Z

During the 1920s worker unrest led to the study of worker satisfaction and its relationship to productivity. The most famous of the studies was lead by Elton Mayo at the Hawthorne Works of the Western Electric Company. He discovered that people respond to the fact that they are being studied and increase whatever behavior they feel will encourage continued attention (Mayo 1953). That response, called the *Hawthorne effect*, led McGregor (1960) to theorize that the attitudes of managers about employees directly affect employee satisfaction. He labeled his conceptual profiles theory X and theory Y. *Theory X* managers believe their employees are lazy, desire security above all else, and avoid work unless coerced; therefore, the managers need a rigid hierarchy to manage and control emplyees. *Theory Y* managers believe their employees enjoy their work, are self-motivated, and are willing to work hard to meet both personal and organizational goals. He felt that theories X and Y were two points on a continuum and that most managers had a mixture of assumptions about people. Maslow (1970) corroborated theory Y by proposing that humans have basic needs that they seek to fulfill, including survival, security, belongingness, self-esteem, and self-actualization.

In 1981, Ouchi proposed a Western adaptation of Japanese management, which he called *theory Z*. Theory Z includes decision making by consensus, fitting employees to jobs, slower promotions, evaluation of long-term decisions, job security, and a holistic concern for workers. Marquis and Huston (1994) note that although theory Z was popular in the 1980s, it lost favor because managers found that the "vast differences in Japanese and American societies, values, and culture hindered the successful adaption of this management style in Western companies."

Participative Management

In spite of the disappointing results of theory Z, many agencies have instituted some form of participative management (PM). Called by such names as group decision making, shared governance, and democratic management, PM has three elements: group decision making, decentralization, and management by objectives (Bower 1990). *Group decision making* is the process by which a formal or informal group makes decisions about specific tasks. For example, primary nurses on a unit mutually decide how and when they will give shift reports. *Decentralization* is the empowerment of subordinates by superiors to make decisions. Decentralization can occur at any level in the organization.

Management by objectives (MBO) is a system for setting organizational objectives for a given period, devising plans to implement the objectives, and providing periodic evaluation of progress. Developed in the early 1950s by Peter Drucker, MBO is built on three basic principles: (1) Results are the primary focus of an institution, and effective managers get results. (2) Application of human motivation and behavioral concepts improves productivity. (3) Stating an objective and measuring its achievement produces orderly growth.

MBO has five steps:

1. Set production objectives. The manager sets clear, concise, attainable, measurable objectives that include target dates for achievement.

2. Plan action. The manager devises objectives with specific plans to attain them.

3. Clarify responsibilities. The manager clearly defines and assigns responsibilities, describing what is to be done, in what sequence, how, when, and by whom, with an estimate of needed resources.

4. Develop a control system. The manager makes frequent reviews to assess progress toward an objective with a focus on solving problems and taking corrective action.

5. Evaluate performance. The manager and workers judge performance relative to the stated objectives and use their findings to plan for the next year.

Shared governance is a type of participative management in which managers and staff members make decisions and set rules together, changing management from an oligarchy to a democracy. While executive authority remains with top managers, professional staff function in a legislative role and have a say in the development of practice policies. Shared governance is a model for professional practice. It requires nurses to assume responsibility for the quality of client care in the whole institution, and to "confront, evaluate, and censor those who do not meet standards. Shared governance permits nurses to become truly accountable for practice" (Bower 1990).

Leadership

Leadership is an interpersonal relationship in which a leader uses specific strategies to influence individuals and groups to accomplish a goal. Leadership is a composite of personal traits, abilities, and circumstances. Although there is no absolute list of traits or behaviors that describes leaders, most of them know where they are going and how to get there; exercise courage and persistence even in the face of danger, opposition, or discouragement; instill confidence; communicate well; and possess qualities and competencies admired by their followers. Bennis (1989) suggests four common traits of leaders. They (1) manage meaning (use communication skills), (2) manage attention (demonstrate a mix of vision and strong personal commitment), (3) manage trust (remain constant and build trust in others), and (4) manage self (develop strengths and reject failure). Hollander (1978) says that leadership effectiveness requires the ability to use the problem-solving process, maintain group effectiveness, have good communication skills, develop group identification, and demonstrate fairness, competence, dependability, and creativity. He notes there are three basic elements in the leadership exchange: (1) leaders, with their perceptions and abilities, (2) followers, with their perceptions and abilities, and (3) situations where leaders and followers function.

The thoughtful reader may ask how leadership differs from management or if the two roles are synonymous. Manthey (1990) says that managers guide, direct, and motivate, whereas leaders empower. Burns (1978) says that there are two types of leaders in management—transactional leaders, who are concerned with day-to-day operations, and transformational leaders, who have a vision and inspire others. Bowers (1994) concludes that "managers are operational agents, while leaders are strategic visionaries." All authorities agree that managers and leaders display two related but different sets of behaviors. Undoubtedly, leaders are more effective when they employ management skills and managers are more effective when they exhibit leadership qualities. See Table 10-1.

Decision Making and Problem Solving

Nurses at every level, and especially nurse managers, are called upon to make decisions and solve problems. The two processes are similar but not identical. *Decision making* is a process of selecting from among alternatives that may or may not pose a conflict, for instance, decid-

TABLE 10-1

Comparison of Leaders and Managers

Leaders	Managers
May or may not be officially appointment to the position	Are officially appointed to the position
Have authority from followers to make decisions that affect followers	Have authority from superiors to make decisions that affect subordinates
Inspire followers to achieve goals and accept leader's decision	Direct others to carry out policies, rules, and regulations of organization
Take risks and explore new ideas	Maintain orderly and equitable structure
Relate to people personally in an intuitive and empathic manner	Relate to people according to their roles and functions within the organization
Pursue personal goals and feel rewarded by their achievements	Feel rewarded when fulfilling mission and goals of organization
May or may not be successful managers	May or may not be successful leaders

Adapted from Douglass LM. *The Effective Nurse: Leader and Manager.* 4th ed. Mosby, 1993.

ing between two styles of stethoscopes. *Problem solving* is the process of addressing a situation that diverges from a desired state of affairs. Both decision making and problem solving follow these steps:

1. Define the decision to be made or the problem to be solved; the more precise the definition, the more exact the result.

2. Gather information about the issue to be decided or the problem to be solved.

3. Analyze the information, categorizing it according to importance, time sequence, cause, and effect.

4. Develop criteria for selecting alternative decisions or solutions.

5. Develop alternative decisions or solutions.

6. Identify advantages and disadvantages of each alternative, considering the cost-benefit results.

7. Make a decision or solve the problem.

8. Consult, confer, and communicate the decision or solution.

9. Implement the decision or solve the problem.

10. Evaluate the decision or solution.

Pearl, whose story begins the chapter, needed to make a decision about client care assignments. Even though she may not have understood the process, Pearl gathered data about the clients who needed care, the abilities and personalities of the staff, and her own needs. With this information, she made a decision to assign herself two patients. By the end of the day Pearl may evaluate her decision and conclude that it did not help meet her goals and that she will not repeat it in the future.

Technological Competence

In an effort to cut costs and improve efficiency, hospitals increasingly rely on technology. As managers, nurses must gain and maintain technological competence. Just as they must learn to use new devices for client care, nurses need to keep abreast with new technology for the storage and retrieval of information. Computer programs provide a immense array of assistance to nurses. One such program, *Patient Care Expert System (PACE)*, was developed at the School of Nursing, Creighton University, Omaha, Nebraska. It provides individualized client care, teaching, and discharge plans and meets the standards of the Joint Commission on Accreditation of Healthcare Organizations (JCAHCO). It gives "an entire library of patient problems and nursing information, eliminates the need for time-consuming research, and increases time for actual patient care" (Kuster 1990).

◆ The Management Process

Planning

The management process begins with planning: deciding in advance what to do. All other management functions depend on planning. To plan effectively, nurse managers identify the purpose and philosophy of an agency, clarify goals, identify objectives, review policies and procedures, prepare budgets, and assess resources.

The Purpose of Planning

The first task of planning is to clarify the reason why an organization exists. For most health care institutions, the primary purpose is to provide quality health care for clients. Other purposes may be to teach, to carry on research, to make money for investors, and to make converts to a belief system. Specialty areas within health care agencies have their own functions, but all must subscribe to the institutional purpose. For example, the purpose of a hospital education department may be to orient new staff members and provide up-to-date inservice education. However, the overriding purpose is to provide quality health care.

Philosophy

A philosophy is a statement of beliefs and values on which an institution is built, for example, "We believe that life begins at conception." Because a philosophy serves as an ethical guide for policy decisions, it needs to be written in clear terms, widely published, and reviewed periodically. Some facilities include the philosophy in the packet given to clients when they are admitted.

Goals and Objectives

Goals and objectives are central to the management process. They state what an institution seeks to do to achieve its purpose. *Planning* defines goals, *organizing* provides a way to accomplish them, *coordinating* provides a staff to carry them out, *directing* uses the staff to attain them, and *controlling* evaluates how well the goals were achieved. *Goals* are general statements of intent that may be short-term or long-term. They should be reviewed periodically to be sure they are still accurate. *Objectives* are specific elements of goals. The more precise an objective, the more likely it is that it will be attained. For example, if a goal is to "provide quality client care," an objective may be to "make accurate assessments."

Policies, Procedures, and Methods

Policies, procedures, and methods are ways to attain goals and objectives. *Policies* serve as guides to define the scope of activities and explain how goals will be achieved. They provide a basis for future decisions and actions. Policies may originate inside an institution at any level or they may come from law-making or accrediting bodies outside the agency. *Procedures* are directions for taking specific action. They are more precise than policies and usually affect a department rather than an entire agency. For instance, the procedure for administering drugs by intramuscular injections (IM) describes actions nurses take to administer IM medications. *Methods* are techniques for performing skills, such as the way to hold a syringe, prepare the skin, and insert the needle.

Budgets

A *budget* is a plan for allocating resources, monitoring expenditures, and controlling costs. Budgeting is part of the planning and controlling functions of management. Although budgets are made on an annual basis, they may be subdivided into monthly, quarterly, or semiannual periods. A fiscal year (financial year) is any 12-month budget cycle. When the cycle begins in January, the fiscal year coincides with the calendar year. Long-term budgets prepared by top managers may be for 3 years or more. Operating budgets prepared by nurse managers are for 1 year and follow the fiscal year of the agency. The four-phase budget process is continuous and cyclical, as follows:

Phase I Top managers determine the requirements for the next fiscal year, anticipating activity levels of departments, such as number of client care days, major surgeries to be performed, and meals to be served. This forecast is based on statistical data about past occupancy levels, proposed changes within the facility, and outside factors such as regulatory changes and population trends. The forecast is given to middle- and first-level managers who translate it into needed personnel, supplies, and facilities, creating a preliminary budget. These budgets go to top managers for review, modification, and approval.

Phase II When a preliminary budget is approved, first-level and middle-level managers develop formal budgets for each quarter of the upcoming fiscal year. These plans take into account the following items:

Salaries and wages. Managers determine staffing levels for each job classification, such as LPN, RN-I, and RN-II. They anticipate changes in wages and staffing patterns, and then add up projected wage and salary costs for each quarter.

Other personnel costs. Managers calculate the cost of items such as disability insurance, fringe benefits, and overtime premiums, taking into account changes in government regulation or policy.

Supplies. Managers calculate projected supply costs based on services and expected costs of new products coming on the market.

Capital expenses. Capital expenses include new construction, physical plant changes, and acquisition of major equipment such a linear accelerator. Capital expenses usually are not included in the operating budget. Instead, they are financed by special expansion campaigns.

Other expenses. Managers include all other expenses in proposed budgets on the basis of forecasted levels of activity. In zero-based budgeting no program is taken for granted. Each must be justified with every request for funds.

Statistics. In the preliminary budget, managers include expense projections and statistics, such as average daily census, direct cost per client day, and hours of work. This information provides a factual base to support budget requests.

Revenue. The estimated income of a health care agency is based on levels of anticipated revenue, changes in billing methods, new or expanded revenue-producing services, and third-party (insurance) reimbursement. Although top managers make these estimates, middle-level and first-level managers also must be alert to social and political changes. Agencies cannot operate if income falls below expenses. When all preliminary departmental budget plans are submitted and approved, the accounting department consolidates them into a total agency budget. The top manager presents the budget to the board of trustees for final approval.

Phase III The third phase of the budget process occurs as part of the controlling function. Managers are held accountable for keeping expenses within projected amounts. If a significant difference between budgeted and actual costs occurs, an exception is declared, and corrective action begins at once; this process is called *management by exception.*

Phase IV As the fiscal year proceeds, managers evaluate and revise the budget for ensuing quarters. With experience, managers are able to forecast expenses and revenues, and begin again with phase I.

Time Management

Perhaps no one appreciates the phrase *tempus fugit* (time flies) better than nurse managers. They must:

Set priorities. When there are several things to be done, ask, "What is the relative importance of each task?" Then ask, "What is its relative urgency?" Doing the most important and urgent tasks first reduces frustration and creates composure.

Clarify objectives. When there is pressure to perform, ask, "What am I expected to do? What action is necessary to achieve the objective? How much time is required for each action? Can these actions occur concurrently or must they be sequential? Can they be delegated to someone else?"

Delegate tasks. Delegation is sharing responsibility and authority with subordinates and holding them accountable for performance. Delegation is not the same as direction. *Direction* is telling others what to do; *delegation* is giving tasks to others and expecting them to do them. Before managers delegate tasks, they determine the amount and limits of authority, define expected behaviors, and hold delegates accountable. Managers who fail to delegate have less time for other tasks and deprive the staff of opportunities for personal and professional growth. When Pearl took Bonnie's clients she had less time to perform her management tasks.

Reduce paperwork. Even with the advent of computerized and telecommunications devices, nurse managers must fill out forms, write memoranda, compose letters, and read and write reports. Here are some ways to reduce paperwork:

- Create a system of file folders or envelopes for sorting incoming papers by urgency and importance

- Throw away things that are no longer valuable

- Use word processors more and handwriting less

- Delegate paper tasks

- Purge files at least once a year

- Combine or eliminate routine forms

- Handle papers only once

- Clear the desk for action: deal with, file, or discard papers.

Eliminate time-wasters. Here are some ways to save time:

- Refrain from duplicating work that others are assigned to do.

- Reduce telephone time by planning calls: minimize small talk, use a timer, ask for preferred call times, and remember that people are more talkative in the afternoon than in the morning.

- Reduce drop-in visitor interruptions by setting limits: encourage appointments, close the door or face away from it, and go to talkative people rather than asking them to come to you so that you can leave when your business is done.

- Become time-conscious: schedule activities.

- Plan time for informal, person-to-person contacts with the people in your setting.

Organizing

The second management function is organizing. Having planned, managers organize work to carry out the plan. Organizing involves installing a structure to accomplish the goals of the institution. To function effectively, managers like Pearl need to know the purpose and process of organizing, organizational structures, staffing, assignment systems, and scheduling.

Purpose and Process of Organizing

Organizing involves creating an orderly mechanism for getting things done. It includes setting up channels for communication, establishing authority relationships, and instituting policies, rules, and regulations. The purpose of organization is to increase productivity. To create such a mechanism, managers: (1) define goals and objectives, (2) establish policies and plans, (3) identify activities, (4) organize them into an efficient system, and (5) delegate responsibility.

Organizational Structures

A structure provides a framework for managerial authority, responsibility, and accountability. Organizational charts graphically portray relationships within an institution. Line authority is the direct responsibility assigned to one position over another. Staff authority usually is the responsibility assigned the lowest position, the staff member. There are two general types of organizational structures: bureaucratic (hierarchical, centralized) and adaptive (participatory, decentralized). Within each type there is a range of applications.

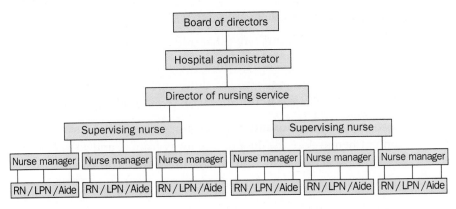

Figure 10-2 Typical bureaucratic hierarchical structure.

Bureaucratic Structures

Bureaucratic structures have a clearly defined chain of command from a few at the top to many at the bottom. Most health care institutions are organized as bureaucratic structures. See Figure 10-2.

Adaptive Structures

Adaptive structures are more flexible than bureaucratic ones because they are based on democratic and humanistic principles. Adaptive structures affirm that job satisfaction and creativity are important, that motivation is more powerful when it is derived from peer pressure and task-related factors, and that leadership is more desirable than control. Several adaptive models have been designed to improve satisfaction and productivity, including free-form, collegial management, project management, matrix, and task force structures.

Free-form structures stress flexibility, using a control center but decentralized operations, profit centers, and risk-taking managers. Open communication, self-regulation, independent judgment, and consensus building are maximized. Organizational charts, position titles, job descriptions, and manuals are minimized.

Collegial management structures restrict single-person authority by maintaining a balance of power among top managers through collective responsibility. Common in Europe, this parliamentary design requires compromise and consensus. Policy decisions are made by a board of directors who have equal power and represent functional areas within the organization.

Project management (PM) structures assign authority to a manager to accomplish a specific project within the existing bureaucracy. Such a design expedites projects but, because it uses employees already assigned to work within the agency, may place workers under two bosses, with potential confusion and conflict. For each project, lines of authority must be clarified.

Matrix structures combine project management and bureaucratic structures, providing clear lines of authority. These structures provide for both hierarchical and lateral coordination across departments and managers. They work best in institutions, such as colleges and universities, where most employees are of relatively equal status.

Task force structures are useful for special projects. They have clear missions, lines of authority, and completion dates. Personnel are relieved of usual duties and given temporary assignments. Although this structure avoids the problem of divided authority, it takes key people from established operations and disrupts normal work patterns.

Coordinating: Staffing

An organizational structure is only an impersonal framework until it is staffed with people. Staffing is the process of analyzing the work to be done; designing and describing jobs; recruiting, selecting, orienting, and developing people to fill those jobs; and assigning and scheduling them to the work.

Job analysis determines three sets of data: (1) principal responsibilities to be assumed, (2) specific tasks to be performed, and (3) knowledge, skills, aptitudes, and personal characteristics needed by the people who perform the tasks.

Job design divides tasks into clusters that become positions or jobs. It assigns monetary value, gives titles, and specifies the relationship of the job to others within the organization.

Job descriptions come from job analysis and design. They specify major duties, relationships, personal characteristics, and the salary range for each position (see the box on page 310).

Recruitment involves attracting qualified applicants to a job. Its purpose is to provide a pool of applicants from which qualified workers can be selected. Although hospital recruiters are assigned this task, first-level managers may be asked to conduct tours and describe the job to prospective applicants.

Sample Job Description

Title: Staff Registered Nurse I

Department: Nursing Service

Reports to: Head nurse

Wage scale: $14.50 to $16.00/hr

Supervises: LPNs, nursing assistants

Date applications close: Open

Position: Provides direct nursing care to clients, including assessment, planning, implementation, and evaluation in a primary care assignment system.

Primary responsibility: Admits and provides ongoing assessment of clients using physical and psychosocial assessment skills, diagnostic data, and medical evaluations. Evaluates effectiveness of care as related to short- and long-term goals. Develops a plan for care, including anticipation of discharge needs. Implements nursing actions and medical prescriptions to meet complex needs of clients and family members. Documents care provided and client responses on appropriate records. Serves as a role model. Demonstrates leadership abilities and skills in communication, consumer relations, problem solving, and decision making. Participates in continuing education and research activities. Performs other job-related duties as assigned. Nurses are required to work day, evening, and night rotating shifts.

Education and credentials: Graduate of a state-approved school of nursing. Current RN license. Current CPR certificate.

Special working conditions: Lifts weights over 25 pounds; often bends, squats, stoops, pulls, pushes; walks and stands for long periods. May be exposed to infectious diseases, toxic drugs, radiant and electric energy.

Experience: None

Application information: Rachel Hemway BSN RN, Nurse Recruiter
Regional Medical Center, Oakville, CA 94560

Employment announcement: October 22, 1995

The Regional Medical Center is an equal opportunity affirmative action employer.

Screening is the process of choosing the best candidate for a given position. Staff nurse selection committees usually include the nurse recruiter, middle-level manager, and first-level managers from the area where the recruit will work. Committee members gather data from written information and interviews, develop criteria, analyze the data, consider alternate applicants, and make a selection.

Application forms, resumés, tests, and letters of reference indicate whether applicants meet minimum job requirements, furnish background data useful for planning interviews, and provide information about the education and work experience of applicants.

Interviews are used to gather information about personal traits, give information about the job, determine if applicants meet minimum standards, and garner goodwill for the institution. They are scheduled at convenient times and places.

To prepare for an interview, managers review applications and resumés ahead of time, and look for a match between a job description and the applicant. The interviewing committee formulates precise questions and writes an interview guide to gather the same information from each applicant.

To conduct interviews, members of the interviewing committee follow these guidelines:

1. Arrive on time.

2. Welcome applicants, using proper names.

3. Establish rapport by sharing something in common to help interviewees relax.

4. State the purpose and structure of the interview and inform applicants that interviewers will take brief notes.

5. Use an interview guide, following the order and content exactly.

6. Probe to obtain details about negative or unclear information.

7. Stay within the law (see Table 10-2).

8. Listen attentively, noting verbal and nonverbal behavior.

9. If applicants look promising, offer realistic information about the position.

10. Ask applicants for comments and questions, answering truthfully.

11. If asked, state the salary range and refer applicants to the personnel office for specifics.

12. Explain the next step in the selection process.

13. Bid the applicant a friendly good-bye.

Selection is the task of choosing the best candidate to fill a job. When the selection committee has interviewed all applicants, it reviews the job description and identifies evidence of qualifications,

TABLE 10-2

Equal Opportunity and Affirmative Action Laws

Law	Description
Title VI and Title VII of the Civil Rights Act of 1964, as amended by the Equal Employment Act of 1972	Prohibits discrimination because of race, color, religion, sex, or national origin in any term, condition, or privilege of employment.
Title IX of the Education Amendments of 1972	Prohibits discrimination on the basis of sex in any educational program or activity receiving federal financial assistance.
Equal Pay Act, as amended by Educational Amendments of 1972	Requires the same pay for men and women doing substantially equal work, requiring equal skill, effort, and responsibility under similar working conditions in the same establishment.
Age discrimination in Employment Act of 1967	Prohibits age discrimination against individuals between 40 and 70 years of age.
Executive Order 11246 as amended by Executive Order 11375	Prohibits all government contracting agencies from discriminating against any employee or applicant for employment; requires that contractors take affirmative action to ensure that minority group applicants are employed and that they are treated equally without regard to race, sex, color, religion, or national origin.
Section 503 and 504 of the Rehabilitation Act of 1973	Prohibits discrimination because of handicap in employment and in programs and activities receiving federal funds; requires contractors to take affirmative action to employ and advance in employment qualified handicapped individuals.
Section 402 of the Vietnam Era Veterans Readjustment Assistance Act of 1974	Requires contractors to take affirmative action to employ and advance in employment qualified disabled veterans, particularly those of the Vietnam era.
Americans with Disabilities Act of 1990	Broadens the protection of handicapped from employment discrimination, forbidding employers from considering a handicap in an employment decision; applies to all health care facilities even if they do not receive any federal funding.

strengths, and weaknesses. The committee then makes a selection. Usually the nurse manager contacts the successful applicant by phone, and the personnel department mails an official employment offer. When the terms of employment are agreed upon, the nurse manager or personnel department write to unsuccessful applicants stating that the position was filled and thanking them for their interest.

Orientation and Socialization

Having made a selection from available candidates, an organization offers orientation and socialization programs to help new employees succeed.

Orientation is the process of introducing new employees to the institution and to their specific jobs. In most health care institutions, this process is coordinated by the education department. Often it prepares an orientation folder containing information about the institution, a job description, an employment contract, and evaluation procedures. Institutional orientation often includes presentations about the history, philosophy, organizational structure, and fire safety measures of the facility. New employees usually receive a tour of the facility during orientation. Unit orientation includes an introduction to coworkers and discussion of work expectations.

Socialization is the process of acquiring the values and accepted modes of behaviors of group members. To facilitate this process, some institutions offer formal internships. Many offer buddy systems, preceptorships, or mentorships.

Internships are formal arrangements between agencies and interns to provide bona fide work experience. Interns may receive a stipend and an offer of employment on completion of the internship. The arrangement benefits both new nurses and health care facilities, providing experience for the neophyte and service at little cost to the institution.

Preceptorships are formal arrangements between a preceptor and a novice, often arranged by hospitals for new employees. The goal is to assist new nurses to acquire the knowledge and skill they need to function effectively in their role. Preceptors serve as orientor, teacher, resource person, counselor, role model, and evaluator for a given time period. They provide on-the-job training for novices.

Buddy systems are modified preceptorships in which a novice is paired for a few hours or days with an experienced nurse. Because no special preparation or contractual agreement precedes the assignment, the buddy usually is not accountable for specific teaching or evaluation. Although new nurses gain some support, the quality of orientation using a buddy system varies considerably.

Mentorships are nurturing relationships between professionals that are not confined to a place or limited by time. Mentors serve as role models, friends, and sounding boards. They give their time, energy, and support, assisting protégés to develop more fully. Mentorships are informal arrangements based on mutual respect and goodwill that develop over time. They usually are not initiated by institutions, but many grow out of preceptor-preceptee relationships.

Staff Development

Staff development provides inservice and continuing education for staff members, inpatients, outpatients, and the general public. Some institutions contract for staff development services with private companies, and others have their own education departments (EDs).

Inservice education is offered by employers to help employees work more effectively. Inservice education begins with orientation and continues throughout employment. It includes general programs for the entire staff and specific programs for selected staff, such as emergency department nurses. Various educational techniques and tools are used, including lectures, computer simulations, demonstrations, discussions, and audiovisual tapes. Videotapes are especially useful because busy nurses can view them at convenient times. For instance, if Pearl obtains a video on how to operate the new infusion pump from the manufacturer, she will not need to schedule a class. The staff will be able to view it during breaks or quiet times.

Continuing education (CE) is much broader than inservice education. It builds on prior skills and knowledge, expanding learning beyond current job functions. Whereas inservice education is offered to improve the work performance of employees, CE is undertaken by individual nurses to achieve career goals. In states with mandatory CE regulations, hospital EDs often design inservice courses to meet state requirements. See Chapter 2 and Chapter 13.

Client (patient) education is a vital part of nursing practice. It gives clients and their families the skills and knowledge they need to assume responsibility for their own health. Many hospital EDs also provide health education for the community, offering classes on such topics as smoking cessation, nutrition, and stress reduction.

Delivery Systems

A health care institution expects its nurse managers to deliver the best client care at the lowest cost, use available staff most effectively, and provide job satisfaction for caregivers. To meet this challenge, managers must find a cost-effective delivery system that matches client and caregiver needs yet gives nurses maximum recognition and autonomy. Some common delivery systems are case nursing, functional nursing, team nursing, patient-focused care, and primary care. Each has advantages and disadvantages.

Case nursing is the oldest delivery system. In this method nurses give total patient care to one or more individuals during a work shift, reporting to a nurse manager. The method is common with student nurses, private duty nurses, and special care unit nurses. Nurse managers make assignments, supervise the activities of the unit, and report to line managers. The advantages of case nursing are that staff nurses gain a holistic view of clients and managers are able to match client needs with caregiver abilities. The disadvantage of case nursing is that continuity of care from day to day is not assured.

Functional nursing is a delivery system that was adapted from industry during the nurse shortage of World War II. It divides nursing into tasks, with different people doing different tasks according to their skills and knowledge. Nursing assistants give personal care; LPNs do treatments and give medications; RNs monitor IVs, do complex treatments, give medications, assess critical clients, and communicate with physicians. Responsibility and authority is delegated from the top. Staff members report to nurse managers who make assignments and supervise. The advantages of functional nursing are that it is efficient and economical. The disadvantages are that care is disconnected and nurses do not gain a holistic view of clients or have much autonomy.

Team nursing is a delivery system that seeks to achieve client care goals through group action. It was developed during the 1960s when there was widespread interest in group dynamics. In this system staff members are divided into teams. Each team consists of a variety of levels of nurses. Team leaders make assignments according to caregiver abilities and do the tasks other team members are not qualified to do. At a daily client care conference, team members review client care plans. Team members care for the same clients each day and report to team leaders, who report to the unit manager. The advantages of team nursing are that it gives leaders a more holistic view of their clients, increases their autonomy and accountability, and maximizes caregiver abilities. The disadvantages are that team leader workloads may be excessive and it is more expensive than other delivery systems.

Primary care is a delivery system in which professional nurses assume total responsibility and authority for the care of several clients 24 hours per day from the time of admission to discharge. On subsequent shifts, associate nurses (LPNs and RNs) follow the nursing care plan developed by the primary nurse and report to the nurse manager. The advantages are that nurses gain a holistic view of clients, nurses have greater autonomy and accountability, and clients have a nurse advocate. The disadvantages are that highly skilled nurses perform unskilled, time-consuming tasks and often carry excessive workloads.

Patient-focused care (PFC) is a delivery system using a team approach, with cross-trained caregivers (Brider 1992). *Cross-training* means that RNs learn to perform tasks that technicians usually perform, such as electrocardiography, and the other team members learn to do traditional RN tasks, such as inserting Foley catheters. PFC is based on the following principles: (1) it is client-focused rather than discipline-focused; (2) it is interdisciplinary rather than multidisciplinary; (3) it is goal-oriented rather than problem-oriented; and (4) its effectiveness is measured from the client's perspective rather than the provider's (Gage 1994). In practice, units are staffed by teams of two or three caregivers (usually headed by an RN) who regularly work together. Each team has complete responsibility for a client's care from admission to discharge. The team communicates directly with physicians, handles client records, arranges for or performs diagnostic tests, performs various therapies, and provides nursing care. The disadvantages of PFC are that costs are high for initial and continuing education and unlicensed assistive personnel must be closely supervised and may jeopardize client safety. The advantages are that over a period of time it is cost effective, nurses have autonomy and accountability, and clients receive holistic care.

Staffing Formulas, Patterns, and Work Shifts

Staffing formulas are ways to calculate the number of people to hire based on the average occupancy rate of nursing units. These formulas take into consideration vacations, holidays, sick leave, and staff development time. For example, if a nurse works 5 days a week in a nursing position where coverage is needed for 7 days, it takes ⁷/₅, or 1.4 nurses to have one nurse on duty for each of the 7 days. Schedulers use more complicated formulas to calculate sick leave and vacation coverage.

Staffing patterns are plans that show the number and mix of care providers needed during a period of time. When managers create these plans, they consider the goals and policies of the agency, client needs, availability and ability of nurses, laws, delivery systems such as team nursing, and other factors such as beds per unit.

Task-level analysis tells what qualifications caregivers need to perform tasks. *Time-and-motion studies* tell how much time it takes to do tasks. *Patient classification systems (PCSs)* tell the acuity of clients by grouping them according to how many hours of care they need per day. There are two PCSs: factor and prototype. Factor PCSs use lists of tasks that nurses must do to provide care, such as incontinent care. Each task is assigned a number according to the time required to provide the care. The total score of each client is calculated, and clients are grouped into four or five categories according to the time it takes to do the tasks. Prototype PCSs use selected tasks, such as maintaining strict isolation, as indicators of care. The total score of each client is calculated, and then clients are grouped into four or five categories according to critical indicators. Both types of PCSs yield data about acuity and nursing care and translate into caregiver hours.

To calculate the number of nurses needed, managers add the direct care time required by all clients on the unit to the indirect time needed for recording, reporting, and break time. They divide that number by the hours in a shift. For example, a group of 16 clients needs a total of 30 hours of direct care plus 2 hours of indirect care during an 8-hour shift, or ³²/₈, or 4 nurses. The number and mix of required staff is then compared to the number and mix of those scheduled to work, minus absences. The key to efficient use of resources is to match required and available staff. If more nurses are needed than scheduled, managers need a float pool of contract nurses or unscheduled employees from which to draw. If more nurses are scheduled than needed, managers must ask them not to work that day or to float to other units with greater need. In the vignette, Bonnie was asked to float to another unit because client acuity on the unit did not justify her presence.

Work shifts historically were 12 to 24 hours, 6 days a week. In the mid-1940s nurses began working five 8-hour shifts per week. Typically shifts were 0700 to 1530, 1500 to 2330, and 2300 to 0730, with a half-hour lunch break and a half-hour overlap. To provide staffing on weekends, evenings, and nights, some institutions mandated that all nurses rotate to evenings, nights, and weekends. Others employed permanent day, evening, night, and weekend staffs. With the advent of intensive care units, primary nursing, and increased nurse autonomy, new work-shift patterns emerged. Today, health care providers use various shift lengths with job-sharing and part-time positions. No longer bound to tradition, managers and staffs decide what will work best, considering quality of care, costs, and availability of nurses.

Scheduling

The final step of the staffing process is scheduling people to fill specific needs. In agencies that operate one shift a day, weekdays only, scheduling is not an issue. In health care institutions that operate 24 hours a day, 365 days a year, scheduling is a major concern. In general, there are two methods of scheduling staff: centralized and decentralized. In centralized scheduling an administrative clerk assumes responsibility for all personnel in the nursing units. The clerk becomes an expert in impartially applying agency policies and observing budgeted nurse-client ratios. Although the process is fair and efficient, it is impersonal and allows for minimal nursing input. Decentralized scheduling is done by nurse managers who are able to take into account client needs and staff abilities. However, the task is time-consuming and thankless, and personal relationships sometimes compromise objectivity. To overcome this problem, some units use self-scheduling with agreed-upon guidelines to ensure fairness.

Directing: Activating

The fourth management operation is directing, the activating function. To carry out this function managers inform workers what is expected of them, enable them to do their jobs, and motivate them to perform efficiently and effectively. Directing requires both technical action and interpersonal skill.

Technical Activities

The technical activities of directing are client-focused, staff-focused, and institution-focused. In client-focused activities first-level nurse managers (1) initiate and update written nursing care plans; (2) main-

Guidelines for Giving a Shift Report of Client Conditions

1. Assemble pertinent data such as intake-output and vital signs.

2. Speak clearly and slowly enough to be understood.

3. Introduce yourself. State your name, title, and room numbers of clients in your report.

4. Report on clients:

    a. State room number, name, physician, medical diagnosis, surgeries or major treatments with dates.

    b. Give pertinent assessment data, nursing diagnoses, and interventions. (eg, fluid volume deficit: intravenous fluids—type, rate, amount; impaired skin integrity; urinary deficit: indwelling catheter—amount, color, clarity of urine).

    c. When clients are scheduled for surgery or other major treatment, state procedure, time scheduled, client's condition, nursing interventions yet to be done (eg, pre-op medications on call to surgery).

5. Do not gossip, state subjective opinions as facts, or discuss personal problems. Speak as a professional to professionals. Maintain ethical standards of behavior.

6. Offer information about expected admissions, discharges, scheduled inservice, and other matters of concern to the staff coming on duty.

7. Conclude report by restating your name and an amiable wish.

tain a healthy, safe, and comfortable environment; (3) accurately and concisely record and report essential information about clients to other responsible health professionals (see the accompanying box); and (4) provide information, assistance, and education to clients and their families.

In staff-focused activities managers (1) give formal and informal direction relative to nursing care; (2) oversee and advise staff regarding work assignments; (3) obtain supplies, equipment, and support services to facilitate quality nursing care; and (4) foster personal and professional growth. In institution-focused activities managers (1) coordinate unit operations with other departments, (2) give information and assistance to other departments, (3) participate in meetings and projects, and (4) represent the staff to middle- and upper-level management.

Interpersonal Skills

Of all the management functions, directing is most dependent on the interpersonal skills of communication, teaching, motivation, conflict resolution, and morale building.

Communication Communication is a process of exchanging ideas and feelings. It occurs when meaning is conveyed from one person to another, verbally and nonverbally. Communication is the key to every other interpersonal skill.

Assertive communication affirms observations, feelings, and needs without attacking or negating others. Passive communication discounts personal needs and yields without question to the needs of others. Passive-aggressive communication senses personal needs and yields to others, disguising true feelings of anger in sweetness, sarcasm, or humor. Assertive communication acknowledges feelings and needs. To communicate assertively (1) state what you believe is true, using "I" rather than "you"; (2) state how you feel, owning your emotions; (3) listen to the other person's point of view, and state what you need or want.

Communication channels are networks through which information flows. They may be formal (official) channels or informal (unofficial) channels, called grapevines. Grapevines transmit information faster than formal channels because they are interpersonal and foster a feeling of comradeship. Savvy managers use both official channels and grapevines to communicate with staff members.

Communication channels carry information down from above, up from below, and horizontally between equals. Downward communication tells subordinates what to do. No matter what its quality, it causes more dissatisfaction than upward communication. Upward communication tells superiors what subordinates are thinking. Though sometimes ignored, it is valuable. When encouraged, upward communication increases morale because it recognizes the value of subordinates to the institution. Horizontal communication connects people at the same level. It includes sharing information, solving problems, and coordinating activities.

Here are some guidelines to help improve communication:

- Identify what you want to communicate before you begin.

- Examine your reasons for communicating.

- Be aware of the nonverbal messages you send.

Principles of Teaching-Learning

Factors that facilitate learning

Acceptance, freedom from fear and condemnation

Active involvement of learner

Comfortable physical and emotional environment

Feedback that is both positive and negative

Logical presentation of information, simple to complex

Motivation, a desire to learn

Physical and emotional readiness

Practice, repetition, and immediate use

Relevance, value, meaning to the learner

Success, mastery

Factors that hinder learning

Anxiety above moderate level

Irrelevance of subject to learner

Physical or emotional discomfort, disease, and disability

Presentation illogical or too complex

Little or no practice or application

Lack of feedback to let learner know progress

Cultural barriers of language, values, meanings, taboos

Failure, lack of success

- Even if the message is negative, find something positive to communicate.

- Follow up on communication to see the effect it produced.

- Be sure your words and deeds are congruent.

Teaching Teaching is an important aspect of directing. It is a deliberate activity aimed at helping another person develop skills, grasp new concepts, and acquire values and beliefs. Because its purpose is to change behavior, teaching is most effective when it focuses on specific learning objectives and meets the needs of learners. A teaching plan includes (1) learning objectives stated in behavioral terms with conditions and criteria, (2) learning activities that facilitate learning, and (3) measurement of the learning objectives. Teaching is the responsibility of all nurses, especially nurse managers. The accompanying box lists some important teaching-learning principles.

Motivation Motivation is an energizing force for action, a powerful force that moves people to act. Nurse managers employ motivation to improve client care, efficiency, job satisfaction, and institutional goals. Understanding that all behavior is caused, and, ultimately motivated by self-interest, managers seek to identify those things that energize staff to act. Some theorists view motivation from a content view, asking what motivates. Others look at it from a process view, asking how to motivate. Freud (1969) proposes that instincts predispose humans to behave as they do and that the pleasure principle motivates them. Maslow (1970) says that a hierarchy of needs motivates people, including physiologic needs and needs for safety-security, belongingness, esteem, and self-actualization. Skinner (1953) suggests that positive and negative reinforcers produce stimulus responses that modify behavior. Nurse managers can use all of these theories to motivate staff members. See the box on page 323.

Self-motivation. Morrison (1993) suggests a five-step process to develop self-motivational skills:

1. Develop positive thinking by replacing negative emotions, attitudes, and opinions.

2. Break the low self-esteem cycle by acknowledging your talents and abilities.

3. Conquer fear and anxiety by remembering that "there are no failures, only outcomes."

4. Find meaning in work by making the ordinary work of client care special for you.

5. Perform self-reviews by identifying your own needs, wants, and expectations.

Motivation of others. To motivate others, nurse managers may take the following actions:

1. Set goals that are clear, specific, and challenging and provide feedback (Straub & Attner 1991).

2. Build trust and integrity by telling the truth and keeping your word.

3. Give honest praise generously (Morrison 1993).

4. Demonstrate respect by listening and exchanging ideas, opinions, and problem-solving ideas.

5. Manifest enthusiasm, anticipation, and optimism; it is contagious.

Motivating Factors in the Work Setting

Physiologic needs

1. Work environment is comfortable and aesthetically pleasing.
2. Scheduling provides time for sleep and recreation.
3. Breaks are adequate for nourishment and stress reduction.
4. Employee health is enhanced by medical care, leave time, and infection control.
5. Salary is adequate to provide food, shelter, and health care.

Security and safety needs

1. Hiring and performance evaluations are fair and growth oriented.
2. Client care assignments are appropriate to ability of staff members.
3. Scheduling provides for regular, dependable work hours.
4. Emergency procedures are practiced with back-up and support.
5. Measures are taken to reduce physical, radiation, and biologic injury.

Belongingness needs

1. Conflict resolution is facilitated.
2. Attention is given to group dynamics to improve interpersonal comfort between staff members.
3. Team work, cooperation, and social contacts between staff members are encouraged.
4. Trust, honesty, assertiveness, and a degree of self-disclosure are modeled by nurse managers.

Self-esteem and other esteem needs

1. Feedback on performance is objective and frequent.
2. Exceptional work is rewarded with timely recognition, merit raises, and promotions.
3. Assignments are individualized to suit abilities and interests of staff.

Self-actualizing needs

1. Staff members are included in planning process.
2. Innovation is acknowledged and encouraged.
3. Professional development opportunities are provided.
4. New project and program testing is encouraged.
5. Staff members are included in decisions about assignments.
6. Staff members are encouraged to become active in professional organizations.

Conflict Resolution Conflict exists when two or more mutually exclusive goals, ideas, actions, roles, values, beliefs, feelings, or attitudes occur within or between individuals or groups. During childhood many people learn that all conflict is bad. In fact, conflict is neither good nor bad. It results from an inherent human drive for self-assertion and survival. Conflict is destructive when it produces hostility, aggression, and intolerable stress. It is constructive when it educates; generates personal growth, ideas, respect, and understanding; and increases group cohesion.

There are many types of conflict: *Intrapersonal conflict* occurs within an individual about allegiances, choices, and motives. *Interpersonal conflict*, the most common type, occurs between two or more individuals. *Intergroup conflict* occurs within established groups about interpersonal issues, roles, and values. *Vertical conflict* occurs between superiors or subordinates about authority issues. *Horizontal conflict* occurs between peers about methods, assignments, and territory. *Interdepartmental conflict* occurs between work groups about values and goals.

Conflict and its outcome is really quite predictable, beginning with a preexisting condition and moving toward a perceived threat, some kind of acting-out behavior, and an aftermath when the conflict is resolved or suppressed and new attitudes and feelings formed. Preexisting conditions that lead to conflict include:

- Differences in beliefs, as between nurses who support collective bargaining and those who do not

- Structural issues, as between bureaucratic levels of authority

- Scarce resources, as when competition develops between departments for available funds

- Incompatible values, as may be found between the social services and the business office

- Role confusion, as when a nurse manager identifies with staff more than with management

- Interdependence issues, as when operating room nurses depend on floor nurses to prepare clients for surgery

- Cultural distance, as when day-shift nurses complain about night-shift nurses.

Expert managers identify preexisting conditions, bring them out in the open, and deal with them before open conflict occurs. When conflict occurs between two members of a group, other group members may take sides, damaging unit cohesion.

People use a number of strategies to manage conflict. They may withdraw, smooth over, avoid, force, declare themselves a winner or loser, negotiate, compromise, or collaborate. Regardless of the strategy used, the outcome of conflict is lose-lose, win-lose, or win-win. In a lose-lose outcome, neither side wins; nobody is happy. In a win-lose outcome, one side wins, the other loses, and bitterness may remain. In a win-win outcome, the needs of both parties are met, and both sides get what they need. The box on page 326 outlines a collaborative strategy for conflict resolution that is useful with both individuals and groups.

Morale Building Morale building is a leadership skill found in the best nurse managers. It is the ability to foster enthusiasm, hope, faith, joy, and confidence. Morale is the attitude workers have toward their job. It is the esprit de corps that develops when people share common goals and experiences. When morale is high, people are able to accomplish extraordinary feats of courage and mastery. When it is low, their discouragement shows itself in reduced effort and efficiency. The box on page 327 lists actions nurse managers can take to build staff morale.

Controlling

Controlling is the fourth management function. It is the action managers take to ensure that outcomes are the same as those that were planned. Controlling entails setting standards and criteria, measuring performance, and making corrections. The watchword of controlling is accountability. Nurse managers are accountable to various degrees for the fiscal budget as well as risk management, quality assurance, and performance evaluations of staff members.

Fiscal Budget

Phase I and phase II of the budget process are part of the planning function of management. Phases III and IV fall within the controlling function. Phase III takes place as an ongoing process throughout the fiscal year as managers strive to keep expenses and revenues within projected limits. If they notice a significant difference between budgeted and actual costs, managers take corrective action. During phase IV they evaluate and revise the budget for ensuing quarters. With

Collaborative Strategy for Conflict Resolution

Listen for understanding

1. The parties commit themselves to negotiate in good faith until an agreement is reached.
2. The parties agree to the following ground rules:
   a. No one walks out of the meeting before it ends.
   b. Everyone uses "I," not accusatory "you" statements.
   c. Everyone takes mutual responsibility for the outcome.
   d. The parties sit facing each other.
   e. Each party has equal time.
   f. The moderator will encourage, restate, maintain control, and enforce rules.
3. Alfa states Alfa's perception of the problem to Bravo.
4. Bravo listens and states it back to Alfa until Bravo "gets" Alfa's point of view.
5. Then Bravo states Bravo's perception of the problem to Alfa.
6. Alfa listens and states it back to Bravo until Alfa "gets" Bravo's point of view.

Define the problem in terms of needs

7. The negotiator helps Alfa and Bravo define the problem in terms of what each one needs:
   "Alfa needs ____ and Bravo needs ____." If the parties get stuck, they go back and repeat steps 1 to 6.

Generate solutions and select one that meets the needs of both parties

8. When the problem is defined in terms of needs, Alfa and Bravo then generate ways to meet their needs.
9. Alfa and Bravo discuss various solutions, assessing how well each solution meets needs.
10. Together the parties decide on a mutually acceptable solution, stated as follows: *Who* is to do *what, when*?

Agree on a follow-up session to evaluate the success of the chosen solution

11. The solution is implemented.
12. At a follow-up session the moderator asks if the conflict was indeed resolved and if the needs of the parties are being met. If not, go back to step 1 and begin again.

time and experience, managers learn to forecast revenues and expenses and to stay within budgeted amounts.

Risk Management

Risk management programs exist to prevent loss and control liability. They identify, analyze, and evaluate risks and develop a plan to reduce

Morale-Building Actions for Nurse Managers

1. Set attainable goals for the staff to accomplish.
2. Address conflicts; do not wait until hostility and frustration destroy group cohesion.
3. Foster supportive behavior by modeling empathy, nonpossessive warmth, and genuineness.
4. When making assignments, consider staff abilities and preferences.
5. Acknowledge individual accomplishment; compliment staff personally.
6. Invite and listen to staff suggestions; serve as a channel for upward communication.
7. Encourage staff to participate in institutional committees where they can be heard.
8. Model assertive communication; give prompt genuine feedback.
9. Maintain high standards and apply rules with absolute fairness.
10. Institute clear lines of authority so that staff will know who is responsible for what and to whom.
11. Defend staff members and serve as an advocate for them.
12. Encourage staff development by adjusting schedules for continuing education, writing letters of recommendation, and applying for educational funds and research projects.
13. Encourage staff to extend to each other the same nonjudgmental caring they give to clients.

the severity and frequency of injuries and accidents. These programs set standards and criteria, measure performance, and take corrective action to reduce incidents that lead to liability suits. Some hospitals hire risk managers to coordinate activities. A large share of responsibility, however, falls on nurse managers and staff because they are the ones who are present or nearby when most incidents occur.

Reportable incidents are any unexpected or unplanned events that affect or potentially affect a client or family member. The most common reportable incidents are (1) medication errors, including errors in administration of intravenous fluids, (2) complications from diagnostic or treatment procedures, (3) falls, (4) dissatisfaction with care by clients or their families, and (5) refusal to sign a consent or to submit to treatment (England & Sullivan 1992).

Incident reports are made on two official documents: client records and incident reporting forms. Nurses who are present write objective descriptions of events in client records. On a separate reporting form, they describe incidents in greater detail than in client records. These reports are made to protect the institution and its nurses from liability. Managers use incident reports to analyze the cause, frequency, and severity of incidents and to plan actions to prevent future incidents. These reports tell what happened, to whom, when, where, under what conditions, who discovered the event, what actions were taken to prevent further injury, who was notified and when, who is reporting the event, and how the event might have been prevented. When reports are incomplete or not written, hospitals are more likely to be sued and more likely to lose.

Many incidents go unreported because nurses fear discipline, feel pressured for time, or lack knowledge of how to document events. Nurse managers can increase the accuracy and percentage of reported incidents by teaching staff members what to do if an unusual event occurs and how to write an objective incident report. See the box on page 329.

Quality Assurance

Quality assurance (QA) describes the process of evaluating the products and services of an institution. QA activities include setting standards and criteria, measuring performance, and correcting deficits. Mandatory standards are set down by state boards of health. Voluntary standards are made by organizations such as the American Nurses Association in its *Standards of Nursing Practice*. Standards set down by the Joint Commission on Accreditation of Healthcare Organizations (JCAHCO) are voluntary, but hospitals that are not JCAHCO-accredited are not reimbursed by third-party payers such as insurance companies and Medicare.

Quality assurance programs aim to maintain quality health care services. In 1982, JCAHCO began requiring that all accredited hospitals have ongoing QA programs to maintain standards of care. Current JCAHCO guidelines state that a quality assurance program should be a systematic, institution-wide, integrated quality review plan for all care-related services, support services, medical staff, and governing boards (Bushy 1992). Although some hospitals hire a QA manager, the responsibility often falls on nurses. Nurse managers must understand and apply JCAHCO nursing service standards to client care, incorporate them in management activities, and familiarize the staff with their interpretation.

An Action Plan for Unusual Events

1. *Discover and report* all unusual events. Anyone can do this.

2. *Notify proper authorities.* Nurse informs physician immediately; if it is a major incident, nurse informs nurse manager or risk manager by phone and completes a reporting form within 24 hours.

3. *Investigate.* Physician, nurse manager, and risk manager investigate the incident immediately.

4. *Consult.* Nurse manager and risk manager consult with the physician and hospital risk management committee.

5. *Take action.* Nurse manager or risk manager explores incident with the client and family:
   a. Listen. Do not respond until client and family have finished.
   b. Avoid reacting defensively. Convey sincere concern.
   c. Ask client and family what solution they expect.
   d. If appropriate, explain actions you can and cannot take.
   e. Agree on steps to be taken within a given time frame.

6. *Record information* in client record and on reporting form; describe conversations with client and family; include agreements that were made.

Adapted from England DA, Sullivan EJ. Quality Assurance and Risk Management. In Sullivan EJ, Decker PJ. *Effective Management in Nursing*, 3rd ed. Addison-Wesley, 1992.

Quality assurance monitoring uses many procedures. Nursing audits are official evaluations of nursing care. Concurrent audits are made while clients are receiving care. Retrospective audits are conducted after clients are discharged. Auditors assess evidence that nursing care meets (or met) expected outcomes of care plans. If it does not, auditors recommend changes. Peer reviews are made by practicing nurses who determine standards that indicate quality care. Their expertise is useful in evaluating the care of complicated cases where a synthesis of knowledge and experience is needed. Utilization reviews are mandated by Title XVIII of the Social Security Act for "maintenance of high quality patient care and assurance of appropriate and efficient utilization of facility services" (Standards 1976). These reviews evaluate medical care and length of patient stays. To receive Medicare reimbursement, facilities must have utilization review plans. Although these plans do not focus on nursing, they affect client care, because they include such things as length of stays. Another measure of client satisfaction is client satisfaction rating scales used to determine the level of client approval. Clients may be asked to fill out a questionnaire before or after discharge. Though not scientific, these surveys help assess the effectiveness of nursing interventions such as client teaching.

Total quality management (TQM), also called continuous quality improvement, is both a philosophy and a program. It has been used with success in Japan and presently is being applied in the United States. TQM seeks to build quality into a service or product throughout its production, instead of relying on inspection and modification afterward (Kirk 1992). TQM means doing the right thing, the right way, the first time, using prevention rather than correction to ensure quality (Marquis & Huston 1994). The philosophy permeates the values, attitudes, and decisions of the organization.

Because TQM is a never-ending process, everything and everyone in the organization is subject to continuous improvement efforts. No matter how good the product or service, the TQM philosophy says that there is always room for improvement. Client needs and experiences with the end product are constantly evaluated, not by a central QA department, but by workers. Because problems are addressed preventatively, crisis management is unnecessary. Ineffective and inefficient policies, procedures, and processes are eliminated. TQM trusts employees to be accountable, responsible, and knowledgeable. They are given positive feedback and provided with ongoing educational programs at all levels (Arikian 1991). The TQM philosophy fits comfortably with nurses who already act as responsible professionals within health care institutions.

Performance Evaluations

The words *performance evaluation* produce strong emotions in almost all nurses. Staff nurses may view evaluations as threats, whereas managers may view them as time-consuming chores. Nonetheless, performance evaluations can be useful for professional growth. They give a formal appraisal of how well a nurse is meeting prescribed standards. Ideally, performance evaluations recognize accomplishments, determine competencies, encourage, motivate, and suggest staff development needs. Like other control functions, performance evaluations set standards and criteria, measure behavior, and correct deficiencies.

The institution gives performance standards to nurses when they are hired. Ideally, these standards mirror job descriptions. Their clarity and specificity make the evaluation process objective, consistent, and job-related. They reduce intimidation and remove the element of surprise. Employee-employer contracts often describe the evaluation process and appeal mechanisms for disputes. When hired, new nurses can expect to be evaluated at the end of the orientation period, in 6 months, and on an annual basis thereafter, unless problems arise.

To facilitate the process, managers keep an ongoing record of both desirable and undesirable behaviors of staff members. Some managers use a tape recorder for immediate use, later writing brief notes in an annotated file, with dates and times. If clients are endangered, managers do not wait for scheduled appraisals but take immediate action. Written evidence objectifies the process and gives managers more power to effect change. As the time draws near for a scheduled evaluation, managers review their annotated file, fill out the evaluation form, and make an appointment with the staff member for a conference when minimal interruptions can be expected.

At the conference nurse managers frame the evaluation as a feedback session for professional growth and career development. They concentrate on objective evidence, are sensitive to human needs, and avoid accusatory "you" statements that create defensiveness. Evaluators use the list of expected behaviors to organize the discussion and address problems. Together, evaluator and evaluatee forge a plan of corrective action with specific conditions and criteria. At the close of the conference, the manager summarizes decisions and confirms the time for the next evaluation.

When staff nurses have a plan to correct deficiencies, managers see that the plan is followed. When it is complete, they acknowledge change. If unacceptable behavior does not stop, managers follow the termination-for-cause policy of the agency.

Some behavior, such as theft and abuse of clients or drugs, calls for immediate dismissal. To protect themselves from liability, managers must have first-hand knowledge, not hearsay. Therefore, they must write detailed notes about incidents and keep superiors apprised of problems. Substance abuse or mental illness may cause a change in the disposition or appearance of a nurse. Managers confront such nurses with their observations and refer them for counseling with compassion but firmness. They report such matters to their supervisor. The institution may report the nurse to the state licensing board. Many states have diversion programs to identify and rehabilitate nurses (see Chapter 3).

◇ Summary

Health care institutions have all the characteristics of open systems, including interrelatedness and input-throughput-output feedback. The management process is involved with the throughput of a system. Management is a set of functions, whereas leadership is a set of abilities. Decision making is the process of selecting from alternatives. Nurses need technological competence to keep abreast of changes in the health care system. The management process has five operations: planning, organizing, coordinating, directing, and controlling. *Planning* includes identifying the purpose and philosophy of the agency, clarifying goals and objectives, reviewing policies, preparing budgets, and assessing resources. *Organizing* involves the structure of the institution. *Coordinating* involves staffing the institution. *Directing* requires technical activities and interpersonal skills. *Controlling* entails setting standards, measuring performance, and making corrections. Nurse managers participate in all these functions.

Critical Thinking Questions

1. What rules or principles appear to determine the order of the management process?

2. Is the management process valuable and necessary for nurses? Why or why not?

3. What are your personal values and beliefs about managing client care? How might these values and beliefs affects discussions of management strategies?

1. Spend a day with a first-level nurse manager. Classify each activity according to its management function (planning, organizing, coordinating, directing, and controlling).

2. Design an orientation program for new employees in a health care agency.

3. Role-play using assertive communication with a physician who is furious because a client was fed breakfast before a fasting blood sample was drawn.

4. Using the conflict-resolution strategy provided in the box on page 326, resolve a conflict you are experiencing in your personal life.

5. Obtain a copy of a staff nurse job description and the performance evaluation form from the local hospital and compare them. Do they match? If not, how would you change them?

6. Invite a nurse manager to speak on the budgeting process and tell how overtime, sick leave, and employing contract nurses affect a budget.

Annotated Reading List

Marquis BL, Huston CJ. *Management Decision Making for Nurses,* 2nd ed. Lippincott, 1994.

This text is a combined textbook-workbook that leads the reader through the decision-making process for nursing management. There are 118 case studies that demonstrate how to apply a problem-solving and decision-making approach to a variety of actual clinical and management situations. The text presents realistic cases that give the reader an opportunity to understand the management process. It is readable, useful, and well-presented.

Morrison M. *Professional Skills for Leadership: Foundations of a Successful Career.* Mosby, 1993.

This practical text is divided into two units. The first unit focuses on people skills needed by nurse leader-managers, including psychosocial, communication, group dynamics, leadership, motivational, conflict-resolution, and management skills. The second unit focuses on the application of those skills to nursing management—applying standards of care, decision making, planning, creating a positive work environment, motivating and building morale, delegating and evaluating—and includes a section on legal implications. The text is well illustrated and strong in interpersonal concepts.

References

Arikian VL. Total Quality Management: Application to Nursing Service. *Journal of Nursing Administration* 1991; 21(6):46.

Bennis W. *Why Leaders Can't Lead: The Unconscious Conspiracy Continues*. Jossey-Bass, 1989.

Bower FL. Personal communication. 1994.

Bower FL. Shared Governance: A Professional Model for Nursing Practice. *California Nursing* Nov/Dec 1990; 29–32.

Brider P. The Move to Patient-Focused Care. *American Journal of Nursing* Sept 1992; 26–33.

Bushy A. Quality Assurance in Rural Hospitals. *Journal of Nursing Administration* 1992; 21(10):34–39.

Douglass LM. *The Effective Nurse: Leader and Manager*, 4th ed. Mosby, 1993.

England DA, Sullivan EJ. Quality Assurance and Risk Management. In Sullivan EJ, Decker PJ. *Effective Management in Nursing*, 3rd ed. Addison-Wesley, 1992.

Freud S (translated by James Strachey). *An Outline of Psycho-Analysis*. Norton, 1969.

Gage M. The Patient-Driven Interdisciplinary Care Plan. *Journal of Nursing Administration* 1994;24 (4):26–35.

Hollander EP. *Leadership Dynamics. A Practical Guide to Effective Relationships*. The Free Press, 1978.

Kirk, R. The Big Picture—Total Quality Management and Continuous Quality Improvement. *Journal of Nursing Administration* 22(4):24–31, 1992.

Kuster J. New Software Could Revolutionize Nursing Industry. *Focus* Aug 1990.

Manthey M. The Nurse Manager as Leader. *Nursing Management* 1990;21(6).

Marquis BL, Huston C. *Management Decision Making for Nurses*, 2d ed. Lippincott, 1994.

Maslow A. *Motivation and Personality*, 2nd ed. Harper & Row, 1970.

Mayo E. *The Human Problem of an Industrialized Civilization*. MacMillan, 1953.

McGregor D. *The Human Side of Enterprise*. McGraw-Hill, 1960.

Morrison M. *Professional Skills for Leadership: Foundations of a Successful Career*. Mosby, 1993.

Ouchi WG. *How American Business Can Meet the Japanese Challenge*. Addison-Wesley, 1981.

Skinner BF. *Science and Human Behavior*. Free Press, 1953.

Standards for Certification and Participation in Medicare and Medicaid Programs. Fed Reg, Vol 39, No 12, Part III, 1974. In Rogers WW. *General Administration in the Nursing Home*, 2nd ed. Cahners, 1976.

Straub JT, Attner RF. *Introduction to Business*, 4th ed. PWS-Kent, 1991.

von Bertalanffy L. *General System Theory: Foundations, Development, Applications*, rev ed. George Braziller, 1968.

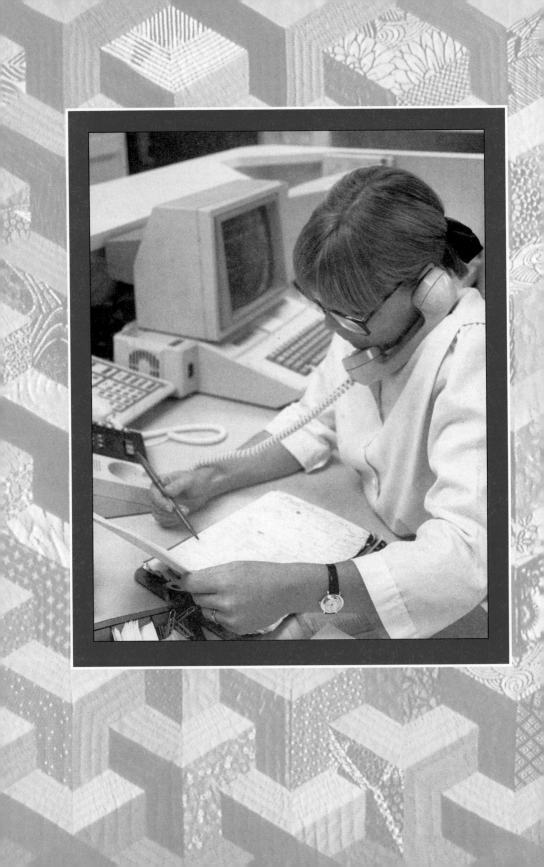

Managing Stress Effectively

◆ Learning Objectives

- Compare the stimulus, response, and transactional models of stress.

- Identify physiologic and psychologic manifestations of stress.

- Explain the causes and dynamics of stress.

- Discuss stress management relative to emotion-focused and problem-focused coping.

- Describe various strategies for coping.

- Discuss networking as a social support resource.

- Examine the concept of emotional exhaustion.

- Discuss how the biologic clock affects the work performance of nurses.

- Describe strategies for successful coping with shift work.

Emily walked into the classroom, dropped her heavy bookbag on the floor, and squeezed her pregnant body under the arm of the desk-top chair. Morning clinical had been a bear, and she'd been afraid to ask for help. Somehow her classmates managed, but she was feeling overwhelmed, working nights and being a single mom. A paper was due on Friday, and there were two midterms next week. The stress was getting to her. Sometimes she couldn't even focus.

Just then a classmate arrived and announced, "Ms Ryle, the unit manager on C-4, wants Emily to call her right away... something about a med." Emily shivered with fear as she hurried to the school office. Finally, she got through to Ms Ryle, a chronically exhausted woman who called patients names like "hippo" and "wacko." There was no record that Emily had given the 10:00 AM antibiotic; she would have to return right away. Emily put the receiver down hard. "Sure, I've nothing else to do!" When Emily returned to the classroom, she tried to ignore her classmates' stares. She didn't have a friend among them; she was just too busy.

Ms Ryle was waiting when she arrived. By the time Emily checked the record and satisfied Ms Ryle that she had given the medication and signed for it, it was too late to return to school. Emily picked up her son from day care, bought some milk at the grocery, and grabbed a handful of bills from the mailbox. She slowly climbed the stairs to her apartment. Her head throbbed and her stomach burned. After all this struggle, what if she failed? Emily desperately wanted to succeed, but right now she felt alone, anxious, and frustrated. In just a few hours she would lift her sleeping boy from his bed, carry him to a neighbor and leave for work.

How could Emily manage stress more effectively? How could she balance so many demands with her resources? How could she avoid the burnout she saw in the unit manager?

◆ Stress

Nurses, teachers, and business executives talk of stress in the workplace. Journalists call this the "decade of stress." But just what is stress, and how can it be managed?

The term *stress* became popular after Hans Selye published his famous book *The Stress of Life* in 1956 and 1976. He defines stress as a measure of the effort it takes to maintain equilibrium and adapt to change. The idea caught on, probably because it gave a name to a universal human experience. Indeed, stress affects the whole person: physically, emotionally, socially, intellectually, and spiritually.

Stress is of special concern to nurses because it is a significant factor in the health-illness continuum, contributing to many common disorders such as hypertension, gastric ulcers, and anxiety states. The phenomenon continues to fascinate both the public and the caregiving professions. The *Cumulative Index to Nursing and Allied Health Literature* cited 4118 articles and abstracts about stress published between 1990 and 1993.

Three models dominate the research. One model views stress as a stimulus, another as a response, and a third as a transaction between an individual and the environment.

Stress as Stimulus

The stimulus model defines stress as a phenomenon that disrupts a person's life. The event or set of circumstances causing a disrupted response is called a *life-change event* or *stressor.* The model proposes that too many life-change events increase one's vulnerability to illness (Holmes & Rahe 1967). It focuses on major life-change events, using a tool known as the Social Readjustment Rating Scale (SRRS), shown in Table 11-1.

The stimulus model is based on three assumptions:

1. Life-change events are similar for everyone and require the same amount of adaptation.

2. A personal view of an event as positive or negative is not relevant.

3. Illness occurs when a common score is reached.

TABLE 11-1

Social Readjustment Rating Scale

Rank	Life Event	Life-Change Unit (LCU)
1	Death of a spouse	100
2	Divorce	73
3	Marital separation	65
4	Detention in jail	63
5	Death of a close family member	63
6	Major personal injury or illness	53
7	Marriage	50
8	Termination of employment	47
9	Marital reconciliation	45
10	Retirement from work	45
11	Major change in health of family	44
12	Pregnancy	40
13	Sexual difficulties	39
14	Addition of a new family member	39
15	Major business adjustment	39
16	Major change in financial state	38
17	Death of a close friend	37
18	Changing to a different line of work	36
19	Major change in arguments with spouse	35
20	Mortgage or loan over $100,000	31
21	Mortgage foreclosure	30
22	Major change in work responsibilities	29
23	Son or daughter leaving home	29
24	In-law troubles	29
25	Outstanding personal achievement	26
26	Spouse starting or ending work	26
27	Start or end formal schooling	26
28	Major change in living conditions	25
29	Major revision of personal habits	24
30	Trouble with employer	23
31	Major change in working conditions	20
32	Changing to a new school	20
33	Changing residence	20
34	Major change in recreation	20
35	Major change in spiritual activities	19
36	Mortgage or loan under $100,000	17
37	Major change in sleeping habits	16
38	Major change in family get-togethers	15
39	Major change in eating habits	15
40	Vacation	13
41	Christmas	12
42	Minor violations of the law	11

Adapted from Holmes TH & Rahe RH. The Social Readjustment Rating Scale.
Journal of Psychosomatic Research 1967; 11: 213–218.

The model portrays a person as a passive recipient of stress. Stress is viewed as a nonchanging, additive phenomenon that can be measured by assigning a score to each life event. People are able to calculate their stress score by counting life events. The score disregards a person's perception of an event, the relationship between events, and the physical and mental disruption caused by an event.

Although the life-change scale may be helpful as a tool to identify people who are at risk, therapists find it is not very useful as a way to understand and manage stress. Because only the total stress score is considered, the model suggests that individuals should avoid additional life-change events, even though such avoidance may not be possible or practical. In some cases, a major life change, such as graduating from college and moving away from an abusive spouse, may be desirable. Furthermore, the model does not account for people who remain well in spite of high scores. It seems reasonable to conclude that viewing stress simply as the sum of stimuli oversimplifies a complex phenomenon.

Stress as Response

The response model defines stress as a nonspecific response of the body to demands placed on it (Selye 1956, 1976). The stress response is represented by the *general adaptation syndrome (GAS)*, shown in Figure 11-1. According to this model, the GAS has three stages: (1) alarm reaction, the first response of the body when exposed to a stressor, (2) adaptation or resistance to demands, called *stressors,* and (3) exhaustion, the result of prolonged exposure to stressors. Every stressful response is characterized by the same three stages. The response model is based on these assumptions:

1. All stressors elicit the same response.

2. Stress is not cognitively mediated.

3. There is a finite amount of adaptive energy.

Selye acknowledged the role of perception in stressful experiences but did not modify his theory to include such things as the cause of the stress, context of the event, or the meaning of an event to a person. He maintained that stress is a nonspecific response of the body to stressors manifested by the general adaptation syndrome.

The response model, like the stimulus model, does not account for individual differences in perception or response. Therapists who

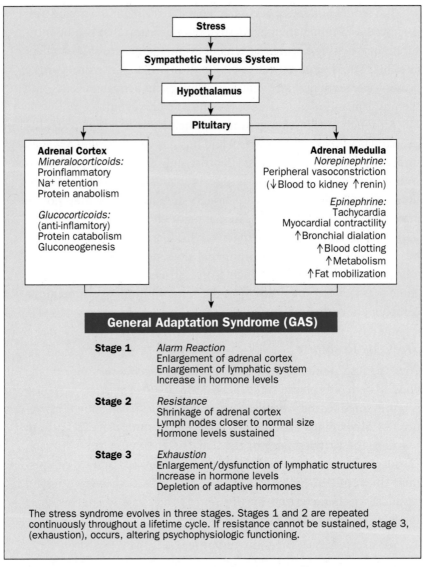

<figure>

Stress

↓

Sympathetic Nervous System

↓

Hypothalamus

↓

Pituitary

Adrenal Cortex
Mineralocorticoids:
Proinflammatory
Na+ retention
Protein anabolism

Glucocorticoids:
(anti-inflamitory)
Protein catabolism
Gluconeogenesis

Adrenal Medulla
Norepinephrine:
Peripheral vasoconstriction
(↓Blood to kidney ↑renin)

Epinephrine:
Tachycardia
Myocardial contractility
↑Bronchial dialation
↑Blood clotting
↑Metabolism
↑Fat mobilization

General Adaptation Syndrome (GAS)

Stage 1	*Alarm Reaction* Enlargement of adrenal cortex Enlargement of lymphatic system Increase in hormone levels
Stage 2	*Resistance* Shrinkage of adrenal cortex Lymph nodes closer to normal size Hormone levels sustained
Stage 3	*Exhaustion* Enlargement/dysfunction of lymphatic structures Increase in hormone levels Depletion of adaptive hormones

The stress syndrome evolves in three stages. Stages 1 and 2 are repeated continuously throughout a lifetime cycle. If resistance cannot be sustained, stage 3, (exhaustion), occurs, altering psychophysiologic functioning.

</figure>

Figure 11-1 Physiologic Response to Stress: The General Adaption Syndrome. Adapted from Smith MJ, Selye H: Reducing the Negative Effects of Stress. *American Journal of Nursing* Nov 1979; 79(10).

use this model advise people who are at risk to take a vacation or relocate to reduce their stress. Such advice does not address life-change events or coping mechanism. Wherever these people go, stress is likely to follow.

Stress as Transaction

The transactional model views stress as a concept that is neither in the environment nor in the person, but a product of their interplay (Lazarus 1991). The person and environment are seen as constantly intertwined, each affecting the other and affected by the other. Stress includes cognitive, affective, and adaptational factors that arise out of person-environment transactions. Unlike the stimulus and response models, the transactional model allows for individual differences in perception, response, and outcome. It acknowledges that some environmental demands produce stress in most people. The transactional model emphasizes that people differ in sensitivity and vulnerability, as well as interpretation of and reaction to demands.

Assumptions of the transactional model are:

1. Stress is not measurable as a single concept.

2. Cognitive appraisal modifies stressful experiences.

Cognitive appraisal is a valuative process that determines why and to what extent particular transactions are stressful. Stress, according to Lazarus (1991), is an interactive process between individuals and their internal and external environments. The transactional model is useful for nurses, both as a way to assist others and to manage their own stress. Interventions focus on exploring how people appraise a potentially stressful event, assessing what coping mechanisms they possess, and helping them develop more effective coping strategies.

Manifestations of Stress

Stress is manifested by physiologic and psychologic symptoms and behaviors. These vary according to the perception of an event and the effectiveness of the coping strategies. Typical physiologic manifestations include those identified by Selye, including increased heart rate, blood pressure, muscle tension, and blood flow to the brain and decreased blood flow to the digestive organs, as well as headache, sweating, dilated pupils, and insomnia.

Psychologic symptoms include feelings of anxiety and anger, verbal and motor responses, cognitive behaviors, and unconscious ego defense mechanisms. Anxiety, a common reaction to stress, is an emotional response to a nonspecific threat. It is experienced at the conscious, subconscious, and unconscious level and is displayed in a continuum from mild anxiety to panic. Anger is an emotional response to an obstacle. In its mild form, anger is manifested as boredom or frustration; in its strongest form, as rage. When individuals fear reprisal, they may exhibit passive-aggressive behavior, such as delaying, ridiculing, or making sarcastic remarks. Motor responses to stress include behaviors such as finger-tapping and tensing of muscles. Cognitive behaviors include intrusive thoughts and the inability to focus on a topic. Unconscious ego defense mechanisms include behaviors such as denial (rejection of reality), rationalization (justifying), and projection (ascribing to another one's own feelings).

Causes of Stress

Stress occurs when demands exceed resources and a person feels overwhelmed and threatened, unable to meet requirements and endangered by circumstances. Such demands may be extrapersonal, interpersonal, or intrapersonal. *Extrapersonal demands* include such things as bright light, noise, odor, air current, temperature, and aesthetics. *Interpersonal demands* come from other people. *Intrapersonal demands* are based on values and beliefs the person holds. Emily, whose story begins this chapter, experienced all three: extrapersonal demands from the environment; interpersonal demands from her unit manager, clients, instructors, and son; and intrapersonal demands from internal beliefs and values about her need to succeed. Emily's perception that she wasn't meeting these demands made her feel anxious and frustrated. As her stress increased and her peripheral blood vessels constricted, she felt cold. As the vessels in her brain dilated, she developed a throbbing headache. She had difficulty focusing and she felt overwhelmed.

Self-Awareness

Self-awareness is the ability to assess realistically one's external behaviors and internal feelings, especially those that indicate stress-related tension. These include behaviors such as finger-tapping, teeth-grinding, procrastination, and fist-clenching and feelings of impatience, inadequacy, and detachment. Friedman and Rosenman (1974) identify two personality types: type A and type B, noting that type A personalities are more prone to cardiovascular disease than type B personalities. They describe type A personalities as hurried, impatient, and sometimes hostile, and under constant pressure to perform. They describe type B personalities as relaxed, free from the urgency of time, and able to enjoy work or play. Nuernberger (1981) identifies a third type, which he calls type C, the coping personality. The development of self-awareness involves noticing bodily sensations, inner thoughts, and feelings. Such self-awareness opens the door to constructive change.

Dynamics of Stress

From a transactional viewpoint, stress is not an environmental stimulus, a personal characteristic, or a response. It is a relationship, a balance between demands and the capacity to respond to demands without unreasonable cost. People interpret situations with respect to the effect the situations will have on their well-being. Then they consciously or unconsciously decide whether they are able to deal with those demands and what they should do about them. The two-step interpretation process goes like this:

1. An evaluation of the significance of an event to oneself: "Does it matter to me? Am I in trouble?"

2. A judgment concerning options, coping responses, and constraint: "Can I handle this? If so, what can I do about it?"

Stress interpretation includes the potential for future harm or loss. This constitutes a threat. The most frightening life events are those that threaten loss of or harm to the self or significant others. When such a threat is anticipated, a person must do something to manage the situation and reduce the danger. Therefore, what might be done becomes critical. The person must decide what coping strategies are available and what the consequences of each will be.

The potential for stress exists in any situation where a person asks, "Does it matter to me? Am I in trouble?" If the answer is, "No. There is no possible gain or loss," the effect on the person's well-being is minimal and so is the stress. However, if the answer is, "Yes it matters; I am in trouble," the person interprets the situation as threatening and negative because it may cause harm or loss. Equilibrium and balance are disrupted, and stress levels rise. For instance, Emily interpreted her clinical performance as a critical test. This was an important part of the nursing program, and she desperately wanted to succeed. Other students managed similar assignments, and she felt she must prove that she could manage, too.

The second part of stress interpretation regards the person's resources. When confronted with a threatening situation, a person asks: "Can I handle this? If so, what can I do about it?" If the person has a history of prior success and a large repertoire of coping strategies, the answer may be, "Yes, I can handle this. I have in the past, and I know what to do." However, if the answer is, "No, I don't think I can cope; I don't know what to do," the situation produces even greater stress. For instance, Emily recognized that she was in trouble and that she didn't know what to do about it. As a result, her stress increased, and she developed a throbbing headache.

Some researchers have said that the ability to handle stress is related to a personal quality called *hardiness*, an innate or learned capacity to cope with stressors. Kobassa (1979) defines hardiness as a composite of commitment, control, and challenge. Pagana (1990) found that nursing students who scored high on a hardiness scale viewed their work as a challenge rather than a threat. Somehow, they had learned to use a variety of coping mechanisms to manage stress. With a history of past success, they viewed intense situations as challenges rather than threats. Emily needs to appreciate her success to date and realistically appraise her physical and emotional resources.

Stress Management

Stress management begins with self-awareness. It proceeds with balancing demands and resources, regulating feelings, and if need be, changing something in the situation. The person who is managing stress is said to be *coping*. *Coping strategies* imply an ability to manage both the physiologic responses portrayed in Figure 11-1 and the psychologic responses of the emotions. By formulating the questions, "Can I handle this? If so, what can I do?" the person addresses the issue of available resources. The way people cope depends on the strategies they bring to a situation. The greater their store, the greater their ability to handle demands. Thus, coping is a crucial variable in a person's efforts to adapt successfully.

Coping has two functions: (1) to manage the somatic and subjective components of stress-related emotions, called emotion-focused coping, and (2) to change the situation for the better, called problem-focused coping (Lazarus 1991). *Emotion-focused coping* addresses the emotional response to a stressful situation. *Problem-focused coping* addresses the situation itself. When a person uses emotion-focused coping, the troubling situation remains the same, but the emotional response may change. When a person uses problem-focused coping, the situation changes and the threat dissipates; in this way, the person avoids emotional responses.

Emotion-Focused Coping

Emotions are powerful forces that humans develop to help them survive. Plutchik (1980) defines an emotion as a complex sequence of events involving cognitive appraisal, feelings, impulses to action, and overt behaviors. He identifies eight primary emotions: fear, sadness, anger, disgust, joy, acceptance (love), anticipation (hope), and surprise (shock). Although fear is a common emotion in stress, the other emotions also may create disequilibrium. Emotion-focused coping strategies address the sequence of events that makes up an emotion, namely, cognitive appraisal (thinking), feeling, and behaving.

Cognitive appraisal involves using the mind to assess a situation. For example, Emily experienced stress as a result of the demands made on her. Had she used the emotion-focused strategy of cognitive appraisal, she would have assessed and identified her feelings of *fear* of failure and *anger* at her situation, the unit manager, and herself for blocking progress towards her goal.

Feeling is the intense subjective experience of an emotion. Emotion-focused strategies involve acknowledging and allowing yourself to experience the feelings generated by demanding situations. For example, Emily felt the uncomfortable distress of frustration, a form of anger. Had she acknowledged the anger, she could have dealt with it more directly.

Impulses to act are strong urges to help a person survive. They are acts to protect oneself from harm, explore the unknown, orient oneself to the environment, reintegrate after injury, incorporate nurturance, overcome opposition, reproduce, and reject harm. Emily wanted to ignore the unit manager's demands and go on with what she saw as her primary responsibility, to attend class. She did not want to deal with yet another demand.

Behaving is acting to manage an emotion. Emotion-focused strategies involve acting to reduce the intensity of an emotion, or gain control of it. These strategies include self-talk, deep breathing, physical exercise, biofeedback training, and self-hypnosis. For example, had Emily identified her feelings of fear, she could have paused and taken a minute to relax and gain control.

Problem-Focused Coping

Problem-focused coping is directed toward defining a problem, generating alternative solutions, weighing the costs and benefits of alternatives, choosing among them, and acting. Problem-focused coping embraces a wider array of strategies than problem solving alone. It involves an objective, analytic process focusing on the internal and external environment.

To *define a problem,* you must become aware of the manifestations of stress and identify the cause. When Emily noticed her feelings, she needed to stop and define the problem. She felt overwhelmed by her assignment and was afraid to ask for help. She was fearful of what she might find when she arrived at the hospital, and she was angry that the unit manager expected her to leave class and go to the hospital immediately. The overall problem, however, was that Emily was overextended. Attending nursing school, working nights, being pregnant, and being a single parent was more than she could handle.

To *generate alternative solutions,* you must create various ways to solve stressful situations. You can do this by decreasing demands, increasing resources to meet demands, or by changing the way you view demands. During her clinical practicum Emily might have asked for help or given herself permission to accomplish only essential tasks. When confronted by the need to return to the hospital immediately, she might have assertively told the unit manager that she would come right after class or assured the woman that she had given the medication and would sign the record by nightfall. Regarding the fact that she was overextended, Emily might consider reducing her workload, taking an incomplete in one of her courses, or asking a trusted relative to care for her son until the semester ended.

To *weigh the costs and benefits of alternatives,* you need to identify the pros and cons of each solution. Emily needed to weigh the risks of each solution. Would she be judged more incompetent for asking for help than for not asking? Would the unit manager make an issue of a delay in signing the record, or would she accept it? Could Emily feel good about herself if she decided to cut back on her work, take an incomplete in one of her courses, or ask a relative to care for her son for the rest of the semester?

To *choose from alternative solutions,* you make a decision and act. Emily might decide the best solution is to ask for assistance when she needs it. She may decide to use assertive communication to make her needs known. She may decide to take a leave of absence from school and concentrate on parenting.

To *act* means to do what one has proposed to do to solve a problem. To act, Emily will carry out some alternative solutions.

Effective Coping

To deal effectively with a stressful encounter requires both emotion-focused and problem-focused coping. People who manage to change a situation only at great emotional cost cannot be said to be coping effectively. Neither can people who regulate emotions successfully but do not deal with the cause of a problem. Effective coping involves both regulating emotions and managing situations.

Strategies for Coping

Coping strategies are purposeful, thoughtful methods of managing stress. These strategies help people balance demands and resources, change stress-producing factors, and regulate their feelings.

Balancing Demands and Resources Here are some strategies to help you balance demands and resources:

Use cognitive rehearsal. Cognitive rehearsal is the use of imagery to visualize successful coping and self-talk during stressful events. Long distance runners and others who endure long periods of stress use this tactic. For instance, when you are learning to use assertive communication, you may rehearse saying what you see, how you feel, and what you want and then visualize how you think the exchange will go.

Use delaying tactics. Take time to gain perspective by putting off tasks that produce overload. Wait until you have enough information to make a decision, one that is not based on emotions alone. Using delaying tactics is not procrastination. It is a conscious decision to deliberate.

Set limits. Setting limits helps you gain control over your life. You may need to limit interruptions, the number of tasks you agree to accomplish, and the amount of time you spend doing an activity. The question here is *who sets the limits*. When you take charge of your life, *you* set the limits, reducing the likelihood that demands will overpower your resources.

Plan ahead. Planning ahead helps you set limits. Although spontaneity may be pleasant when demands are few and resources are great, impulsive responses often get people into trouble. Planning ahead allows you to match resources with demands.

Control the timing of activities. Controlling the timing of undertakings makes it possible for you to keep them at a reasonable pace, thus reducing the stress produced by flurries of activity.

Develop personal assets. By developing personal assets such as aesthetic talents, financial assets, skills, experience, creativity, and spirituality, you increase your store of resources. When demands come along, these resources will be available as a balance.

Develop environmental assets. Environmental assets are such things as a cheerful home, a support system, and a network of professional and personal associates on whom you can depend. These all increase your store of available resources.

Take responsibility for your choices. Adults have the right to make choices about their lives; they do not have to be victims of circumstances. By taking responsibility for your life you become empowered to act in your own best interest and need not fall into a victim role.

Emily can use all of these coping strategies to balance the demands of her life as a pregnant woman, mother, student, and employee. By planning ahead, prioritizing tasks, and setting limits, she can reduce her stress. By developing a collegial relationship with her classmates, she can call upon them for help when she needs it. By taking responsibility for the choices she makes, Emily will be empowered to act in her own best interest.

Changing Situational Factors Here are some ways to change the threatening aspects of a situation:

Reappraise the situation. Reappraisal means taking a second look. By doing so you may change your view of an event, decrease its importance, modify expectations of yourself and others, and find something good or humorous in a complex situation.

Modify values from absolutes to relatives. Absolutism is black-and-white thinking that creates win-lose situations. By modifying their values, people become more realistic and less judgmental. When Emily recognizes that she can modify her goal and does not have to carry a full course load or work full time, she may not be as overwhelmed.

Talk through concerns with others and seek their feedback. Discussions with others who understand a situation gives new perspectives. Such conversations help you objectify problems and reach better solutions. You can remove some of the threat of unexpected censure by proactively seeking feedback from others. If Emily asks for feedback from her classmates or clinical instructor, she may learn more efficient methods of managing her assignment and reducing her level of stress.

Identify and acknowledge emotions. By identifying and honestly acknowledging feelings, you will find it easier to resolve issues that produce emotional responses. Denying how you feel is self-defeating and prevents reality-based problem solving.

Focus self-talk statements on accomplishments and abilities. By focusing your self-talk on accomplishments and abilities rather than failures, you are more likely to feel successful. As Emily considered her life, she might have given herself credit for all that she had accomplished so far, but instead, she focused on her aloneness and her fear of failure.

Managing Anger and Frustration We feel anger when we are blocked from accomplishing a goal or objective. The emotion ranges in intensity from mild boredom to frustration, anger, and rage. Although conventional wisdom advises people to vent their anger, research shows that anger is magnified by venting, not lessened (Lazarus 1991, Travis 1983). Here are some ways to manage anger:

- Acknowledge your feelings of anger and frustration; others don't make you angry, you make you angry.

- Discover what goal is being blocked.

- Identify who or what is blocking your goal.

- List assumptions about your right to achieve your goal.

- Decide how important your goal is.

- Use assertive rather than passive-aggressive communication.

- Decide to fight for the goal, abandon the goal, or compromise graciously.

When you do these things you are able to let go of anger and move on with your life. The boxes on pages 352 and 353 give some exercises to help you manage anger and frustration.

Managing Guilt, Blame, and Shame Guilt is an experience of sadness, self-anger, and fear of the consequences of doing, thinking, or feeling something that is inconsistent with internalized ideals or values. Blame is the experience of feeling anger toward others when they fail to behave in ways that fit your ideals or values. Shame is the experience of feeling sad, angry, and fearful of rejection when you fail to behave in ways that fit society's ideals and values. Here are some

Exercise to Manage Anger

Directions: Answer each question "Yes" or "No":

1. Is my expectation a self-expectation?
2. Is my expectation an expectation of another?
3. Is my expectation realistic?
4. Have I verbalized my anger?
5. Have I attempted to change my expectations?

Strategies:

A. If you answered "Yes" to questions 1 and 4, then you need to work on changing unrealistic aspects of your self-expectations.
B. If you answered "Yes" to questions 2 and 4, then you need to work on changing unrealistic aspects of your expectations of others.
C. If you answered "Yes" to question 2, then you need to work on changing unrealistic expectations.
D. If you answered "Yes" to questions 2 and 3, you need to learn to verbalize your anger appropriately.
E. If you answered "Yes" to questions 2, 3, 4, and 5, you are well on your way to managing anger.

Adapted from Lyon BL. *Stress Management, an Essential Ingredient for Good Health,* 1984.

ways to manage guilt, blame, and shame:

- Acknowledge feeling angry toward yourself and others.
- Apologize and make restitution to those you have damaged.
- Recognize that ideal behavior is not always possible in nonideal situations.
- View shame-producing events as learning experiences.
- Recognize that the intensity of feelings lessens with time.
- Forgive yourself or others.
- Go on. The past cannot be changed. Life is an experience of the present—not the past, not the future.

Exercise to Manage Frustration

Directions: When you find yourself blocked, answer the following questions.

1. What is my goal?
2. What is the time-frame for accomplishing my goal?
3. What ingredients does it take to accomplish my goal?
4. Is the goal realistic for me?
5. Am I able to provide the ingredients to ensure accomplishment of my goal?
6. Am I able to manipulate my environment so that I can facilitate accomplishing my goal?
7. Am I capable of developing over time necessary ingredients to accomplish my goal?
8. Is the time-frame for goal accomplishment realistic?
9. If not, have I broken the goal down into accomplishable steps?
10. As I move toward accomplishing my goal, do I need to experience early gratification?
11. What blocks prevent me from accomplishing my goal?
12. Is the block an internal one, such as lack of skill or knowledge, fear of success, or unwillingness to spend the necessary time, effort, and energy?
13. Is the block an external one, such as institutional policies, or funds, or other persons?
14. Have I imagined that there is a block without concrete evidence that it actually exists?
15. If the block is real, have I tried to overcome the block?
16. Do I need to consider modifying my goal?
17. Would failure to accomplish my goal have negative consequences on what I think of myself?
18. Have I had similar experiences of frustration in the past?
19. Was I able to deal with those experiences successfully?
20. Can I use similar strategies in the current situation?
21. Am I expending a lot of energy responding to this situation?
22. Do I experience frustration as an opportunity to problem-solve in a creative way?
23. In what ways can I facilitate successful management of my frustration?

Adapted from Lyon BL. *Stress Management, an Essential Ingredient for Good Health,* 1984.

Exercise to Manage Guilt

Directions: Answer "Yes" or "No" to questions 1 to 7, then answer
questions A to D.

1. Is your self-expectation realistic?
2. Is your self-expectation part of your value system?
3. Was someone hurt as a consequence of your actions?
4. Can you correct the situation?
5. Are you punishing yourself for your actions?
6. Can you learn something from the situation?
7. Have you attempted to correct the situation?

A. If you answered "Yes" to questions 2, 5, and 6, re-examine your expectations in relation to your values and the situation.
B. If you answered "Yes" to questions 1, 2, 4, 5, and 6, attempt to correct the situation.
C. If you answered "Yes" to questions 1, 4, 5, 6, and 7, refer to the anger management exercises.
D. If you answered "Yes" to questions 2, 3, 5, 6, and 7, identify what you can learn from the experience, avoid repeating such actions in the future, accept the reality of the situation, forgive yourself, and go on.

Adapted from Lyon BL. *Stress Management, an Essential Ingredient for Good Health*, 1984.

The accompanying box gives some exercises to help you manage guilt, blame, and shame.

Nurturing Self-Esteem People with low self-esteem are especially vulnerable to the stress-related emotions of fear, anger, guilt, blame, and shame. Therefore, strategies that build self-esteem help prevent damaging levels of stress. Some of these include: (1) setting realistic personal goals and expectations, (2) engaging in positive self-talk, (3) viewing "failure" as a learning experience, and (4) focusing on positive aspects of difficult situations.

Accepting the Givens People who base their expectations and actions on the ideal rather than the real set themselves up for failure and frustration. Here are some coping strategies to help you avoid unrealistic expectations:

- Learn what is possible and is not possible in the real workaday world.

- Accurately assess your values, beliefs, limitations, abilities, competencies, priorities, experience, and energy levels.

- Make a factual appraisal of the work environment and the people who work there.

- Make the best use of the real, not the ideal.

Learning to Relax Relaxation is an effective way to reduce stress. Relaxation helps reduce tension and rest muscles, promote peripheral blood flow, and normalize heart and breathing patterns. It provides psychologic calm and spiritual peace. There are many methods for producing a relaxed state of mind and body. Some people use prayer; others, meditation. The box on pages 356 and 357 gives an exercise you can use to begin to relax.

Developing a Social Support Network A network is a group of people to whom we can go for support, information, and guidance. We find these people in our neighborhood, at work, in various organizations, at school, in the stores where we shop, and among the members of our family. One of the great advantages of a network is that it is made up of people with a variety of talents, experiences, and points of view. Networks change over time and differ from person to person. A network provides (1) esteem support, (2) instrumental support, (3) informational support, and (4) social companionship. *Esteem support* fosters productivity and creativity and gives a sense of belonging, acceptance, and encouragement. *Instrumental support* provides material aid, financial assistance, and services. It offers concrete help when it is needed most. *Informational support* provides facts and guidance for decision making. *Social companionship* offers pleasurable activities and recreation. A social support network is a resource we can use to balance demands and reduce stress.

Networking is the process of communicating with members of your network for the purpose of sharing resources and information. Networking is not all take and no give. A network makes demands on its members. It is dynamic and reciprocal in nature; members expect

Relaxation Exercise

Directions: Choose a quiet area, assume a comfortable position, and repeat each statement several times as you passively concentrate on a particular part of your body.

My feet feel warm.

My feet feel heavy.

My feet are warm and heavy.

> *I feel very much at ease.*
>
> *I feel comfortable and relaxed.*

My right leg feels warm.

My right leg feels heavy.

My right leg feels warm and heavy.

My left leg feels warm.

My left leg feels heavy.

My left leg feels warm and heavy.

Both my legs feel warm and heavy.

> *I feel very much at ease.*
>
> *I feel comfortable and relaxed.*

My right arm feels warm.

My right arm feels heavy.

My right arm feels warm and heavy.

My left arm feels warm.

My left arm feels heavy.

My left arm feels warm and heavy.

➤

assistance and support in return for what they give. A network functions because its members identify with and feel positively toward one another. If one member becomes overly dependent, aggressive, or competitive with other members, mutuality is destroyed and the connection ceases to exist. If Emily had a social support network, she might not have felt so alone and fearful.

Communicating Assertively Assertive communication is honest, straightforward exchange of information. It enables individuals to act in their own best interest, to stand up for themselves without undue anxiety, to express honest feelings comfortably, and to exercise personal rights without denying the rights of others. Assertive communi-

Both my arms feel warm and heavy.

My hands feel warm.

My hands feel heavy.

My hands feel warm and heavy.

I feel very much at ease.

I feel comfortable and relaxed.

My abdomen feels warm.

My abdomen feels heavy.

My abdomen feels warm and heavy.

My chest feels warm.

My chest feels heavy.

My chest feels warm and heavy.

I feel very much at ease.

I feel comfortable and relaxed.

My shoulders feel warm.

My shoulders feel heavy.

My shoulders feel warm and heavy.

My head and neck feel warm.

My head and neck feel heavy.

My head and neck feel warm and heavy.

I feel very much at ease.

I feel comfortable and relaxed.

Adapted from Lyon BL. *Stress Management, an Essential Ingredient for Good Health*, 1984.

cation is the opposite of passive-aggressive communication, in which anger is clothed in sarcasm or vented in libelous gossip. Assertive communication involves an objective, nonemotional, nonjudgmental exchange of information, based on respect of oneself and others.

To communicate assertively, (1) state what you believe to be true, using "I" rather than "you" statements, (2) state how you feel about the situation, owning your emotions, and (3) state what you want or need relative to the situation. For example, when the unit manager demanded Emily's immediate return, Emily might have made these statements: (1) "I remember giving the 10:00 AM antibiotic and appreciate how important it is to keep accurate records." (2) "I am upset about the oversight and will not let it happen again." (3) "I need to be in class until 3:00 PM, but will return to sign the record just as soon as class is over."

Assertive communication is not a one-way dialogue. It includes a willingness to listen to another point of view. When people listen to another perspective, they gain new information. This information opens the door to compromise. As a result, emotions as well as wants and needs may change. For example, in response to Emily's assertive communication, the unit manager might have responded this way: (1) "I realize that your assignment this morning was heavy, but antibiotics must be given on time and as scheduled." (2) "I feel uncomfortable asking you to come back to the hospital." (3) "Even so, I must insist you do so as soon as possible because the patient is being transferred and his record must be complete."

Assertive communication is especially useful as a coping strategy to reduce stress. It helps objectify issues by stating clearly what the problem is and what emotion is being experienced. Assertive communication provides a tool to either change a situation or alter negative feelings about the situation. It affirms respect for oneself and others.

◆ Emotional Exhaustion (Burnout)

Emotional exhaustion (burnout) occurs when members of the helping professions lose concern and feelings for those they are trying to help, treating them in detached, dehumanized ways. Some writers attribute this exhaustion to "an attempt to cope with the stress of intense interpersonal work by distancing oneself from the source of painful experiences" (Wilson & Kniesl 1992). Schlomann (1993) suggests replacing the term *burnout* with *exploitation*: she would solve the problem by giving nurses greater autonomy through empowerment.

The unit manager shows symptoms of emotional exhaustion when she calls clients "hippos" and "wackos." Nurses who withdraw from clients and hide in a nurses' station are manifesting emotional exhaustion. Such exhaustion may be evidenced in the rigid application of rules that keep nurses from thinking of clients as individuals. Emotional exhaustion changes caring people into mechanical bureaucrats. It is the result of an unsuccessful effort to manage overwhelming demands. Its sufferers experience headaches, fatigue, lack of enthusiasm, and feelings of powerlessness and hopelessness.

Here are some strategies to reduce the likelihood of emotional exhaustion:

- Nurture yourself by getting adequate sleep and recreation and by expanding your interests.

- Use a social support network to express, share, and analyze feelings of frustration.

- Become empowered; work for greater autonomy within the nursing profession.

- Work for respite days to replace guilt-producing "mental health escapes."

- Work for increased nurse-client ratios so that nurses can provide sensitive, humanistic care.

- Explore your personal motives for becoming a caregiver. Are you filling a need to be needed or to control others?

◆ Surviving Shift Work

Most clinical experiences of student nurses takes place during the day. When students graduate, however, they must often work evenings and nights. This change in the work-sleep cycle greatly increases the stress that new nurses experience. Sleep research studies suggest ways to reduce this stress and help nurses successfully cope with shift work.

Sleep and Health

By nature, humans are diurnal creatures; that is, they are awake during hours of light and asleep during hours of dark. North Americans normally sleep about one-third of every 24-hour cycle, or about 6 to 9 hours a day. Very few people can sleep less than 5 hours per day without suffering serious mood and performance deficits. In fact, death rates are higher in people who sleep less than 7 hours or more than 10 hours per day (Coleman 1986). Adequate sleep, therefore, is essential to health and a feeling of well-being.

Sleep and Performance

Not only is the number of hours of sleep important, but the time of sleep is critical to performance. Workers who are sleep-deprived make serious mistakes. The nuclear accident at Three Mile Island, the Union Carbide chemical explosion in Bhopal, and the nuclear disaster at Chernobyl all occurred during the night shift. Because nurses must work at peak performance at all hours of the day and night, they need to sleep when their bodies say it is time to sleep.

Sleep Cycle

Biologic Clocks

The timing of bodily functions is set by biologic clocks, innate physiologic systems in humans that measure the passage of time. Each physiologic function has its own unique pattern that cycles over a 24-hour period. The body temperature cycle is of particular interest to shift workers because mental alertness closely follows its curve. During night hours, the temperature of the body drops by 2 to 3 degrees. As long as people stay on regular day schedules, the biologic clock operates efficiently, and they barely notice its effects. However, when the biologic clock must adjust to a new schedule, either as a result of work shifts or jet travel, the system becomes stressed. Figure 11-2 shows the sleep and alertness cycle of a worker starting a new night-shift rotation after being off for 2 days.

Resetting the Clock

Shift-workers and jet travelers need not despair. Within certain limits the biologic clock can reset itself and run autonomously. Because the internal clock, left on its own, gravitates to a 25-hour day, it is easier for people to stay up later than to go to bed earlier. In general, people can reset the 25-hour clock about 2 hours each day, allowing them to live comfortably on a 23- to 27-hour day. When they wish to adjust to a new sleep cycle, they find it less difficult to move in a clockwise direction than a counterclockwise one. Thus, if you must adjust to a new schedule, the most natural biologic direction is to move from day to evening to night work. The least natural is to move from night, to evening, to day work.

Hospitals do not shut down at the end of the day, and nurses who work during the evening and night need to adjust their lives to reduce the stress such work creates. Here are some things you can do to help you adjust to shift work:

- Remain on one shift, such as evenings, for several months at a time rather than rotating from one shift to another.

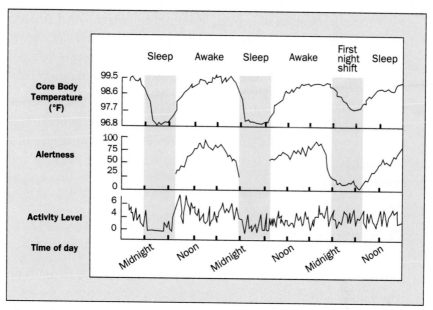

Figure 11-2 Sleep and alertness cycle of a worker starting a new night shift rotation. From Coleman RM. *Wide Awake at 3:00 AM By Choice or By Chance?* Stanford Alumni Association, 1986.

- Follow the same sleep-wake cycle on days off as on work days.

- If rotating schedules are necessary, rotate from days to evenings to nights, resetting the sleep-wake cycle by 2 hours (going to bed two hours later) during days off.

- During sleep, duplicate night-time sleeping conditions as much as possible by reducing light, noise, and interruptions.

- Consider 12-hour shifts, if they are offered, so that you will have 3 or 4 days to adjust the sleep-wake cycle.

- Discuss the need for restful sleep with your family and work out a mutually acceptable plan.

- Make friends with other people who work evenings and nights to reduce feelings of loneliness and isolation.

- When working at night, dress warmly to maintain your body temperature at daytime levels.

- Participate in professional activities and work-related committees to avoid feelings of powerlessness and victimization.

- Count the benefits of working evenings and nights, such as a less harried environment, more chances to meet client needs, opportunities for education or hobbies during the day, more pay per hour of work, and more time with children and significant others.

Undoubtedly, Emily was not getting adequate or restful sleep. Some of these strategies might have reduced her stress. Many nurses enjoy the reduced stress they experience when they work evening and nights, and they find it an excellent schedule for working and rearing children.

◇ Summary

Stress is conceptualized as a stimulus, a response, and a transaction. The stimulus model attributes stress to life-change events. Each life event is given a score; the total score indicates the amount of stress. The response model defines stress as a nonspecific response of the body to demands placed on it. People are advised to reduce their stress before they reach the exhaustion stage. The transaction model attributes stress to cognitive, affective, and adaptational factors arising from people-environment transactions. It emphasizes differences in sensitivity and interpretation of demands. It suggests people develop coping strategies to manage stress by balancing demands and resources, regulating feelings, and changing situations. Coping strategies include management of anger, guilt, blame, and shame; self-nurturance; acceptance; relaxation; networking; and assertive communication. Emotional exhaustion (burnout) is an unsatisfactory attempt to manage stress. It may be due to overwork and feelings of powerlessness. Sleep deprivation is another source of stress. A number of strategies to reduce its detrimental effects are described.

Critical Thinking Questions

1. What new insights did you gain by considering stress from three theoretical positions?

2. What questions arise as you consider various strategies for coping with stress?

3. Is burnout a personal experience or is it shared? Do you think you could ever experience burnout as a nurse? How would it make you feel about yourself?

Learning Activities

1. Using the Social Readjustment Rating Scale, add up your score for the past 12 months. Are you at risk for major life disruption (a score over 100 points)? If so, can you make any changes in your life to reduce the score?

2. Focus on yourself. Are you exhibiting any of the psychologic or physiologic manifestations of stress described by Selye?

3. List the demands placed upon you and the resources you have to meet them.

4. Use the exercises described in this chapter to reduce frustration, anger, fear, and guilt.

5. Use assertive communication to tell another person something you believe she or he needs to hear. Ask that person to do the same for you.

6. Keep a record of your sleep-wake cycle for a week.

7. If you work evenings or nights, take your temperature every 3 hours. Compare your alertness level with your temperature reading.

Annotated Reading List

Pagana KD. The Relationship of Hardiness and Social Support to Student Appraisal of Stress in an Initial Clinical Nursing Situation. *Journal of Nursing Education* Jun 1990; 29(6): 255–61.

This interesting article describes research that examined the stressful nature of the first clinical experience of 246 student nurses. Using the transactional model of Lazarus, the researchers employed hardiness and social support as variables. They found that students who felt challenged rather than threatened by their first clinical experience scored higher on the hardiness scale and had work-related social support.

Schlomann P. Burnout or Exploitation? *Revolution—The Journal of Nursing Empowerment*. Winter 1993.

Declaring that "burnout blames the victim," the author traces the history of the term *burnout* from 1974, when Freudenberger defined it a "condition of over-dedicated and committed caregivers." Because it focuses on the individual, this view overlooks the possibility that burnout may be a functional response to a mechanistic model of health care. The result, Schlomann concludes, is "low self-esteem, lack of identity, horizontal violence, and passive-aggressive syndrome, all responses to oppression!" Rather than being deviant or sick, nurses who experience burnout may be "reflections of a deviant or sick system." Schlomann concludes that "empowerment strategies, rather than stress-reduction exercises, are more appropriate for dealing constructively with burnout/exploitation."

References

Coleman RM. *Wide Awake at 3:00 A.M. By Choice or By Chance?* Stanford Alumni Association, 1986.

Friedman M, Rosenman R. *Type A Behavior and Your Heart*. Fawcett, 1974.

Holmes TH, Rahe RH. The Social Readjustment Rating Scale. *Journal of Psychosomatic Research* 1967; 11:213–218.

Kobassa S. Stressful Life Events, Personality, and Health: An Inquiry into Hardiness. *Journal of Personality & Social Psychology* 1979; 37(1):1–11.

Lazarus RS. *Emotion and Adaptation*. Oxford University Press, 1991.

Lyon BL. *Stress Management, an Essential Ingredient for Good Health*. 1984. (Available from author: Indiana University School of Nursing, 610 Barnhill Drive, Indianapolis IN, 42620.)

Nuernberger P. *Freedom from Stress: A Holistic Approach.* The Himalayan International Institute of Yoga Science and Philosophy, 1981.

Pagana KD. The Relationship of Hardiness and Social Support to Student Appraisal of Stress in an Initial Clinical Nursing Situation. *Journal of Nursing Education* Jun 1990; 29(6): 255–61.

Plutchik R. *Emotion: A Psychoevolutionary Synthesis.* Harper and Row, 1980.

Schlomann P. Burnout or Exploitation? *Revolution—The Journal of Nursing Empowerment.* Winter 1993.

Selye H. *The Stress of Life.* McGraw-Hill, 1956.

Selye H. *The Stress of Life;* 2nd ed. McGraw-Hill, 1976.

Smith MJ, Selye H. Reducing the Negative Effects of Stress. *American Journal of Nursing* Nov 1979; 79(10).

Travis C. *Anger: The Misunderstood Emotion.* Simon & Schuster, 1983.

Wilson HC, Kniesl CR. *Psychiatric Nursing,* 4th ed. Addison-Wesley, 1992.

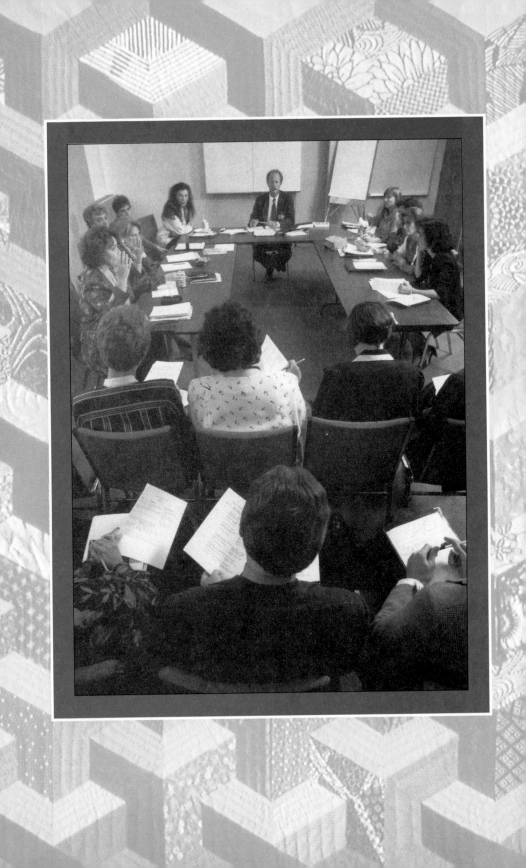

Collective Bargaining

12

◆ Learning Objectives

- List the four essential elements of a legally enforceable contract.

- Compare formal and simple contracts, written and oral contracts, and expressed and implied contracts.

- Discuss the elements of a sound employment contract.

- Trace the history of labor laws in the United States since 1935, naming some of the most significant legislation as it affects nurses.

- Describe some important functions of the National Labor Relations Board.

- Describe unfair labor practices prohibited to labor unions and employers.

- Explain the steps of organizing a union.

- Describe the collective bargaining process to negotiate a contract with an employer.

- Explain the purpose and process of typical grievance procedures.

- Discuss the purpose and process of arbitration.

- Discuss the actions employers can take to prevent discontent among personnel.

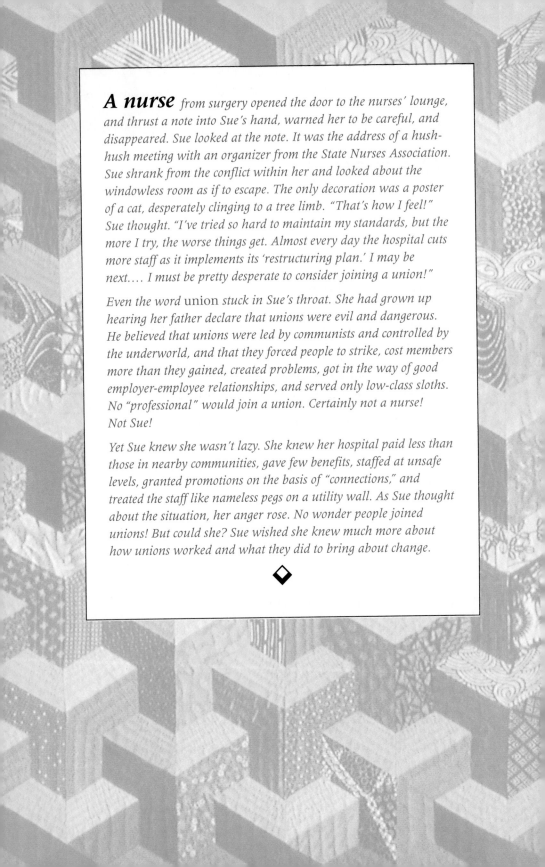

A *nurse* from surgery opened the door to the nurses' lounge, and thrust a note into Sue's hand, warned her to be careful, and disappeared. Sue looked at the note. It was the address of a hush-hush meeting with an organizer from the State Nurses Association. Sue shrank from the conflict within her and looked about the windowless room as if to escape. The only decoration was a poster of a cat, desperately clinging to a tree limb. "That's how I feel!" Sue thought. "I've tried so hard to maintain my standards, but the more I try, the worse things get. Almost every day the hospital cuts more staff as it implements its 'restructuring plan.' I may be next.... I must be pretty desperate to consider joining a union!"

Even the word union stuck in Sue's throat. She had grown up hearing her father declare that unions were evil and dangerous. He believed that unions were led by communists and controlled by the underworld, and that they forced people to strike, cost members more than they gained, created problems, got in the way of good employer-employee relationships, and served only low-class sloths. No "professional" would join a union. Certainly not a nurse! Not Sue!

Yet Sue knew she wasn't lazy. She knew her hospital paid less than those in nearby communities, gave few benefits, staffed at unsafe levels, granted promotions on the basis of "connections," and treated the staff like nameless pegs on a utility wall. As Sue thought about the situation, her anger rose. No wonder people joined unions! But could she? Sue wished she knew much more about how unions worked and what they did to bring about change.

◆

Nurses everywhere are concerned about their economic status. They realize that the shortage of nurses has ended and that health care facilities are "down-sizing" and replacing professional nurses with unlicensed "assistive personnel." Nurses are concerned about the quality of care and professional standards and have banded together with others to bargain with employers for improved RN-patient ratios, control of professional practice, greater autonomy, and improved compensation. For some nurses, the decision to join a union is difficult. Many consider union activity unprofessional, even when the state nurses association represents them. They see negotiations for wages and working conditions as obstructing rather than facilitating quality care. Some nurses hesitate to trust their economic and professional welfare to an organization, preferring to negotiate directly with employers as individuals. Others find the cost of union dues and the commitment of time and effort more than they can handle. Still others are nurse managers or entrepreneurs who prefer a direct relationship with those they manage, without the constraints unions impose.

Securing satisfactory working conditions is a serious matter, one that all nurses need to consider. Joining a union may or may not be the way you choose to achieve your career goals. However, if you know little about contracts, union organizations, collective bargaining, and settling disputes, read on.

◆ Contracts

When a health care facility offers you a position, it enters into an employment contract with you. You will want to read the contract carefully, understand the terms and conditions and notice if crucial elements of the contract are present. See the box on page 370 for key terms used in contracts.

Essential Features of Contracts

Every contract, to be enforceable by law, must have four essential features: (1) promises made between two or more legally competent parties to do or not to do something, (2) mutual understanding of the terms and obligations of the contract by all parties, (3) compensation in the form of something of value in exchange for an action or inaction, and (4) a lawful purpose (Creighton 1986).

Key Terms Used in Contracts

Breach of contract: Failing to perform all or part of the contracted duty without justification.

Contract: Legally binding agreement between two or more people to do, or not do, something.

Contract violations: Actions that break mutually agreed-on rules.

Expressed contract: Verbal or written agreement between two or more people to do, or not do, something.

Implied contract: Verbal or written agreement, inferred rather than expressed, between two or more people to do, or not do something.

Invalid contract: An agreement involving illegal or impossible actions; no legal obligation exists.

Terminate: To fulfill all contractual obligations or absolve oneself of the obligation to fulfill them.

Reprinted with permission from Nurse's Reference Library: *Practices.* Springhouse, 1984.

As a legally binding agreement between two or more people to do or not do something, a contract can be enforced by court action. Of course, if fraud, coercion, or an illegal act is involved, the contract is invalid or void, and the courts will not enforce it. If either party to a legal contract fails to perform its part of an agreement, the damaged party can seek relief in the courts. The damaged party also can seek penalties for noncompliance with the contract. For instance, if a nurse borrows money from a bank but fails to make the agreed-upon payments, the bank can take the nurse to court to enforce the contract. If a hospital agrees to pay a nurse $18 per hour but actually pays a different rate, the nurse can take the hospital to court to force it to fulfill the agreement.

Types of Contracts

Formal and Simple Contracts

A *formal contract* is one required by law to be in writing. To prevent fraudulent practices, each state has a statute of frauds that requires that certain contracts, such as deeds and mortgages, be written. Some formal contracts also must be under seal, that is, they must be written on paper imprinted or stamped with an official seal. All other contracts are called *simple,* whether they are written or oral.

Written and Oral Contracts

Oral contracts are just as binding as written contracts, but they may create problems. Because the terms and conditions of oral contracts are not written down, they are subject to memory and interpretation. The passage of time and changes in policies or personnel of an institution may blur the original meaning, causing disagreement between the parties about the terms of the contract. As a result, most state courts do not consider oral contracts valid unless the terms can be fulfilled within a year (*Nurse's Handbook* 1992).

Expressed and Implied Contracts

An *expressed contract* may be written or oral. For example, during a job interview Luz is offered a position as a staff nurse for a certain shift at a certain salary. If she agrees verbally to the offer, she enters into an *oral expressed* contract. If she signs a contract, she enters into a *written expressed* contract. On the way home Luz stops by a hair salon. Even though she does not sign an agreement or discuss the price, Luz, by having her hair cut, enters into an *implied contract* and must pay for the service she receives.

Most contracts contain implied conditions, elements of agreement that are not explicitly stated but are assumed to be part of the contract. For example, hospitals assume that registered nurses will practice in a safe, competent manner, as defined by the state nurse practice act. Nurses assume that the hospital will staff the units with qualified personnel and will provide necessary supplies and equipment for them do to their job (Creighton 1986).

Individual and Collective Contracts

Contracts with employers may be *individual* (those negotiated personally by individuals) or *collective* (those negotiated by a labor union for employees). Most individual contracts are negotiated informally, and the nurse accepts without question the contract offered by the agency. Collective contracts, by contrast, are negotiated formally, spelling out specifics in detail. Such precision leaves less room for interpretation but also leaves less room for flexibility in real-life situations involving the delivery of nursing care.

After deciding to accept an employment contract, a nurse can sign the contract, verbally agree to it, provide a written acceptance of it, or simply report for work. By reporting for work the nurse gives implied agreement to the terms of the contract. However, if a nurse fails to respond in any way to an employment offer, no contract exists. The employer is free to withdraw the offer without penalty at any time before it is accepted (*Nurse's Handbook* 1992).

Termination and Breach of Contract

It is important for nurses to know how to end, or terminate a contract. One way is for each party to fulfill all the terms of a contract or for both parties to agree to end it. Another way is for one party to release the other from further obligation to the contract. Some contracts provide for termination at the end of a fixed time or on the occurrence of an event, such as completion of a project. Most individual employment contracts do not state termination dates. They may be ended by either party by following procedures prescribed in the contract.

When people breach a contract, they have unjustifiably failed to perform all or part of their contractual duty. A substantial breach of contract is never lawful. If Joe signs a contract agreeing to work the night shift for a minimum of 6 months but after 2 months refuses to do so, he is breaching his contract. The hospital can discharge him and seek an injunction against him. An *injunction* is a court order to refrain from some specific act, such as working for any other hospital. Because obtaining an injunction is complex and expensive, hospitals rarely seek injunctions against nurses. Even so, such a breach may damage Joe's reputation and make it difficult for him to get a job at another hospital.

Elements of a Sound Employment Contract

When you go to work for an institution with a union contract, you sign an individual contract with the agency, agreeing to a work assignment, to a beginning classification, and to the terms of the union contract in effect at that time. It is important for you to recognize the features of a sound employment contract. If you go to work for a nonunion agency, such knowledge is even more vital. In that situation, to protect yourself, you may want to hire an attorney to explain the implications of the proposed contract before you sign.

Collective contracts are written by the representatives of organized employees and their employers. Each contract looks different from any other. Even the names vary. One may be called an agreement, another a memorandum of understanding, and still another a contract. Although the items may appear in a different sequence and be called by different words, a sound employment contract includes certain items:

1. *Date and parties to the agreement.* The contract declares who is entering into a contract and when: "This Memorandum of Understanding was made and entered into September 1, 1995, by and between the Illinois Nurses Association...and the Petaluma Valley Hospital District...and covers all Registered Nurses...in those classifications specified in Article II."

2. *Preamble or purpose.* The contract states the overall reason for the contract: "Both parties recognize that it is to their mutual advantage and for the protection of the patients to have efficient and uninterrupted operation of the Hospital. This agreement is for the purpose of establishing such harmonious and constructive relationships between the parties that such results shall be possible."

3. *Recognition of representatives.* The contract states that the employer formally recognizes the legal authority of union representatives: "The Hospital recognizes the Association as the exclusive representative of the nurses covered by this Agreement for the purpose of establishing mutual satisfactory conditions of employment."

4. *Coverage.* The contract stipulates which employees are covered by the contract: "This Agreement covers all Registered Nurses, excluding Head Nurses and Supervisors, as defined in the National Labor Relations Act." First-level nurse managers are usually covered unless specifically excluded.

5. *Hospital rights.* The contract affirms areas of authority reserved by the institution: "The Hospital retains all the rights, powers, and authority exercised or had by it except as may be limited by a specific provision of the Agreement."

6. *Association rights.* The contract affirms specific rights of the union regarding membership, dues collection, and access to members. In a *closed shop*, membership in the union is mandatory. New hires must join within a specific period of time if they are to continue working. The employer may also agree to deduct membership dues from employee paychecks, as authorized, to remit the money to the union, and to permit the union to visit the agency, post notices, and to use meeting rooms as available.

7. *Classifications of nurses.* The contract describes the various levels of nurses, such as Staff Nurse I, II, and III, and how to advance from one level to the next.

8. *Scheduling categories.* The contract states how full-time, part-time, per diem, on call, call-back, and other categories are defined, how nurses may change from one category to another, and how fringe benefits are calculated. This section may be long and detailed.

9. *Compensation.* The contract addresses wages and salaries, often with a grid of classifications, scheduling category, and years of service, stating specific dollar amounts. It may have subsections stipulating credit for tenure, academic degrees, special certification, certain shifts, holidays, special services, and relief for higher classifications and on-call differentials.

10. *Hours of work.* The contract describes procedures governing normal shift schedules, mandatory shift rotation (if any), weekends off, extra shifts, rest periods, lunch periods, overtime, double shifts, late calls, posting the schedule, reporting pay, guaranteed hours of work per pay period, the right to object to a work assignment, and the method to register that objection.

11. *Education and training.* The contract addresses educational leaves, inservice education, and mandatory recertification.

12. *Holidays.* The contract lists recognized holidays and specifies compensation for working on those days.

13. *Vacations.* The contract states accrual rate of vacation hours and addresses the issue of holidays and sickness during vacations and vacation time carry over.

14. *Sick leave.* The contract states how sick leave is accrued, when it begins, and when it can be used.

15. *Leaves of absence.* The contract recognizes that bereavement, medical, maternity, military, parental, jury duty, and personal leaves may be needed and stipulates procedures to apply for them.

16. *Insurance.* The contract describes available dental, vision, medical, disability, and life insurance, stating the amount or the percentage of the premiums paid by the agency.

17. *Retirement and pension.* The contract describes retirement and pension plans available through the agency and amounts paid by the

agency. Desirable features are pension plans that are transferrable if the nurse moves and retirement accounts that have immediate vesting and portability.

18. *Seniority.* The contract defines seniority: how it is accrued, how it affects temporary and permanent work reductions (lay-offs) and advancement, and how it is lost. An affirmation of the principle of "last hired, first fired" is desirable.

19. *Posting and filling of vacancies.* The contract describes the method of announcing staff vacancies, criteria for filling them, and means for employees to bid for work assignments.

20. *Professional performance committee (PPC).* The contract authorizes the formation of a PPC and defines its composition, meetings, purpose (to improve patient care), and role, if advisory. If the PPC is empowered, the contract defines its limits of power and the enforcement process.

21. *Discipline for cause with due process.* The contract describes the procedure for discipline, suspension, and discharge of nurses who do not meet performance criteria. "For cause" ensures that discipline is not frivolous. "Due process" provides a mechanism for correction of deficiencies and endorses rehabilitation programs for impaired nurses. Managers must follow these procedures precisely when they discipline staff.

22. *Grievance procedure.* The contract defines a grievance as "Any dispute, claim, or complaint involving the interpretation or application of any of the provisions of this Agreement, except of those Articles or provisions which state that they are not subject to the grievance procedure." The contract states that individuals or the union may file a grievance. It affirms that individuals may be represented at any meeting or hearing they think may lead to disciplinary action and describes the grievance procedure in detail.

23. *No strike or lockout.* The contract stipulates that there will not be a strike, slowdown, or other work stoppage by the nurses or a lockout by the hospital during the life of the agreement.

24. *Terms of agreement.* The contract states the effective dates of the contract, often "extending it from year to year thereafter without change or amendment unless either party serves notice in writing to the other party."

◇ Union Organizations

Historical Background

The history of unions in Europe can be traced to medieval guilds when tradesmen banded together for economic and social welfare. The factory system of the Industrial Revolution largely replaced the guilds and lead to widespread abuse and growing worker unrest. In 1884, the British House of Commons recognized the "desirability of relieving tensions" and conceded the right of workers to "form combinations for collective bargaining with their masters" (Wells 1956). See Table 12-1 for a historical summary of collective bargaining. By the early twentieth century, trade unions in the United States grew in number and strength. Violent clashes disrupted society and cried out for legal intervention. In response, the US Congress passed the National Labor Relations Act (NLRA) of 1935, known as the Wagner Act. It gave workers the legal right to organize for better working conditions and required employers to bargain with labor unions. Unfortunately, the act used the term *labor organization*. At that time, the term was interpreted as excluding professionals such as nurses, physicians, and teachers. The act created a quasijudicial body called the National Labor Relations Board to administer and enforce its provisions. More will be said about this important body later in the chapter.

In 1946, the American Nurses Association (ANA) launched its Economic Security Program, setting up national salary guidelines. It passed a resolution encouraging state nurses associations to act as exclusive bargaining agents for members. However, *professional collectivism* was not widely accepted, and in 1950 the ANA adopted a no-strike policy that remained in effect until 1968.

In 1947, the National Labor Management Relations Act, known as the Taft-Hartley Act, established the Federal Mediation and Conciliation Services and expanded some employee rights. Unfortunately, it excluded nonprofit hospitals from the legal obligation to bargain with employees. In 1962, by presidential order, federal employees gained the right to bargain collectively. In 1964, the Civil Rights Act forbade job and wage discrimination based on religion, race, sex, or ethnicity, and in 1967, the Age Discrimination in Employment Act added age to the list. During the 1960s several states passed laws granting bargaining rights to employees of nonprofit hospitals. In 1974, amendments to the Taft-Hartley Act gave employees of nonprofit hospitals throughout

TABLE 12-1

Landmarks in the History of Collective Bargaining in the United States

1850s	Horace Greeley, publisher, reformer, and politician, writes sympathetic accounts of worker issues in *New York Tribune.*
1929	Stock market crashes; Great Depression begins; widespread poverty and low economic activity.
1932	National Industrial Recovery Act creates National Recovery Administration to administer codes of fair practice in industry; establishes a work week of 35 to 40 hours, sets minimum pay at 30–40 cents per hour, and prohibits child labor.
1935	National Labor Relations Act (Wagner Act) passes; gives workers right to organize; requires employers to bargain with labor unions; excludes nurses and other professionals; creates National Labor Relations Board (NLRB) to administer and enforce law.
1946	The ANA launches Economic Security Program; sets national salary guidelines; encourages state nurses associations to act as exclusive bargaining agents for members.
1947	National Labor Management Relations Act (Taft-Hartley Act) passes; Federal Mediation and Conciliation Service begins. The Taft-Hartley Act expands some employee rights; excludes federal employees and nonprofit hospitals from obligation to bargain with employees.
1950	The ANA adopts a no-strike policy (rescinds policy in 1968).
1959	Landrum-Griffin Act regulates internal affairs of unions; gives union members bill of rights.
1960s	Several states pass laws giving collective bargaining right to employees of nonprofit hospitals.
1962	Kennedy Executive Order 10988 gives federal employees, including nurses, right to join unions.
1964	Civil Rights Act forbids discrimination on the bases of religion, race, sex, or ethnicity.
1967	Age Discrimination in Employment Act adds age to list of forbidden discrimination bases.
1974	Taft-Hartley Act amendments give employees of nonprofit hospitals right to bargain collectively.
1991	US Supreme Court upholds NLRB regulation giving nurses the right to organize in separate, all-RN bargaining units.
1994	US Supreme Court rules that nurses who direct the work of others may be considered "supervisors" and thus deprived of collective bargaining rights.

Key Terms Used in Collective Bargaining

Agency shop: A business where employees covered by a contract may or may not join the union and pay dues; however, after joining, an employee must maintain union membership until the next contract period.

Amnesty agreement: An agreement between the union and the employer to drop unfair labor practice charges and to reinstate employees to their former jobs.

Arbitration: Procedures for settling labor disputes using the services of a third party. See *binding arbitration.*

Arbitrator, arbiter: Person chosen by agreement of two parties to decide a dispute between them.

Authorization cards: Cards employees sign to authorize representation by a specific union (Figure 12-1).

Bargaining agent: A group or person who is chosen by members of a bargaining unit to represent them in collective bargaining.

Bargaining unit: An employee group that the state or NLRB recognizes as eligible and an appropriate division for collective bargaining.

Binding arbitration: Arbitration that two parties agree to abide by, in advance. See *arbitration.*

Certification: Official recognition of a labor organization by the NLRB as the exclusive bargaining agent for employees of a specific bargaining unit.

Closed shop: A business where all employees covered by a contract must be members of the union.

Collective bargaining: A legal process by which representatives of organized employees negotiate with an employer about wages, benefits, and working conditions, resulting in an employment contract.

Contract violations: Actions that break the terms of a contract.

Deadlock: A stall in the negotiation process because of an issue about which neither party will compromise.

the United States the right to bargain collectively. In 1991, nurses gained the right to all-RN bargaining units; however, in 1994, the Supreme Court ruled that nurses who direct the work of others may be considered "supervisors," thus depriving them of collective bargaining rights (Ruling 1994). The effect of this ruling is not yet known.

Decertification: Withdrawal of recognition by the NLRB of a union as the exclusive bargaining agent for a group of workers.

Grievance: Any complaint by an employer or union concerning any aspect of the employment relationship.

Grievance procedures: Steps both sides agree to follow to settle disputes.

Injunction: A court order that requires a person to take or refrain from taking a specific action.

Mandatory bargaining issues: Issues such as wages and working conditions about which employers must bargain in good faith.

Mediation: A process for settling labor disputes whereby a mediator assists the parties to reach their own decision.

Mediator: A person chosen by both parties to help them agree.

Open shop: A business where employees are not required to become members of a union as a condition of employment; the opposite of agency shop.

Professional collectivism: The concept of members of a profession joining together to bargain about wages and working conditions.

Supervisor: Any individual having authority, in the interest of the employer, to hire, transfer, suspend, lay off, discharge, recall, promote, assign, reward, or discipline other employees, or responsibility to direct them or adjust their grievances, or effectively to recommend such action if, in connection with the foregoing, the exercise of such authority is not of a merely routine or clerical nature but requires the use of independent judgment (Public Law 93-360, Sec. 2, 1974).

Unfair labor practices: Illegal strategies employers or unions may use against each other to harass or punish.

Union steward: An employee who assumes a leadership role among peers regarding collective bargaining and union concerns.

Voluntary bargaining issues: Issues such as noneconomic fringe benefits, about which employers are not obliged to bargain.

From: Mary Foley RN & The Center for Labor Relations. Personal communication, 1992.

Terminology

Many of the terms used by labor organizations are foreign to nursing because unions began in the manufacturing industry rather than the service industry. The accompanying box gives some of the most common terms used in collective bargaining.

Union Representation for Nurses

After nurses throughout the United States won the right to bargain with their employers, a number of unions wanted to represent them. However, many nurses wanted their professional organization to become their bargaining agent and proposed that the ANA assume that role. Others thought the proposal would create a conflict of interest because both staff nurses and supervising nurses are ANA members. Today, state nurses associations serve as bargaining agents for more than 140,000 of the 240,000 organized nurses in the United States (*Nurse's Handbook* 1992). Some of the other organizations that act as bargaining agents for nurses are the National Union of Hospital and Health Care Employees, AFL-CIO; Service Employee International Union, AFL-CIO; American Federation of State, County, and Municipal Employees, AFL-CIO; and American Federation of Teachers, AFL-CIO. Although the door is now open for nurses to organize, only about 18% of all employed RNs are members of any labor union.

The National Labor Relations Board

The National Labor Relations Board (NLRB) administers and enforces national labor laws. It decides appropriate bargaining units for employee groups, conducts elections for bargaining agents, protects the rights of both employees and employers, and resolves disputes between labor and management. In 1989, the NLRB voted to recognize the following bargaining units within health care agencies: (1) RNs; (2) MDs, excluding house staff; (3) all other professionals such as pharmacists; (4) technical workers, such as LPNs; (5) skilled maintenance personnel, such as plumbers; (6) business clerical staff; (7) nonskilled maintenance and service employees, such as aides; and (8) security guards. The NLRB action was blocked by a US district court ruling, but in 1991, on an appeal, the US Supreme Court decided in favor of the NLRB (Supreme Court 1991).

Employer Protection

The NLRB protects both employers and employees from unfair labor practices. It ensures that employers have the freedom to explain election rules to employees, tell them about union drawbacks, and encourage them to vote against unionization. Specifically, unions may not (1) restrain or coerce employees from exercising rights guaranteed by labor laws; (2) refuse to bargain collectively with an employer if the union is the certified representative; (3) attempt to cause an employer to discipline an employee who is out of favor with the union; (4) engage in unlawful strikes; (5) require employees to pay excessive membership fees; and (6) attempt to coerce an employer to pay the union for services not performed (Sloane & Witney 1991).

Employee Union Protection

The NLRB ensures that labor unions have the freedom to explain election rules, extol the advantages of union membership, and encourage employees to vote for the union in an election. Specifically, employers may not interfere, dominate, discriminate, or refuse to bargain in good faith.

Interfere means to (1) threaten to close down a facility if a union is elected, (2) make intimidating statements to employees regarding participation in union activities, (3) question employees about union activities (4) spy on union meetings or suggest that spying may occur, and (5) unilaterally improve benefits or wages during a union campaign to sway employees to vote against a union.

Dominate means to (1) give union leaders special benefits or compensation, (2) organize a competing union, and (3) to pay the expenses of a certain union.

Discriminate means to (1) enforce rules unequally between employees who are involved in union activities and those who are not; (2) refuse to hire anyone who belongs to a union or has been a union organizer; (3) discharge, discipline, or threaten an employee for joining a union or for encouraging others to join; and (4) refuse to reinstate or promote employees who testify at a NLRB hearing.

Refuse to bargain in good faith means to (1) refuse to meet for negotiation at regular times with the intent to resolve disputed issues, (2) demand to negotiate a voluntary issue, (3) refuse to negotiate a mandatory issue, and (4) take unilateral action affecting employment conditions that are covered by an existing contract or included among legally mandated areas of bargaining (Sloane & Witney 1991).

◆ Collective Bargaining

Organizing a Bargaining Unit

You may ask, "How, then, do people go about organizing a bargaining unit so that they will be recognized by the NLRB?" The process is as follows:

1. A group meets informally and decides to form a bargaining unit in their institution and to ask an established employee union such as a state nurses association (SNA) to represent them. The economic and general welfare division of the SNA, not local regions, provides this service. When invited, the union determines the level of interest and then may assign an organizer-representative to the group of nurses.

2. Union representatives provide nurses with authorization cards (Figure 12-1). If they are not already members of the union, the nurses join, sign authorization cards, and recruit others. If 50% of eligible nurse members sign the cards, the nurses meet NLRB requirements for representation. If only 30% of eligible members sign cards authorizing a union to represent them, whether a competing union has entered the picture or not, an election to select a representative union must be held.

3. The nurses deliver the signed authorization cards to the union. When sufficient cards are collected, the union petitions the NLRB for recognition. If necessary, the NLRB appoints a representative to referee and organize an election.

4. If either the employer or a competing union challenges the eligibility of certain nurses to be counted as employee members of a union and not supervisors, the NLRB representative schedules a hearing. Disputed eligibility is settled by reviewing the job description and the actual supervisory functions of those in question. The regional director of the NLRB makes the decision and declares the percent of eligible members who authorized a particular union.

5. If an election is necessary, the NLRB representative announces a date and place. Within 7 days the employer must give the NLRB representative a list of the names and addresses of all eligible nurses. The NLRB forwards this list to all competing unions.

6. The employer and other competing unions begin campaigning to

---

State Nurses Association

AUTHORIZATION TO REPRESENT

I hereby authorize the State Nurses Association to be my exclusive representative with my employer for the purpose of negotiating all matters related to salaries, hours of work, and other terms and conditions of employment.

Signature _____ Hospital _____

Date _____ Position _____

Name _____ Area _____

Soc. Sec.# _____ Shift _____

Mailing address _____

Home telephone _____

Figure 12-1 Typical authorization card. Adapted from: California Nurses Association, 1992.

gain the vote of eligible nurses. On election day the nurses vote by secret ballot for one of the competing unions or for no representation. Two representatives from each competing union and the NLRB representative supervise the election.

7. NLRB representatives count the ballots in the regional office and send the tabulation to the NLRB General Council in Washington, DC. No matter how many nurses were eligible to vote, only actual votes count. Failure to vote counts as a "no representation" vote. The winner is decided by simple majority. If "no representation" gets the most votes or ties with a union, the "no representation" (the employer) wins. Another election is prohibited by law for 1 year.

8. If any one of the competing unions receives the most votes, the NLRB certifies the winner as the official representative of employees. That representative is then legally bound to represent all eligible employees, regardless of their loyalty prior to the election. An election to decertify a union follows the same process as the one to certify a union.

The Negotiation Process

Formation of a union is just the beginning. A satisfactory contract is yet to be negotiated through the process of collective bargaining. It proceeds as follows:

1. Immediately after the election, contract negotiations begin. Both the union and the employer select a negotiating team. The employer team of a health care facility often includes a labor law expert, a nursing administrator, a personnel director, a hospital administrator, and heads of departments where union employees work. The employee team includes union representatives, an attorney, and employees selected to serve on the negotiation team.

2. In consultation with its members, the union creates a list of desired conditions of employment, called "demands," which it gives to the employer prior to the first negotiation session. The list includes mandatory bargaining issues such as wages and working conditions, as well as voluntary issues such as fringe benefits. Likewise, the employer presents a counterproposal to the employee team, usually at the first or second meeting.

3. Face-to-face meetings of the two sides begin. Negotiations may be item-by-item or all-or-none. The all-or-none system gives negotiators more room to bargain right up to the final agreement. The process may move along smoothly or may be long and arduous. Each side keeps its constituents informed. If all goes well, the parties reach agreement on every issue, and negotiating team members initial the proposed contract.

4. The proposed contract is printed and distributed to union members, and a vote is scheduled. If a majority of union members accept it, the contract is ratified. The negotiating teams sign the document, and on a specific day the contract goes into effect.

When Negotiations Break Down

Mediation

If negotiations break down and neither side will compromise, bargainers have several options. The least coercive way to resolve disputes is through mediation. The two sides may invite a mediator to facilitate negotiations. In fact, because of a desire to shorten the process to meet needs of the public for hospital care, the parties may invite a mediator to be present from the beginning of negotiations. Professional mediator-arbitrators may be requested from several sources. The American Arbitration Association is a nonprofit, non-partisan agency that for a nominal fee provides a list of qualified persons. Various state mediation and conciliation services and the Federal Mediation and Conciliation Service (FMCS) also provide mediation services.

Strikes and Lockouts

If mediation fails to bring about agreement, employees may undertake a number of strategies to convince the employer to make concessions, such as working to rule (following the exact rules of the contract; taking no shortcuts to expedite work), calling a sick-out (taking sick leave), refusing to work overtime or extra shifts, undertaking informational picketing, and striking. The employer may decide to lock out or lay off employees to convince them to make concessions. Because of the critical nature of health care, the NLRB requires many more steps for these institutions than for non-health care institutions before a strike can be called or a lockout imposed, as follows:

1. If the employees or the employers wish to modify or terminate an existing contract, they must notify the other side of intended changes 90 days before the contract is due to expire. During that time the two sides meet to negotiate a new agreement.

2. If after 30 days the two sides have not reached agreement, or if the parties are negotiating a contract for the first time and have reached an impasse, the parties must notify the FMCS and the appropriate state agency.

3. Within 30 days, the FMCS appoints a mediator-arbitrator to gather information from both sides and to submit the findings to the FMCS regional director for evaluation. The FMCS may then appoint a board of inquiry (BOI).

4. Within 15 days of appointment the BOI conducts hearings and issues a written report with its findings and recommendations for resolution of the dispute. The report is given to both sides.

5. If after 15 more days the parties still do not agree, the employees may plan to strike or the employer may plan to lock out the employees.

6. If a strike vote has not yet been held, it is conducted at this time. If a majority of employees vote to strike, the union must send the employer a notice at least 10 days before, stating the exact date, time, and place of the strike.

7. A strike cannot be scheduled before a contract expires. If employees ignore the rules and engage in an illegal strike, they lose NLRB protection and may be fired by the employer. The NLRB can decertify a union that sanctions an illegal strike.

8. After scheduling a strike, a union may delay it for up to 72 hours if it feels the extra time will help resolve the impasse.

9. To delay a strike, employees must give employers written notice at least 12 hours before a strike is scheduled to begin. If an initial strike date passes during negotiations, the union must issue another 10-day strike notice. If a contract expires during negotiations, the parties remain bound by the old contract.

10. If a strike is called, both sides must abide by strict rules of conduct. They cannot threaten nonstriking employees, attack employer representatives, or physically block other nurses and personnel from entering or leaving the facility.

11. Negotiations may be broken off for a time, but they eventually must be reinstituted and continue until a settlement is reached. When negotiators reach an impasse, they may submit the disputed issue to binding arbitration, using the services of a private or FMCS arbitrator. Settlements often include an amnesty agreement whereby both sides agree to drop unfair labor practice charges and employers agree to rehire employees who were involved in the strike. This agreement to rehire is called *reinstatement privilege.*

Strikes cause serious disruptions of services to clients, deep divisions between staff members, and lost income for both employers and employees. Strikes and lockouts are measures of last resort, undertaken only when all else fails. For this reason, contracts may include "no-strike, no-lockout" clauses whereby both sides agree to follow grievance and arbitration procedures throughout the life of the contract.

◆ Grievances and Arbitration

When an employer and employee bargaining agent sign a contract, they agree to follow the specific provisions of the contract. Because they cannot anticipate every possible difficulty, they agree on grievance procedures to resolve disputes. Often arbitration is the final step in the grievance procedure.

Each contract defines a grievance. Most describe a *grievance* as any dispute, claim, or complaint that involves violations of any part of a contract, of past practice, or precedent. A grievance may also be a complaint of an unfair labor practice, such as interference, domination, discrimination, refusal to bargain in good faith, or encouraging employees to do any of these things.

Contract violations are actions that break mutual agreements stipulated in the contract. For instance, Lou is working under a contract that states that if two or more equally well qualified nurses bid for an open position, the one with most seniority will be chosen. Although she is equally well qualified and the most senior nurse, Lou is not selected for the open position. She files a grievance on the basis of a contract violation.

Violations of precedent or past practice are unilateral changes in established policies or procedures. For example, although work shifts are not mentioned in the contract, for at least 10 years normal work shifts in a local hospital have been 8:00–4:30, 4:00–12:30, and 12:00–8:30. One day the director of nurses announced that beginning in 1 week, normal work shifts would be 7:00–3:30, 3:00–11:30, and 11:00–7:30. The nurses filed a grievance based on a past practice violation.

Both employers and employees may file grievances against the other. Employers file grievances against employees in the form of disciplinary action for such things as failure to perform assigned tasks, chronic tardiness, excessive sick leave, and negative relationships with coworkers. Employees file grievances against supervisors for unequal or unfair treatment. These complaints often involve issues such as promotion, vacation time, shift assignment, and merit pay raises. Many grievances result from unwitting contract violations, such as poorly thought-out workload decisions of nurse managers. Nurse managers can avoid some of these disputes by gaining a thorough knowledge of the contract, consulting with resource persons, and using a participatory rather than an authoritarian management style.

Grievance Procedures

Because the purpose of grievance procedures is to resolve disputes, they usually provide (1) time limits for filing a grievance and making a decision, (2) opportunities for both sides to investigate complaints, (3) procedures for appealing to higher authority with a plan for ultimate resolution, and (4) assignment of priority to more serious complaints. The one who files the complaint, the grievant, has a right to be assisted by legal and union counsel at each step of the grievance procedure.

Grievance procedures typically follow a series of steps:

1. The grievant discusses a claim, complaint, or dispute with the immediate supervisor. The supervisor renders a decision within a specified number of days.

2. If not satisfied with the decision, the grievant may submit the issue in writing to the next level of authority, often the nursing service administrator. The nursing service administrator meets with the grievant to try to resolve the matter and renders a written decision within a specified number of days.

3. If not satisfied with the decision, the grievant may submit a written appeal to the highest level of authority, often the hospital administrator. The hospital administrator meets with the grievant to try to resolve the issue and renders a written decision within a specified number of days. If the grievant is not satisfied with the decision, the next step is arbitration.

Arbitration Process

Arbitration is a process that settles a labor dispute by presenting evidence to a neutral labor relations expert, usually an employee of a private or government agency. The process may be clearly defined in the contract, but since an arbitration clause is not required, not all labor contracts include it. Without such a clause, all these arrangements must be negotiated at the time of a dispute.

When the process is defined in the contract and a grievant is not satisfied with the outcome of step 3 of the grievance procedure, the grievant, in consultation with the union, may submit a written request for arbitration to the employer. The contract stipulates the source of an arbitrator, such as from a list supplied by the Federal Mediation and Conciliation Service, and the method of selection. A date, time, and place for the arbitration hearing is set.

The arbitration hearing is similar to a court case, but not as formal. The side requesting the arbitration has the burden to prove that a contract has been violated, except in cases of disciplinary action, in which the employer must prove its case. Both sides may call witnesses and cross-examine them. After the hearing, the arbitrator can issue a summary judgment shortly after the proceedings or a written decision within a month (Marriner-Tomey 1988). Often, both parties share the costs of arbitration.

Both employers and unions prefer arbitration to a court trial because it is faster and less costly. However, when a dispute goes to arbitration, both sides lose control of the outcome. In the United States the arbitrator's decision is binding. Either side may challenge the decision in court, but courts rarely overturn an arbitrator's decision.

Amicable labor relations require that both sides honor the contract and demonstrate goodwill in using grievance procedures. Both sides must carefully consider when to retreat, press forward, or compromise. Union representatives must distinguish between a substantive complaint involving a contract violation and a personal problem of an employee. Employers must separate contract violations from personal problems of supervisors. Both unions and employers may pursue groundless complaints to harass the other or to pursue an immediate political goal. In the long run, however, it is to their advantage to respect one another and resolve disputes with minimum conflict.

Enforcement of the contract is assured through the settlement of grievances and arbitration decisions. This process truly assures that the contract is more than a piece of paper. Enforcement of the contract through the grievance procedure is as important as, or more important than, the actual negotiations because this is the area where precedent (past practice) creates a body of unwritten law, governing the day-to-day interpretation of the contract.

Other Grievances

Most grievances arise from contract violations and are settled through the grievance process. When either employers or unions believe the other has engaged in "unfair labor practices" as described earlier, they can complain to the NLRB. After a preliminary investigation, the NLRB may conduct a hearing to review the evidence and issue a decision. The decision may be challenged by either the union or the employer in court.

All employees, whether union members or not, have a right to file complaints with the Equal Employment Opportunity Commission (EEOC) and comparable state agencies if they believe they have been discriminated against because of race, religion, national origin, age, or sex. Union members also may file grievances as stipulated in their employment contract. The EEOC handles violations of a number of antidiscrimination laws, including: (1) the Equal Pay Act of 1963, forbidding wage discrimination based on sex; (2) the Civil Rights Act of 1964, forbidding job and wage discrimination on the basis of religion, race, sex, or ethnic background and sexual harassment; and (3) the Age Discrimination in Employment Act of 1967, forbidding discrimination based on age.

◆ Preventing Discontent

You may ask, "Why do nurses join labor unions?" Nurses join labor unions because unions provide a means of collective activity. They enable nurses to gain some control over their practice, to improve working conditions, and to secure adequate compensation. Some nurses may have tried other approaches for change, but have been frustrated. In desperation they turn to a union for help. If employers, nurse entrepreneurs, and nurse managers want to avoid the intervention of unions in their relationships with employees, they must pay attention to the reasons people become discontented. Marquis and Huston (1994) say that people join unions to increase the power of the individual; to communicate their aims, feelings, complaints, and ideas to others; to eliminate discrimination and favoritism; and to achieve acceptance. Sloane and Witney (1991) say it is because employers fail to meet the need for nurses "to have a voice," to have leadership opportunities, to achieve self-fulfillment, and to gain economic benefits. Othman and Chaney (1987) list actions employers take or fail to take that create discontent. Turning that list around, the accompanying box suggests ways employers can prevent discontent.

Twelve Ways to Prevent Employee Discontent

1. Treat all employees fairly and equally.

2. Offer opportunities for advancement.

3. Recognize people as valued individuals.

4. Make the workplace safe and pleasant.

5. Offer special training and education.

6. Provide adequate supervision and leadership.

7. Institute grievance procedures.

8. Open two-way channels of communication.

9. Give opportunities for self-expression.

10. Maintain high standards of client care.

11. Encourage autonomy and innovation.

12. Give economic security with adequate and competitive wages and a full range of benefits.

◇ Summary

Work contracts, like other legal contracts, contain promises, mutual understandings, compensation, and a lawful purpose. A sound employment contract includes specific elements. Nurses turn to employee unions for help in obtaining employment contracts that give them economic security, improved working conditions, and greater autonomy. The NLRB administers and enforces national labor laws, ensuring that both employers and employees abide by the rules and avoid unfair labor practices. Unions organize workers in a prescribed sequence, culminating in official recognition by the NLRB. State nurses associations serve as union representatives for most organized nurses. When disputes arise, the parties use prescribed grievance procedures. If these fail, arbitration may be necessary. Amiable working relations require that both sides honor the contract and demonstrate goodwill.

Critical Thinking Questions

1. In addition to what you have read in this chapter, what additional information would you need to attain full understanding of contracts?

2. Given the current rise in unemployment, how do you account for the fact that only 18% of nurses are members of labor unions?

3. What is your opinion of nurses who belong to unions and go on strike? Explain how you came to hold this view. For example, what personal experiences have you had with other kinds of unions? What attitudes might you have acquired from your family or friends?

Learning Activities

1. Visit the regional office of a state nurses association; ask to see copies of employment contracts of hospitals in your area and compare them.

2. Go to the personnel office of a local hospital and request a copy of the employment contract that is currently in force.

3. Interview a nurse administrator or hospital administrator and ask about the disadvantages of labor organizations.

4. Interview a state nurses association labor representative or a member of a bargaining team and ask about the advantages of labor organizations.

5. In a group discussion, list what the group believes an ideal employment contract would contain; then prioritize the items on the list.

6. Debate the proposition: "Professional collectivism is an oxymoron."

Annotated Reading List

Joel L. Collective Bargaining, A Positive Force in the Workplace. *Revolution, A Journal of Nurse Empowerment* Winter 1993; p. 26.

In this lively article, the author says that collective bargaining is rarely, if ever, portrayed by management consultants as a positive force in the workplace. She says that few managers are willing to admit constructive resolution of significant issues at the bargaining table. She affirms that there is concrete evidence that constructive change for health care workers, providers, and patients can take place through the bargaining process. Dr. Joel goes on to support her contention with specific arguments. A brief but pithy article.

Nurses' Rights As Employees. Chapter 7 in *Nurse's Handbook of Law and Ethics.* Springhouse, 1992.

In their typically succinct fashion, the editorial writers of this chapter present the essence of employee rights. They describe employee contracts, unions, legal issues in collective bargaining, and grievances and arbitrations. Several graphic features, such as "Recognizing Unfair Labor Practices" and "The Perils of Not Bargaining," group information together. Subjects are presented from neither a "for" nor "against" stance. Therefore, the chapter is a valuable source of factual information.

References

Creighton H. *Law Every Nurse Should Know,* 5th ed. Saunders, 1986.

Marquis BL, Huston CJ. *Management Decision Making for Nurses,* 2nd ed. Lippincott, 1994.

Marriner-Tomey A. *Guide to Nursing Management,* 3d ed. Mosby, 1988.

Nurse's Handbook of Law and Ethics. Springhouse, 1992.

Othman JE, Chaney HS. Labor Relations in Union and Nonunion Environments. In Vestal, KW. *Management Concepts for the New Nurse.* Vestal KW, Lippincott, 1987.

Ruling Questions NLRA Protection for Nurses. *The American Nurse* June 1994; p. 10.

Sloane AA, Witney F. *Labor Relations,* 7th ed. Prentice Hall, 1991.

Supreme Court Okays All-RN Unit. *American Nurse,* June 1991.

Wells HG. *Outline of History,* 5th ed. Volumes I and II. Doubleday, 1956.

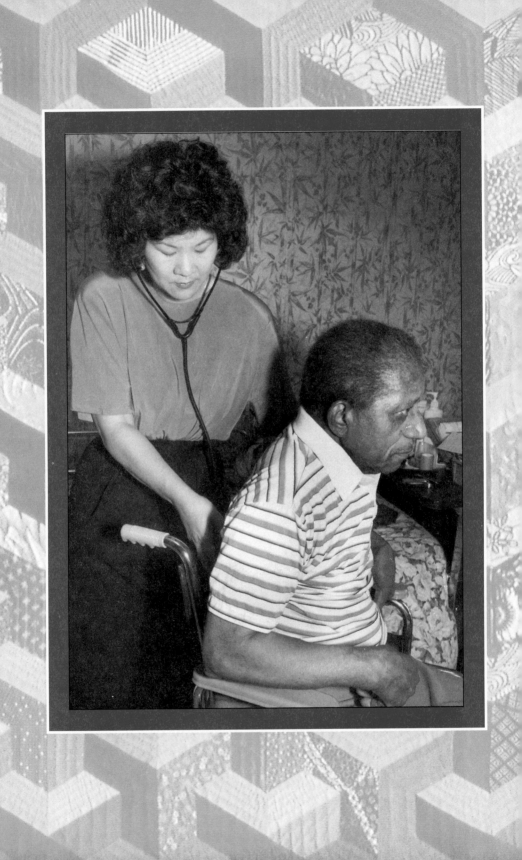

Career Management

13

◇ Learning Objectives

- Compare a job perspective with a career perspective.

- Explain how personal characteristics and aspects of the profession relate to planning a career in nursing.

- Discuss the implementation phase of career management, describing specific actions.

- Explain the value of management strategies and the concepts of marketing, relationships, production, and control strategies.

- Compare resumés with curricula vitae as to content and purpose.

- State the purpose of cover letters and the rules for writing them.

- Discuss the interviewing process and its follow-up from an interviewee's perspective.

- Describe some strategies for negotiating, networking, and maintaining collegial relationships.

- Explain why continuing education and occupational health and safety are production strategies.

- Discuss the value of control strategies in helping nurses manage their careers and survive in the real world of nursing.

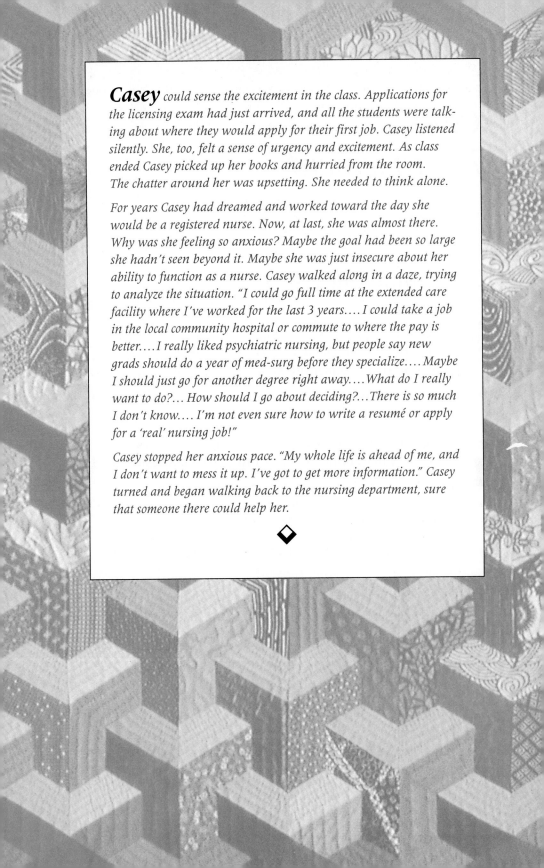

Casey *could sense the excitement in the class. Applications for the licensing exam had just arrived, and all the students were talking about where they would apply for their first job. Casey listened silently. She, too, felt a sense of urgency and excitement. As class ended Casey picked up her books and hurried from the room. The chatter around her was upsetting. She needed to think alone.*

For years Casey had dreamed and worked toward the day she would be a registered nurse. Now, at last, she was almost there. Why was she feeling so anxious? Maybe the goal had been so large she hadn't seen beyond it. Maybe she was just insecure about her ability to function as a nurse. Casey walked along in a daze, trying to analyze the situation. "I could go full time at the extended care facility where I've worked for the last 3 years.... I could take a job in the local community hospital or commute to where the pay is better.... I really liked psychiatric nursing, but people say new grads should do a year of med-surg before they specialize.... Maybe I should just go for another degree right away.... What do I really want to do?... How should I go about deciding?...There is so much I don't know.... I'm not even sure how to write a resumé or apply for a 'real' nursing job!"

Casey stopped her anxious pace. "My whole life is ahead of me, and I don't want to mess it up. I've got to get more information." Casey turned and began walking back to the nursing department, sure that someone there could help her.

◆

Graduation from the nursing program is something you work hard to achieve and look forward to for a long time. It marks the end of one phase of your life and the beginning of another. It is an ideal time to make a personal and professional work-life plan. Making such a plan is quite different from finding a job. Finding a job, a *job perspective*, is short-term; it meets immediate needs. A *career perspective* is long-term; it involves use of the management process to make a work-life plan and achieve personal and professional goals. Coordinating career management involves planning, organizing, directing, and controlling.

◆ Managing Your Career

Assessing Your Personal Values and Goals

Before you rush ahead with your career, take time to ask yourself, "Who am I? What do I believe? What do I value? What do I want to do with my life?" To help you find answers to these questions, do Exercises 13-1 to 13-7.

EXERCISE 13-1

Assessment of the Physical Self

Directions: Stand in front of a full-length mirror dressed as you are at work. Rate yourself on a scale of 1 (unkempt) to 5 (well-groomed). When you have done this, go back and look at the features you marked 1 or 2. Ask yourself, "Is that the picture I want to portray to others?" Though you cannot change genetics, you can change behaviors.

	Unkempt	Well-groomed
Appropriateness of dress for practice area	1 2 3 4 5	
Cleanliness of clothing, including shoes	1 2 3 4 5	
Cosmetics and jewelry	1 2 3 4 5	
Energy level	1 2 3 4 5	
Facial expression	1 2 3 4 5	
General size and shape of body	1 2 3 4 5	
Grooming, neatness	1 2 3 4 5	
Posture	1 2 3 4 5	

Assessment of Values

Directions: First, select the 10 items that are of HIGH value or need for you. Then, from those 10, select the 5 that are of HIGHEST value for you.

	High	Highest
Achievement, accomplishment, recognition	_____	_____
Adventure, risk, exploration	_____	_____
A meaningful love relationship	_____	_____
Authenticity, genuineness, honesty	_____	_____
Beautiful home in a choice setting	_____	_____
Being a change agent	_____	_____
Education, self-growth, development	_____	_____
Equal opportunity for everyone	_____	_____
Expertness, skillfulness in a task	_____	_____
A happy, contented family	_____	_____
Independence, personal freedom	_____	_____
Intelligence, a bright mind	_____	_____
Leadership, influence, power	_____	_____
Leisurely life without pressure	_____	_____
Long life	_____	_____
Meaningful, purposeful work	_____	_____
Physical appearance that brings pride	_____	_____
Physical health	_____	_____
Security, stability	_____	_____
Self-confidence, emotional strength	_____	_____
Service, contributing to others	_____	_____
Spirituality, religious beliefs	_____	_____
Unlimited wealth	_____	_____
Wisdom, maturity, insight	_____	_____

Assessment of Personal Characteristics

Directions: Consider how often each of the characteristics listed below describes you. In the space write a 0 (never or not at all), 1 (sometimes or somewhat), or 2 (continually).

Then go back and look at the items that you marked with a 0 or a 2. You may want to hold on to these traits and choose a career where they are assets. You may conclude that they are a detriment and decide to change them. The decision is yours to make.

_____ Arrive on time for work and other appointments

_____ Believe I am treated fairly

_____ Consider myself a rebel

_____ Cry when I am angry

_____ Display a hot temper

_____ Enjoy speaking out, being in the spotlight

_____ Experience numerous physical symptoms

_____ Fear authority figures

_____ Feel angry and misunderstood

_____ Feel anxious and tense

_____ Feel discouraged and hopeless

_____ Feel inferior to others

_____ Feel left out of things

_____ Feel shy, hesitate to voice an opinion

_____ Get along with everyone

_____ Have an intense need to be perfect

_____ Identify with "underdogs" and unfortunates

_____ Like to manage other people and activities

_____ Prefer to work alone, independent of others

_____ Say "yes" when I really want to say "no"

_____ Seek out and enjoy taking responsibility

_____ Suffer migraine headaches or a nervous stomach

_____ Talk less than anyone else in a group

_____ Talk more than anyone else in a group

_____ Think of myself as unworthy or ugly

_____ Use sarcasm and indirect ways to express anger

_____ Vacillate when I need to make a choice

EXERCISE 13-4

Assessment of Interests

Directions: For each of the activities listed below indicate your interest as: 1 (low), 2 (moderate), or 3 (high). Add the scores for each category of activity and write the total in the space provided.

Activities	Score	Activities	Score
Creative-artistic		*Ordering*	
Acting	_____	Classifying data	_____
Composing music	_____	Filing	_____
Designing	_____	Finance record keeping	_____
Drawing	_____	Following directions	_____
Generating ideas	_____	Inventorying	_____
Photographing	_____	Managing budgets	_____
Sculpting	_____	Organizing records	_____
Writing	_____	Processing forms	_____
Creative-artistic score	_____	*Ordering score*	_____
Investigative		*Physical*	
Assessing	_____	Biking	_____
Analyzing	_____	Dancing	_____
Clarifying	_____	Hiking	_____
Diagnosing	_____	Running	_____
Evaluating	_____	Sailing	_____
Experimenting	_____	Singing	_____
Researching	_____	Skiing	_____
Using logic	_____	Swimming	_____
Investigative score	_____	*Physical score*	_____
Management		*Social*	
Assigning tasks	_____	Care giving	_____
Coordinating	_____	Counseling	_____
Competing in games	_____	Entertaining	_____
Implementing policies	_____	Group sports	_____
Planning change	_____	Listening	_____
Managing conflicts	_____	Meeting in groups	_____
Leading meetings	_____	Telephoning	_____
Scheduling events	_____	Writing letters	_____
Management score	_____	*Social score*	_____

➤

EXERCISE 13-4 *(continued)*

Assessment of Interests

Scoring Summary		Scoring Key	
Interest		*Scoring range*	*Interest level*
Creative-artistic	_____	0–8	Low
Investigative	_____	9–16	Moderate
Management	_____	17–24	High
Ordering	_____		
Physical	_____		
Social	_____		

Adapted from Henderson FC, McGettigan BO. *Managing Your Career in Nursing,* 2nd ed. National League for Nursing, 1994.

EXERCISE 13-5

Assessment of Proficiency Level

Directions: Assess your level of nursing proficiency (ability, competency, skill) based on the five levels identified by Patricia Benner.

Level I Novice: No experience in situations where a nurse is expected to perform; relies on rules to guide actions.

Level II Beginner: Limited recurring experience; relies on concrete guidelines from experience of others; performs basic assessment skills but has limited ability to discern importance.

Level III Competent: Minimum of 2 years experience in stable situations; systematically solves problems and analyzes situations.

Level IV Proficient: Minimum of 3 to 5 years experience with similar patient population; demonstrates ability to perceive situations as wholes with speed and flexibility due to reflection on previous experience.

Level V Expert: More than 5 years experience with similar patient population and setting; demonstrates immediate and intuitive grasp of situation due to experience and mastery of previous complex situations.

My experience level is _____

From Benner P. *From Novice to Expert.* Addison-Wesley, 1984, pp. 20–30.

Assessment of Education, Credentials, and Experience

Directions: Although retention of knowledge varies, one way to assess and verify your knowledge is to compile a list of formal and informal learning experience. You will use this information to write your resumé.

Education List all schools where you have studied since high school, major area of study, and the certificate or degree earned in each.

Special Knowledge and Skills Describe special knowledge and skills; state where they were learned; indicate locations, dates, and circumstances.

Licenses, Credentials, and Certificates List licenses, credentials, and certificates you possess; indicate the official number and expiration date.

Organizational Memberships List the names of professional and personal organizations to which you belong if they might be an asset; indicate the offices you held and the committees on which you served.

Publications List articles, books, papers, videos, and computer programs you have created such as teaching modules, procedures, and policies; indicate the title, date, and formal publisher.

Special Achievements List significant professional or personal awards, honors, and unique projects in which you have participated. Name, describe, and give date of each one.

Documentation Collect and preserve in a safe place the following:

All past or present resumés

Applications for nursing positions and schools

Awards and letters of commendation

Certificates of completion

Course descriptions of higher education courses from college

Catalogs and continuing education brochures

Current continuing education certificates

Performance evaluations

Published materials you have authored

Transcripts from educational institutions

Summary of Personal Characteristics

Directions: Summarize your findings from Exercises 1 through 6:

My physical appearance is_____

My highest values and needs are_____

My persistent psychosocial behaviors and attributes are_____

My primary interests are_____

My proficiency level is_____

My areas of greatest knowledge and skill are_____

Assessing Options in the Nursing Profession

After you have appraised your personal characteristics, the next step is to assess aspects of the nursing profession relative to your needs and preferences. Some of the important areas to consider are health problems and nursing specialties; nursing functions, services, and levels of prevention; nursing roles and settings; clients; and compensation and working conditions. There are no right or wrong, good or bad answers, just honest ones. You are planning *your* career. Your plan should fit your unique mix of attributes, skills, and aptitudes. Exercises 13-8 to 13-15 will help you assess options in the nursing profession.

Health Problems and Nursing Specialties

Health problems can be classified as acute, chronic, developmental, and environmental. Acute conditions demand immediate action; work is exciting and ever-changing. Chronic and developmental disorders call for great patience and deliberate actions. Cultural and environmental problems require holistic approaches and often require involvement with social service agencies. Health problems are described by medical and nursing specialties, such as oncology and neonatology. You will want to consider which category of health problems best suits your personal interests and aptitudes. Exercise 13-8 helps you identify health problems of particular interest to you.

EXERCISE 13-8

Health Problems and Specialties

Directions: Place an X by the type of health problems and medical specialties you find most challenging.

Category: _____Acute _____Chronic

_____Developmental _____Environmental

Medical/nursing specialty:

_____	Allergy	_____	Obstetrics
_____	Cardiology	_____	Oncology
_____	Dermatology	_____	Ophthalmology
_____	Endocrinology	_____	Orthopedic surgery
_____	Gastroenterology	_____	Otorhinolaryngology
_____	General surgery	_____	Pathology
_____	Geriatrics	_____	Pediatric disorders
_____	Gynecology	_____	Physical medicine and rehabilitation
_____	Hematology		
_____	Infectious diseases	_____	Plastic and reconstructive surgery
_____	Infertility		
_____	Internal medicine	_____	Preventive medicine
_____	Neonatology	_____	Psychiatry
_____	Nephrology	_____	Pulmonary disorders
_____	Neurology	_____	Radiology
_____	Neurosurgery	_____	Rheumatology
_____	Nutrition	_____	Urology

Human Responses to Health Problems

The unique concern of nursing practice is to promote adaptive and effective human responses to health problems. Nursing diagnoses are the terms used to describe potential and actual responses to health problems. Since its beginning in 1973, the North American Nursing Diagnosis Association has been creating a taxonomy of diagnoses. The 11 categories into which they have been sorted will give you a means to sort your professional areas of special interest. Those categories are: activity-exercise, cognitive-perceptual, coping-stress tolerance,

Human Responses to Health Problems

Directions: Place an X beside the category of human responses that particularly interests you.

_____   Activity-exercise

_____   Cognitive-perceptual

_____   Coping-stress tolerance

_____   Self-perceptual and self-concept

_____   Elimination

_____   Sexuality-reproductive

_____   Health-perception/management

_____   Sleep-rest

_____   Nutrition-metabolic

_____   Value-belief

_____   Role-relationship

---

elimination, health-perception/management, nutrition-metabolic, role-relationship, self-perceptual/self-concept, sexuality-reproductive, sleep-rest, and value-belief (Gordon 1982).

Although nurses view humans holistically, you may find one category of human responses more interesting than another and may wish to focus your practice in that area. For example, you may be interested in activity-exercise and may prefer working in a neuro-rehabilitation unit. You may be more interested in sexuality-reproduction and may choose to work in a women's health clinic or labor and delivery. Exercise 13-9 helps you assess which category of human responses most interests you.

Nursing Functions, Services, and Levels of Prevention

Nursing functions are actions that comfort and sustain the sick, prevent and treat health problems, and teach and encourage healthful living. Nurses carry out these functions by applying the nursing process to client problems and providing service at various levels of prevention. Because the nursing process can be shared, nurses can

Preferences of Nursing Functions, Services, and Levels of Prevention

Directions: Place an X beside the nursing functions that interest you the most.

Nursing process	Services	Prevention
_____ Assessment	_____ Direct	_____ Primary
_____ Diagnosis	_____ Semidirect	_____ Secondary
_____ Planning	_____ Indirect	_____ Tertiary
_____ Implementing		
_____ Evaluating		

choose to perform those functions they find most challenging. For example, a nurse who enjoys assessment and diagnosis may choose to work in triage in an emergency department. A nurse who prefers planning, implementing, and evaluating may choose to work in an inpatient care unit.

Services to clients may be direct, semidirect, or indirect. *Direct services* to clients include all those direct care functions nurses do for and with clients. *Semidirect services* include functions such as supervising or educating others to give direct care to clients. *Indirect services* include functions nurses perform working administratively and politically to influence client care.

Levels of prevention are termed primary, secondary, and tertiary. In *primary prevention,* nurses promote health and prevent health problems by such action as providing prenatal care. In *secondary prevention,* nurses treat health problems by such action as administering antibiotics. In *tertiary prevention,* nurses help people cope with disability and chronic problems. Exercise 13-10 helps you identify nursing functions that give you the most satisfaction.

Nursing Roles

A role is a set of behaviors expected of a person holding a position. Nurses function in one or more of four roles: administrator, clinician, educator, and researcher. Although the roles overlap, in general,

Preferences of Nursing Roles

Directions: Place an X by the role that particularly appeals to you.

Role	Expected Behaviors
_____ Administrator	Manages nursing service, establishes budgets, collaborates with other units, oversees implementation of standard policies and procedures, evaluates personnel, provides leadership, and represents the institution in the community
_____ Clinician	Provides and manages client care, using the nursing process to assess, diagnose, plan, implement, and evaluate that care
_____ Educator	Develops learning objectives, activities, and measurement; develops curricula; maintains clinical and educational currency; participates in professional activities
_____ Researcher	Develops proposals for funding; plans and carries out research within theoretical frameworks; presents findings for critique

administrators lead and manage nursing services, clinicians manage and provide nursing care, educators teach, and researchers conduct scientific studies. Aptitudes and expected behaviors vary for each of the roles. All nurses begin as clinicians. They must have additional education and experience to assume other roles. As you plan your career, you may want to consider other roles, such as a nurse educator, administrator, or advanced nurse practitioner. Exercise 13-11 helps you identify the roles you would like to assume.

Clients

Clients are the focus of all nursing care. To be effective, nurses must enjoy people. They cannot allow personal preferences to interfere with ethical, competent practice. However, nurses experience greater satisfaction when they work with certain kinds of people. While these

Preferred Client Characteristics

Directions: Place an X beside characteristics you prefer in clients.

Age

_____ Premature infants   _____ Adolescents (13 to 19)

_____ Infants (birth to 1 yr)   _____ Young adults (20 to 39)

_____ Young children (1 to 5)   _____ Middle-aged adults (40 to 64)

_____ School age (6 to 12)   _____ Older adults (65+)

Sex

_____ Female   _____ Male

preferences change with time and life experience, these preferences are legitimate and deserve recognition. For example, some nurses enjoy working with children, others prefer young adults, and others prefer older adults. These preferences reflect personal values, interests, and psychosocial traits. Exercise 13-12 helps you identify the characteristics of clients you prefer.

Settings

Nurses practice in many different settings: hospitals, nursing homes, extended care facilities, clinics, and clients' homes. As you plan your career, you need to consider several aspects of settings that contribute to your personal satisfaction and professional success. These include the type of industry, kind of care, union affiliation, organizational profile, autonomy, and orientation and socialization programs available to new employees.

Type of Industry The type of industry has to do with whether a setting is or is not part of the health care industry. Hospitals, nursing homes, clinics, and companies that sell health care products or services are part of the health care industry. Schools, government agencies, recreational facilities, and most businesses are not part of that industry. Autonomy and opportunity often are greater in agencies not associated with the industry. Supervision and mentoring often are more available in agencies associated with the health care industry.

Kind of Care Kind of care refers to whether health care is provided through an inpatient facility, ambulatory center, or home care agency. The role of nurses is significantly affected by the kind of care. Inpatient institutions provide 24-hour care; clients are sicker and more dependent, but there are more support services. Ambulatory centers serve clients for shorter periods, and clients tend to be more independent and not as ill. Home care agencies serve clients for longer periods of time, and clients are relatively self-reliant or have home attendants. Nursing practice in home care agencies tends to be holistic, less structured, and more independent than in health care facilities.

Labor Organizations Labor unions provide collective bargaining services for their members. Nurses may enjoy higher salaries, more autonomy, and better working conditions in institutions with collective bargaining agreements. In return, however, they must pay dues and abide by union rules. (See Chapter 12.)

Organizational Profile The organizational profile has to do with the size, type of service, structure, management style, and ownership of an institution. Size reflects the location and resources of a facility and often influences the atmosphere and organizational structure of an agency. The structure affects its ability to change. Management style influences the degree of independence staff members enjoy. Ownership affects every aspect of an institution, including its philosophy and management style. Ownership may be vested in religious groups, charitable organizations, investors for profit, educational institutions, or governments. Because owners have ultimate control, you, as a potential employee, need to know who they are.

Autonomy for Nurses Autonomy for nurses increases as the profession more clearly defines its roles and functions and as the health care system undergoes change (Morrison 1994). More and more nurses provide leadership for nursing care teams, are self-employed, and work as nurse practitioners, midwives, clinical specialists in private practice, and independent contractors. Autonomy for nurses, however, varies widely from setting to setting and even from unit to unit. For this reason, you need to assess whether the degree of autonomy in each setting fits your needs.

Work Setting Preferences

Directions: Place an X beside characteristics of work settings you prefer.

Type   _____ Associated with the health care industry

            _____ Not associated with the health care industry

Kind   _____ Inpatient (clients more dependent, sicker)

            _____ Ambulatory (clients less dependent, brief contact)

            _____ Home (clients sometimes less dependent, nursing

                   functions are holistic, innovative, less structured)

Labor organizations   _____ State nurses association

                 _____ Other organization

                 _____ Not organized

Organizational profile

Ownership   _____ For-profit corporation

                _____ Government

                _____ Nonprofit corporation

                _____ Community

Profit motive   _____ High _____ Moderate _____ Low

Size   _____ Small (100 or less employees)

                _____ Medium (101 to 600 employees)

                _____ Large (601 to 1500 employees)

                _____ Very large (1501 or more employees)

Resources   _____ Extremely limited

                _____ Somewhat limited

                _____ Almost unlimited

➤

Work Setting Preferences

Structure

_____ Informal   _____ Formal   _____ Highly codified

Autonomy of nurses

_____ Great   _____ Moderate   _____ Little

Orientation and socialization programs for new staff members

_____ Less than 2 wks. _____ 3 to 8 wks. _____ More than 8 wks.

_____ Preceptorship   _____ Mentorship _____ Buddy system

Management style

_____ Authoritarian   _____ Democratic   _____ Laissez-faire

Orientation and Socialization Programs   Orientation and socialization programs for new staff members are indicators of the commitment an institution has to quality care. Generally, the longer an orientation, the greater the commitment. Morale is usually higher in institutions that assist staff to succeed. Chapter 10 describes orientation and socialization programs in greater detail. Exercise 13-13 helps you identify your needs and preferences in the work setting.

Compensation and Working Conditions

Payment for nursing services is an indication of the value an employer places on nursing care. Nurses have a right to economic reward based on responsibility and qualification. Within a geographic area, their pay should be comparable to that of other professionals of like preparation and responsibility whose work involves similar risk. You can expect differential pay for evening, night, and overtime work. Employers may offer, in addition to wages, benefits such as health care, sick leave, vacation time, disability insurance, and continuing education. You need to assess the benefits a prospective employer offers in the light of your personal needs. Sometimes such benefits are more important than wages.

EXERCISE 13-14

Compensation and Working Conditions

Directions: Fill in the wages, hours, and benefits you consider minimum requirements. Remember to be realistic. Consider the current wage scales of your community.

Wages per hour _____

Evening/night differential _____

Weekend/holiday differential _____

Overtime pay _____

Health care _____

Dental care _____

Salary increments _____

Vacation credits _____

Sicktime credit _____

Disability insurance _____

Career-ladder options _____

Continuing education _____

Shift: days, evenings, nights _____

Hours per shift _____

Shifts per week _____

Other benefits (for instance, child care) _____

In ambulatory and home care agencies that provide health care during normal working hours, most nurses work five 8-hour days per week. In hospitals and long-term care facilities providing 24-hour, 7-day-a-week care, some nurses must work evenings, nights, and weekends. Some agencies require nurses to rotate shifts so that all nurses work the less desirable ones equally. Others give nurses a choice of shifts. When not enough people choose to work the less

Summary of Preferences in the Nursing Profession

Directions: Summarize your finding from Exercises 13-8 to 13-14 in the following statements.

Health problems and nursing specialties I find most challenging

_____

Human responses to health problems I find most interesting

_____

Nursing functions I prefer

_____

Nursing roles I find most appealing

_____

My preference of client characteristics

_____

My preference of setting characteristics

_____

My requirements for compensation and working conditions

_____

_____

desirable shifts, agencies often use seniority to decide who works these shifts. Consequently, new employees often work evenings and nights. Some facilities offer four 10-hour shifts and three to four 12-hour shifts per week. Exercise 13-14 helps you assess compensation and working conditions in health care settings.

Summary of Preferences in the Nursing Profession

Before going on to set goals and make a work-life plan, use Exercise 13-15 to summarize your preferences relative to the nursing profession.

Goal Setting

Goals are as essential to career plans as destinations are to a journey. They serve as guides for a work-life plan. Without goals nurses are vulnerable to economic pressure and employment expedience. Set-

General Statement of Intent

Directions: Fill in the following statement of intent.

Based on my assessment of various aspects of the nursing profession, I see myself...

focusing on these health problems:

_____

in these nursing specialties:

_____

caring for clients with these human responses:

_____

performing these nursing functions:

_____

in these roles:

_____

for these clients:

_____

in these settings:

_____

for this compensation:

_____

Adapted from Henderson FC, McGettigan BO. *Managing Your Career in Nursing.* 2nd ed. National League for Nursing, 1994.

ting goals involves making a general statement of intent and checking it against personal characteristics. You devise a general statement of intent from information collected during the assessment process. Now that you have identified significant aspects of the nursing profession that you prefer, it is time to make a general statement of intent. Exercise 13-16 provides a framework for this statement.

The next step is to check your statements of intent against the personal characteristics you identified earlier to see if they match. Ask yourself, "Do my intended goals match my values, needs, interests, psychosocial behaviors, proficiency level, and physical capacities? Are my goals realistic?"

Case Study 1. *Connie sees herself in an acute care obstetrics unit, concerned with sexuality-reproductive human responses, providing direct service to young women as a nurse midwife in private practice, with an income equal to that of other advance practice nurses. Connie has an associate degree in nursing and is a single mother supporting three young children. She believes parenting is her God-given responsibility and places high value on spending maximum time with her children. To fulfill her tentative goal, Connie needs several more years of education. To do this she will need to work full time and go to school evenings and weekends, leaving her children in the care of others. As a result Connie will probably experience conflict between her role as a mother and her role as a student. Her tentative goal is not realistic at this time. Connie decides to modify her goal until her children are older and to become a proficient clinician in the maternity unit of her local hospital.*

Case Study 2. *Harvey sees himself focusing on developmental psychiatry and cognitive-perceptual human responses, providing indirect service to people as an administrator of a mental health facility, with an income equal to that of other top-level managers. Although Harvey is bright and motivated, he has difficulty with authority figures and assertive communication and calls himself a "loner." To fulfill his tentative goal, Harvey will need to deal with his authority problem, to learn to communicate assertively, and to work with people. Even if Harvey undergoes psychotherapy and enrolls in an assertiveness class, he may feel more successful if he alters his career goal and becomes an independent nurse practitioner.*

Case Study 3. *Celeste sees herself focusing on preventive care, environmental health, and management, providing direct services to employees in a large industrial plant as an occupational health nurse practitioner, with an income equal to that of other like professionals. Celeste is grossly overweight, has a serious self-esteem problem, and avoids leadership roles. To fulfill her tentative goal she needs to become a role model of health and to learn management skills. Even if Celeste initiates therapy to deal with her lack of self-esteem and obesity, she may find greater satisfaction if she alters her career goal to become a clinician in a health care agency, where she can function as a team member rather than a leader.*

Making Changes

It is important to recognize that personal characteristics can and do change. For example, after Connie's children were reared she decided to return to school. As a result of Harvey's psychotherapy and course work, he learned to deal with authority and to communicate assertively. Because of Celeste's resolve, she lost 95 pounds. Her self-esteem increased, and she decided to pursue her goal of becoming an occupational health nurse.

Some personal characteristics change coincidentally, causing a change in career plans. For instance, one of Connie's children developed leukemia. Because of her involvement in his care, Connie became interested in pediatric oncology. When she returned to school, she became a pediatric nurse practitioner instead of a midwife. One summer Harvey took a job at a camp for developmentally disabled boys. Until then he had never enjoyed outdoor activities. He found the experience exhilarating. Over time, Harvey became an avid outdoorsman and decided to start a ranch for developmentally disabled children. When Celeste lost so much weight, she needed new clothes. To save money she learned to sew, became involved in fashion design, and developed a fulfilling avocation. Thus, both deliberate and coincidental changes affected the work-life plans of each of these nurses just as they may affect yours.

Planning

Once you have clarified your goals, you can begin planning. The first step of planning is to identify necessary education and experience. This information can be obtained from the American Nurses Association (ANA) and various specialty organizations (see Chapter 4). For example, Celeste contacted the Council on Primary Health Care Practitioners of the ANA and the American Association of Occupational Health Nurses. She discovered that the preferred education for top-level occupational health positions is a master's degree in community health nursing with a specialty in occupational health and a minimum of 1 year each of medical-surgical nursing, emergency care, and community health nursing (AAOHN 1992).

When you know the requirements of a goal, you can then compare your education and experience with the requirements and identify what more you need. These needs then become specific objectives in your career plan. Celeste had an associate degree but needed bachelor's and master's degrees in nursing. She had worked a year in acute medical-surgical nursing but needed a year of emergency and a year of community health nursing experience.

Besides education and work experience, you should consider other interests that contribute to a well-rounded life and fit these into your work-life plans. For example, Celeste wanted to do some traveling and to develop a love relationship. She included these personal goals in her career plan.

The final step in the planning process is to make a timeline to accomplish specific objectives, including education, work, and social activities. Celeste decided to combine school, work, and recreation rather than do only one thing at a time. She calculated that she could achieve all of her objectives and reach her goal in 7 years. Exercise 13-17 on page 418 helps you summarize your career plan.

It is never too late to make a work-life plan. Whether you are 18 or 80 years of age, the process is the same. Begin where you are, assess yourself and your work, identify your goals, and create a career plan.

Implementing a Career Plan

The beginning date of a career plan is important. It signals the end of dreaming and the beginning of doing, a time for action. After a while, however, the excitement of implementing a career plan may dwindle. Returning to school or acquiring new experience requires sacrifice. Discouragement is common. Here are some tips for reducing fatigue and maintaining enthusiasm: (1) Post your goals somewhere. (2) Take time to sleep, exercise, and eat. (3) Develop a support system. (4) Periodically reward yourself. You deserve it.

Evaluating Your Career Plan

As you go about implementing your career plan it is important to evaluate not only the goal but also your progress toward that goal. If the job market is tight, you may have to revise your plan, taking a position that is not quite your ideal for a while. Be ready to compromise, but don't give up. Make the most of every twist and turn in your life. Stay in charge of your life. For example, Celeste found that returning to school and working part-time was more difficult than she anticipated. After a month of working 20 hours a week and taking 12 units at the university, she decided to drop 3 units and revise her timeline accordingly. The adjustment made her life more manageable.

A Career Plan

Directions: Fill in the blank spaces with your career plan.

My professional goal is

_____

Educational requirements

_____

Experiential requirements

_____

Educational needs (objectives)

_____

Experiential needs (objectives)

_____

My personal goal is

_____

Personal needs (objectives)

_____

Cost of living

_____

Sources of funding

_____

Timeline to achieve specific objectives

_____

Date I will begin implementing my plan

_____

Accomplished by the end of 1 year

_____

Accomplished by the end of 2 years

_____

Accomplished by the end of 3 years

_____

Accomplished by the end of 4 years

_____
_____

Things went well and Celeste completed her bachelor's degree on the revised schedule. When she applied for graduate school she found that federal money had become available for graduate students in the mental health major. Celeste thought carefully about modifying her major because such a change would alter her career plan. After checking the job market and consulting with people in mental health, she decided to become a clinical specialist in mental health nursing. The revised goal eased her financial burden, gave Celeste a chance to explore her interest in eating disorders, and allowed her to use her experience to help others.

◆ Management Strategies

Management strategies are tactics people use to achieve their career goals. They include marketing, relating, producing, and controlling.

Marketing

Marketing is the process of selling goods or services to prospective buyers. This means convincing them to buy what they want from you because you provide what they need. You may feel uncomfortable with the idea of selling yourself to an employer, yet that is exactly what you do to market yourself. You may think of nursing care in altruistic terms, but the health care industry thinks in terms of market value, asking, "What can this nurse do for our organization? What is this nurse's expertise worth to us?" Some professionals, such as actors and athletes, hire agents to market their services. Usually nurses serve as their own agents. Therefore, you need the essential written communication and interviewing skills of marketing.

Written Communication

Resumés and Curricula Vitae

Resumés and curricula vitae are valuable instruments in the marketing process. Both provide a summary of the qualifications of a nurse, but they have different uses and formats. A *resumé* is a summary of education and experience most relevant to a specific career objective. It is written to attract attention and obtain an interview. Formats of resumés vary, depending on the position for which they are written. Some resumés use a chronological format, listing positions held, education, experience, special accomplishments, and skills, beginning with the most recent. Some resumés use a functional format, stating a career objective and then giving a summary of education and experience. Still others combine the features of chronological and functional formats to fit special circumstances.

A *curriculum vitae (CV)* is a precise formal account of scholarly achievements and activities. It is most often used by educators when they apply for academic appointment, promotion, tenure, or honor. *Curriculum vitae* means "life story," and it is meant to engender respect. Its format is relatively fixed. Here are some general rules for both resumés and CVs:

1. Decide on a format that presents you to your best advantage and is appropriate for the position you are seeking.

2. Use precise phrases with action verbs, such as *directed, solved, led, built,* and *taught;* avoid wordy descriptions and explanations.

3. Use numbers to show quantitative results, for instance, "nosocomial infections dropped by 52%."

4. Omit personal information such as your birth date, marital status, religion, health status, and politics; *never use* "I," "me," or "my" in a resumé or curriculum vitae.

5. Never use gimmicks such as smiling faces, and avoid trying to be clever; these devices trivialize your marketing efforts.

6. Do not be afraid to use the vocabulary of nursing, such as *primary nursing,* or *triage.*

7. Never mention the salary of prior positions or the salary expected in a new position; salary is discussed during negotiation.

8. Be prepared to give names and addresses of references by asking colleagues and supervisors for their permission in advance.

9. Be aware that employers may ask questions about long gaps of unemployment or numerous, brief periods of employment.

10. Use high-quality white, gray, or cream-colored paper of letter size. Center the content on the page, and use only one side of the paper. Select a simple, legible typeface. Word processors produce flawless copies at little cost and make updating easy.

11. Proofread your document to eliminate misspelled words, typographical errors, and grammatical mistakes; never underline for

Framework for a Chronological Resumé

Name: (First, middle initial, and last. Do not state birth date.)

Address:

Home Phone:

Education: (Degrees or certificates earned; school, beginning with the most recent. Do not include high school.)

Licenses and Certificates: (eg, RN #07235, California.)

Other Skills: (eg, fluent in Spanish.)

Professional Experience: (Begin with the most recent. State the dates, employer, position, and a brief job description, using action verbs in words such as "managed a 20-bed burn unit." Do not use "I," "me," or "my.")

Special Accomplishments and Honors: (Go ahead, brag. List recent or outstanding achievements, eg, 1995 Nurse of the Year Award, Seton Hospital, Albany, NY.)

Continuing Education: (Recent or relevant)

Other Activities: (Show your specialness, eg, coordinator, Health Faire 1994; volunteer, Meals-on-Wheels, 1994–96.)

References Available on Request (Never include names in resumé.)

---

emphasis or make corrections in ink after the resumé has been printed.

12. Never attach transcripts, letters of recommendation, or photographs to a resumé or CV; do include your resumé or CV with your cover letter.

13. Make resumés brief, preferably one page long, so that employers can scan them in 30 to 45 seconds. Make CVs as long as it takes to list the complete "story of your life."

Exercises 13-18, 13-19, and 13-20 provide frameworks for writing resumés and curricula vitae.

Framework for a Functional Resumé

Name: (First, middle initial, last. Do not state birth date.)

Address:

Home Phone:

Professional Objective: (Optional. Stress employer-valued benefits rather than applicant-valued benefits, eg, to demonstrate creative leadership as nurse manager.)

Summary of Qualifications: (eg, RN, BSN, Certified Cardiac Rehabilitation Nurse.)

Significant Qualifications: (eg, six years experience in cardiac care: set up cardiac step-down unit; nurse manager for 2 years in cardiac step-down unit; staff nurse for 4 years in cardiac rehabilitation.)

Professional Development: (List your work experience, beginning with your most recent job. State title, dates, name and address of each institution.)

Education: (Beginning with the most recent, state each school and degree or certificate earned.)

Professional Affiliations: (eg, American Nurses Association, Illinois Nurses Association.)

References Available on Request (Never include names in resumé.)

Framework for a Curriculum Vitae

Name: (First, middle, last. Do not state birth date.)

Address: (May use academic address.)

Phone: (At given address.)

Education: (Begin after high school. State degree, major, and school, but no dates; eg, BS, Nursing, Stanford University; MS, Community Mental Health Nursing, University of California, San Francisco; EdD, University of San Francisco.)

Credentials: (Licenses and certificates; eg, RN California: #73102, PHN California: 16495, Psychiatric Mental Health Nurse Certificate #206, Community College Instructor, Lifetime.)

Experience: (Begin with the most recent position. Give dates, showing time span, title, institution.)

9/93–6/95	Instructor, VN program, Laney College, Oakland, CA
11/90–6/93	Staff nurse II, oncology, Peralta Hospital, Oakland, CA
8/85–9/90	Staff nurse I, oncology, Peralta Hospital, Oakland, CA

Honors and Awards: (eg, Outstanding Teacher Award, Laney College.)

Professional Memberships: (eg, California Nurses Association, Sigma Theta Tau, Lambda Gamma Chapter.)

Publications: (List alphabetically as in a bibliography.)

References Available on Request (Never include names in CV.)

Cover Letters

The purpose of a cover letter, or letter of inquiry, is to introduce yourself, to express interest in a position, and to point to the enclosed resumé. It is written for a certain job, and when possible, addressed to a specific person. Cover letters accompany resumés, personalize them, and allow you to draw attention to an area of expertise or interest. Employers use cover letters as screening tools, to get a "feel" for applicants. Here are some general rules for writing cover letters:

1. Whenever possible, address the letter to a specific person.

2. State why you are writing the letter and where or how you heard of the position; you may use "I," "me," and "my."

3. Explain your interest in the position in terms of what the employer values rather than what you value (for instance, challenge and growth, rather than location and money).

4. Highlight major career accomplishments and refer the prospective employer to your resumé for further details.

5. Indicate a desire for an interview and suggest a plan for arranging it.

6. Close with appreciation for consideration of your application and a final statement of enthusiasm and interest.

7. Use high-quality, letter-size stationery, and a legible, simple typeface. Center the letter on the page; proofread for errors of spelling, grammar, or punctuation. See Exercise 13-21.

Job Application Forms

Even though you send a cover letter and your resumé to a prospective employer, you should expect to fill out the application form of the agency. These forms vary in length, detail, and format. They often ask for information not included on resumés, such as the names and addresses of references. Although it may seem redundant to copy data from a resumé onto an application, doing so has a valid purpose. A form provides employers with a standardized means to compare candidates, thus simplifying the selection process. It is acceptable to attach a resumé to an application form, but it is not acceptable to line through the form and write "see attached," at least, not if you are serious about the position.

Record Keeping

It is helpful to keep a copy of every resumé, cover letter, application form, and letter of resignation you write throughout your career.

Framework for Cover Letter

Nancy Preven, BS, RN, C (*your name and degrees*)
24 Aledo Dr. Napa, CA 94558 (*address*)
(707) 555-1234 (*phone number*)

February 7, 1996 (*date*)

Paul Walden, RN (*person responsible for employing or recruiting
    nurses, If unknown, call agency for name and correct spelling*)
Director of Nursing Recruitment (*title, if unknown, obtain from
    agency*)
Camp Laurelwood (*name of institution*)
360 Amity Rd., Woodbridge, CT 06525 (*address*)

Dear (*Mr., Ms, or Dr. and last name*):

I (*say how you heard or read of a position in the institution*) read
your advertisement for a camp nurse at Camp Laurelwood in the
February, 1995 issue of *AJN* with great interest. My career includes
(*tell of special experiences that relate to the position*) 5 years in
pediatric nursing, the past 2 working with diabetic children and their
parents in an outpatient clinic. I am (*tell of special knowledge and
education as it relates to the position*) knowledgeable of current
treatment protocols for childhood diabetes and teaching techniques
for children. I have a BS in nursing and an ANA certificate as a
pediatric nurse.

I (*suggest a plan to follow up on this letter*) will call you a week from
today at 3:00 PM to set up a time to meet with you.

Thank you for your consideration of my application. I am eager to
put my talents to work for (*clients and staff of the institution*)
Camp Laurelwood.

Sincerely,

(*full signature*)
Nancy Preven, RN, BS (*type name and degrees below signature*)

When it is time to revise your resumé or to write another cover letter, you will find the old ones useful. They include names, addresses, and dates of education and experience.

Interviewing

If a resumé or CV accomplishes its purpose, you are invited to a job interview. The resumé or CV persuaded the agency that the person it described had the knowledge and skill the agency is seeking. The interview confirms and reinforces that impression. An interview is a purposeful, goal-directed interaction between people aimed at determining if the abilities and skills of the applicant match the needs of the agency. The goal of both interviewees and interviewers is to learn more about the other, to present themselves in the best light, and to determine if there is a match. Success for both parties requires careful preparation, skillful participation, and energetic follow-up.

Preparation

To prepare for a job interview, gather information about the agency, take stock of yourself, and reduce as much stress as possible. You can obtain information about a prospective employer from informal conversations with employees and from published material available from the personnel department, such as newsletters, official histories, and policy manuals. When you take the time to gather such information you demonstrate interest in the agency and are able to ask more insightful questions in the interview.

A good way to take stock of yourself is to use the personal assessment exercises in this chapter. Take time to develop a vocabulary of key words and short phrases that describe your accomplishments and personal strengths, such as *reliable, energetic, conscientious, objective, tolerant, resourceful, logical, productive, discreet, forward-thinking,* and *perceptive*. You can reduce your stress by doing the following:

1. Role-play answering standard questions ahead of time, such as: What are some of your accomplishments at your present job? What is your greatest strength, weakness? What are your short-range and long-range career objectives? Why are you leaving your present job?

2. Avoid last minute crises. Make a practice trip to the agency, noting the route, driving time, and parking facilities. Try on the clothes you plan to wear. Gather together and take: a job descrip-

tion, your resumé, your cover letter, all correspondence, and a list of your questions.

3. Bring a list of questions to ask interviewers, such as: How would you characterize the management style of this agency? Is professional growth encouraged and rewarded? What opportunities are there for advancement? What happened to the last person in the position? How would you describe ideal behavior in the position? What is the best thing about this institution? What is the worst thing?

4. Go to bed early the night before; start the day by eating easily digested food; just before the interview, go to the restroom and take a few moments to gain composure and control. You know who you are, what you can do, and what you want.

Participation

You may be interviewed by one person, a series of individuals, or a group of people. The opening of an interview includes introduction of participants to one another, clarification of the purpose of the interview, and agreement on guidelines, such as the allotted time and screening process. Here are some suggestions for a successful job interview:

1. Arrive no more than 10 minutes early. If you are unavoidably delayed, phone and ask for another appointment time. If you are kept waiting more than 20 minutes, ask for another appointment and excuse yourself.

2. Dress well, but conservatively. A suit is a good choice for both men and women, although in some areas more casual attire is acceptable. Avoid faddish clothes, excessive jewelry or make-up, and strong perfume. Torn or soiled clothing, dirty hair, body odor, and bad breath are unacceptable. Avoid fumbling with a heavy coat or packages. Ask to place them in an out-of-the-way place before the interview begins. Remember, your appearance speaks louder than words. When you feel good about your appearance, you will be more confident.

3. Remain calm and cordial. Speak clearly and slowly. Be brief, positive, and enthusiastic. Think before speaking. Avoid "and-ahs," "you-knows," and other nervous noises.

4. Take brief notes to help you remember names or information.

5. Be truthful. If your background includes substance abuse or a felony offense, volunteer only what you must reveal legally. If asked, tell the truth without defensiveness. You are now a healthy, competent professional. Title VII of the 1964 Civil Rights Act as amended by the 1972 Equal Employment Opportunity Act requires that employer inquiries be position-related. This means you can respectfully decline to answer questions unrelated to job performance, such as age, religion, race, handicaps, and marital status. Chapter 10 lists questions interviewers cannot ask.

6. Use a soft sell. Underplay your need for the job, and emphasize your assets and accomplishments.

7. Maintain professional dignity and emotional control. Do not criticize, condemn, complain, or divulge confidences of your present employer.

8. Be a good listener. Avoid showing impatience or boredom. When a period of silence occurs, ask questions that demonstrate your knowledge and experience.

9. The interview is as much for you to "get a feel" for the agency as for the agency to "get a feel" for you. Ask your prepared questions and any others that occur to you.

10. The initial interview is rarely the time to negotiate wages; however, salary is always part of the discussion. Do not initiate the subject too early; you may appear overeager. Before the interview ends, ask about the salary range, benefits, employee-employer contract, and requirements for membership in a labor union. If the institution offers you a position at the interview, give yourself time to consider it. For middle- and higher-level positions, salary is never discussed with a search committee. It is negotiated later with other officials.

11. At the close, thank the interviewers, by name. Confirm when you can expect to hear their decision, and make sure that the interviewers know when, where, and how to contact you.

Evaluation

Evaluating your performance at an interview helps you learn from the experience so that you will be more skillful the next time. Soon after the interview ask yourself these questions:

1. Did I reduce stressors sufficiently? What else could I have done to bolster my composure and sense of control?

2. Was I dressed appropriately? Did I talk too much, too little? Did I present my knowledge and skill accurately? Did I watch for non-verbal or verbal clues and adjust my behavior accordingly? What will I do differently in the future?

3. Did I gather enough information about the agency ahead of time? What did I lack?

Evaluation of the position and institution involves comparing it to an ideal one and to others you have visited. Exercise 13-13, Assessment of Settings, and Exercise 13-16, General Statement of Intent, may help with this task.

Follow-Up

Follow-up of an interview is vital. It is done to demonstrate social skills, to confirm interest in the position, and to remind interviewers of your qualifications. A follow-up letter should be written after every interview. If you are highly interested in a position, telephone interviewers as well as writing to them. Make follow-up messages brief and focused. Express appreciation for the interview, indicate continued enthusiasm and interest in the position, and remind interviewers of your qualifications. See Exercise 13-22 on page 430.

Relationships

Relationship strategies pave the way for nurses to achieve career goals. They include negotiating, networking, maintaining collegial relationships, and discriminating.

Negotiating

Negotiating is a mutual discussion of disputed issues aimed at reaching an agreement. It is open communication between parties for the purpose of reaching an accord. If there is no union contract, you may need to negotiate with the prospective employer about salary, benefits, and working conditions.

Until recently, it was rare for nurses to have open discussions about salary. The topic was deemed unprofessional because the primary reward was supposed to be personal satisfaction. Today, nurses view discussion of compensation a normal part of professional

Framework for an Interview Follow-up Letter

Priscilla Perez, RN, C (*your name and degrees*)
27 Webster St., Oakland, CA 94117 (*address*)
(510) 555-1234 (*phone number*)

August 29, 1995 (*date*)

Muriel Halvorson, PhD, RNC, NP (*name of person who conducted
   the interview with degrees*)
Director of Nursing Services (*title*)
San Francisco General Hospital (*name of institution*)
2100 Potrero Ave., San Francisco, CA 94110 (*address*)

Dear (*Mr., Ms, Dr. and last name*):

It was a pleasure to meet with you and the members of the screening committee on (*state the day and date*). I found the interview
informative and (*state any other positive experience or idea with
which you agreed*) enjoyed the tour of the new wing.

I am enthusiastic about (*state anything you wish to emphasize about
the institution and how you would fill its needs*) the challenge available at General Hospital in interdisciplinary care of developmentally
disabled children. I would welcome the opportunity to (*whatever it is
you want to do*) be involved in setting up the new unit.

I look forward to hearing from you in the near future.

Sincerely,

(*full signature*)
Priscilla Perez, RN, C (*type your name and degrees below signature*)

considerations. Here are some strategies for negotiating salaries and benefits:

1. Before negotiations begin, learn what the employer needs and find out what other institutions are paying for the same work.

2. Set realistic goals; when you change positions, it is unrealistic to expect a salary increase of more than 20%. In fact, if you move from one region of the country to another with a lower economic standard, your new salary may be lower than your old one.

3. Start with a range, not a specific figure; the employer will negotiate down from your figure.

4. Avoid negotiating from your present salary. Instead, emphasize the unique credentials (past achievements, experience, education) you will bring to the position.

5. Be positive about everything except salary; express both enthusiasm and sincerity about your salary needs.

6. If the salary is fixed and seems low, try for other things, such as automatic pay increases, tuition and educational leave, reimbursement for moving expenses, and medical insurance.

7. When you have their "bottom line," make written notes in the presence of the employer representative and suggest a time when you will give your answer.

Networking

Networking is the cultivation of relationships with others for the purpose of sharing information and resources. The overriding function of networking is to help people build their careers. A network provides a sense of belonging and acceptance, social companionship, concrete assistance, information, and advice. It is made up of a variety of people in and out of nursing. In practice, networking means sharing information, listening to a story, contributing to a special need, and giving advice to neophytes. When people need mutual assistance to build their careers, networking can help. Develop a network wherever you go.

Maintaining Collegial Relationships

Collegial relationships are based on a professional connection but are closer than those found in networks. Colleagues are coworkers, allies, collaborators, teammates, peers, and mentors (as discussed in Chapter 10). They share knowledge, provide support, and challenge one another to new ways of thinking. Colleagues respect one another. They may have varying experiences and education or even belong to different professions, but you can count on them to give advice and assistance when asked. Colleagues write letters of reference, listen when you need a sympathetic ear, and explain something you don't know.

Discriminating

To *discriminate* means to make a distinction on a categorical basis rather than according to particular merit. Discrimination can be helpful or harmful. It is helpful when it aids decision making. For example, the career goal of Ulla is to become an educator. She is offered two positions, one in education and one in administration. Ulla chooses the education position because it matches her career goal, not because education is better than administration. When discrimination denies people equal opportunity to pursue career goals, it is harmful. In the United States it is unlawful to discriminate in the workplace on the basis of age, sex, religion, race, politics, physical disability, and marital status. Sexual preference is not yet specifically protected.

Production

Production strategies are tactics that increase your skill, knowledge, and effectiveness. Two such strategies are continuing education and occupational health and safety.

Continuing Education

In many states continuing education (CE) is mandatory for relicensure. (See Chapter 2.) Even when it is not required, nurses need continuing education to refocus, remediate, or advance. Isabel wants to move laterally from a medical to a rehabilitation unit. To support her goal, she is taking a series of CE courses in rehabilitative nursing. Jan wants to move vertically into management. To do this she is pursuing a master's degree in nursing administration.

Occupational Health and Safety

Maintaining personal health and safety is an essential production strategy for nurses. If you don't have health, career planning is futile.

As you care for the sick and injured, you may forget to safeguard your own health and safety. As a nurse, you are exposed to potent chemicals, dangerous pathogens, physical strain, assaultive patients, hazardous radiation, and emotional stressors. Compliance by employers to national and state codes is not enough. Nurses must assume responsibility for their own health. You can do this by getting adequate rest, exercise, and nutrition; reducing stress; and getting regular physical checkups and immunizations.

Control

Control strategies are mechanisms that measure how well a process meets its goals. These strategies include setting standards, evaluating performance as compared to standards, and correcting behavior that does not meet standards.

Setting Standards

To manage your career effectively, you need to set standards by which you can measure your progress toward your goals. Here are some suggestions:

1. Collect data systematically and continuously.

2. Include long-term goals and short-term objectives in your career plan.

3. Define and prioritize the actions you need to take to achieve your career plan.

4. Make periodic checks to evaluate progress toward your career goals.

5. Revise your career goals to reflect progress and changing circumstances.

Evaluating Performance

When you accept employment you can expect the employer to evaluate your performance. Often new employees are hired with probationary status for 2 to 6 months. At the end of probation, performance is evaluated. Thereafter, agencies evaluate performance at designated intervals unless special problems arise. Various methods are used to evaluate performance, including self-review, peer review by coworkers, and administrative review by supervisors. Because performance evaluations affect salary, professional advancement, and self-esteem, they produce immense anxiety. Here are some guidelines to help you improve your performance and reduce your fear of evaluation:

1. During orientation to the agency, obtain a list of evaluation criteria. Learn exactly what you are expected to do and by what standards you will be measured. Ideally, evaluation criteria are stated as behaviors, such as, "communicates pertinent client information at shift change."

2. During the probationary period, review evaluation criteria to remind yourself of the behaviors your employer expects.

3. When it is time for an evaluation interview, or if your supervisor sets a "counseling session" with you because of a problem, take a moment to relax and become centered. View negative comments as a way to grow and become a better nurse.

4. No matter what is said or written, do not exhibit hostility or become defensive. Do listen carefully to what is said. If you feel the feedback is exaggerated or untrue, say so in a matter-of-fact way. Without admitting fault, assure the evaluator that the errant behavior will not happen in the future. Your goal is the same as that of your supervisor: to deliver high-quality nursing care. If you are deficient in some way, enlist the help of the evaluator to change.

Only you can evaluate progress toward your career goals. However, performance evaluations may open new career options. For example, in several reviews, Ulla's supervisor commended her for her teaching ability. Until then, Ulla had never seriously considered a teaching career. The evaluations encouraged her to consider enrolling in a master's degree program for nurse educators.

Termination and Resignation

Control strategies involve terminating old positions and moving on to new ones. Like the feedback loop of the nursing process, where evaluation serves as reassessment, terminating one position serves as the beginning of a new employment cycle. Terminations may be initiated by an employer as a firing or layoff or by the nurse as a resignation.

When performance evaluations identify behaviors that do not meet standards, employers follow the process spelled out in the employer-employee contract. Often the steps include counseling and written warnings, with opportunities for change. If these measures fail, the nurse is terminated (fired). Common reasons for nurse terminations include substance abuse, poor job performance, tardiness, absenteeism, inappropriate behavior, and staff reductions. Reasons for immediate terminations include abuse of a client or visitor, drug possession, intoxication, theft, disorderly conduct, falsification of records, willful destruction of property, and sleeping on duty.

Termination is especially difficult when nurses are laid off through no fault of their own. Nurses who are hired into highly visible and vulnerable positions sometimes anticipate layoffs and make "termination agreements" in advance, stipulating continuation of benefits or salary for a certain time. Many hospitals follow the lead of industry, offering "outplacement counseling" for terminated staff members. The purpose of this counseling is to help nurses deal with their loss and grief and find other employment. Rituals such as going-away parties facilitate the process.

No job lasts forever. Eventually all nurses resign or are terminated. Even so, resignation should not be impulsive or precipitous. Neither should it be delayed endlessly because of guilt or misplaced loyalty. Moving on toward goals means saying good-bye to the old and familiar. Nevertheless, before you talk or write to anyone about leaving, consider these suggestions:

1. Check your employee-employer contract regarding benefits, accrued sick leave, and vacation time. It is important to comply with legal agreements and ethical commitments. Give advance notice for at least the number of days of the pay period; give more notice if you have an especially responsible position.

2. Check with personnel to determine current accrued time.

3. Be considerate of coworkers; try to complete projects you have begun and prepare helpful guides to assist your successor.

4. Write a letter of resignation using these guidelines: (a) State your intention to leave, the effective date of resignation and last working day, a reason for leaving, some sincere positive experience in the position, and an offer to assist in the transition. (b) Use precise wording; avoid being maudlin or malicious; mention by name people who have been especially helpful. (c) Address the letter to the unit manager, with a copy to your immediate supervisor.

(d) Proofread your letter for correct spelling, punctuation, and grammar. (e) Use high-quality, letter-size paper; center the text on the page; and use one side only with a legible typeface. (f) Remember that resignation letters are like epitaphs on tombstones. They leave a final impression of the writer; better to say nothing than make bitter or inappropriate statements.

5. Before you deliver a resignation letter to the administrator, courtesy dictates that you meet with your immediate supervisor. Give the essential facts stated in the letter of resignation and express your personal appreciation. See Exercise 13-23.

◆ Sources of Information

Audiovisual Media

Each year professional nursing organizations and publishers produce periodicals, books, AV tapes, and computer programs to help with career planning. Nursing periodicals such as the *American Journal of Nursing, RN Magazine,* and *Nursing* publish classified sections listing particular employment offerings. Information about specific topics is indexed in references such as the *International Nursing Index, Cumulative Index to Nursing* and *Allied Literature, Index Medicus,* and *Hospital Literature Index,* and in computerized databases such as the *National Library of Medicine (NLM Medline)* and *Educational Resources Information Center (ERIC).*

Individuals and Organizations

Individuals and organizations are a rich source of information about careers in nursing. These include (1) staff nurses, mentors, nursing leaders, and instructors; (2) representatives of professional organizations; (3) offices of the state nurses associations affiliated with the ANA; (4) placement agencies; (5) recruitment offices of the United States armed services; (6) career fairs where health care providers set up exhibits to recruit nurses; (7) bibliographies of workshop speakers; (8) networks of other nurses at conferences and workshops; (9) National League for Nursing placement center; (10) World Health Organization, Avenue Appia, 1211 Geneva 27, Switzerland;

Framework for a Letter of Resignation

Tina Certa, BS, RN (*your name and degrees*)
2301 Harrison St., Denver, CO 80818 (*address*)

May 10, 1996 (*date*)

Sandra Haber, RN, MS (*name of top nursing service administrator and degrees*)
Vice-President of Nursing Services (*title*)
Denver General Hospital (*name of institution*)
150 Evans Ave., Denver, CO 80820 (*address*)

Dear (*Mr., Ms, Dr. and last name*):

I have decided to (*state plan of action*) return to school for a MS degree in nursing at the University of Texas. Therefore, I wish to resign effective (*state the date that will include all accrued leave days*) _____. Since I have _____ accrued vacation days, my last working day will be (*state the date*) _____.

Working with the patients and staff at (*name of institution*) has been a satisfying personal and professional experience. I have (*say something positive*) learned so much about pediatric nursing care. I particularly appreciate (*name someone, if true*) because (*state act or attitude*). I am proud to have been a part of (*name of institution*) because (*state why*). (*Omit the last sentence if it is not true.*)

If there is something I can do to help in the transition, I will be happy to do so.

Sincerely,

(*full signature*)
Tina Certa, BS, RN (*type your name and degrees below signature*)

---

and (11) Nursing Abroad, ^c/o The International Council of Nurses, Box 42, 1211 Geneva 20, Switzerland; and Intercristo, Box 33487, Seattle, WA 98109; (12) recruitment offices: the Peace Corps, Washington, D.C. 20525, (800) 424-8580.

◇ Summary

Career management means making a work-life plan to provide self-fulfillment and realize personal and professional goals. To make such a plan, nurses collect and assess data about themselves and their profession. With this information they set goals, make plans, implement them, and evaluate progress. To sell themselves to prospective employers, nurses use the marketing strategies of written communication and interviewing and use relationship, production, and control strategies to succeed in their selected profession. With a work-life plan, nurses experience successful, fulfilling careers.

Critical Thinking Questions

1. As you completed the assessment exercises in this chapter, what did you discover about yourself that might influence your career plans?

2. Did this chapter cover everything that is important to you regarding career planning? What other information, if any, might be important for you to have?

3. As you begin making a career plan, what single issue is most important to you? Does anything hold you back from making a commitment to a career path at this time? If so, what?

Learning Activities

1. Make a personal and professional assessment using Exercises 13-1 to 13-15.

2. Write your career goals and tentative plan using Exercises 13-16 and 13-17.

3. Write a resumé or curriculum vitae using Exercises 13-18, 13-19, or 13-20 as a guide.

4. Write a cover letter to accompany your resumé or curriculum vitae using Exercise 13-21 as a guide.

5. Visit a career center at a college or university. Find out the services they offer to students and graduates.

6. Visit a recruiting office of a military service; report your findings in a group discussion.

7. Interview the nurse recruiter or personnel manager at a local hospital or long-term care facility. Ask what that person looks for in nurse applicants.

8. Interview a new graduate. Ask what that person would recommend to others beginning a nursing career.

9. Write a letter of resignation using Exercise 13-23 as a guide.

Annotated Reading List

American Journal of Nursing, Job Focus and Career Guide, 1994.

Each issue of the magazine includes a "Career Guide" and a "Job Focus" section. Each month, the "Career Guide" has articles to stimulate your thinking about making your work more satisfying. For example, the June 1994 article, "Six Ways to Take This Job and Love It," tells nurses how to choose not to be victims, but rather to create ways of giving clients high-quality care and at the same time enjoy their work. In the "Job Focus," the magazine highlights various sections of the country each month, listing institutions that have openings for nurses. In today's tight job market, this section fills a definite need.

Minority Nurse Summer/Fall 1994. 16030 Ventura Blvd., #560, Encino, CA 91436.

This entire publication is devoted to career options for both new graduate nurses and those with many years of experience. Titles of some of the articles in this issue are: "Peace Corps: The Toughest Job You'll Ever Love," "New Directions in Orientation," and "Employer Profiles." The advertisements in this biannual publication are almost as interesting as the articles. They describe employment opportunities nurses might not otherwise consider, such as in insurance companies, the National Institutes of Health, and the Department of Veterans Affairs. A valuable help for beginning as well as seasoned nurses.

References

American Association of Occupational Health Nurses. *Guidelines for Developing Job Descriptions in Occupational Health Nursing.* AAOHN, 1992.

Benner P. *From Novice to Expert.* Addison-Wesley, 1984.

Gordon M. *Nursing Diagnosis.* McGraw Hill, 1982.

Henderson FC, McGettigan BO. *Managing Your Career in Nursing.* Addison-Wesley, 1986.

Marriner-Tomey A. *Guide to Nursing Management,* 4th ed. Mosby, 1992.

Morrison M. *Professional Skills for Leadership: Foundations of a Successful Career.* Mosby, 1994.

Appendix A

◇ Members of the National Council of State Boards of Nursing

Alabama Board of Nursing
RSA Plaza, Suite 250
770 Washington Ave.
Montgomery, AL 36130

**Alaska Board of Nursing,
Department of Commerce
and Economic Development**
Division of Occupational Licensing
3601 C St., Suite 722
Anchorage, AK 99503

**American Samoa Health
Service, Regulatory Board**
LBJ Tropical Medical Ctr.
Pago Pago, American Samoa 96799

Arizona State Board of Nursing
1651 E. Morten Ave., Suite 150
Phoenix, AZ 85020

**Arkansas State Board
of Nursing**
University Tower Bldg., Suite 800
1123 S. University St.
Little Rock, AR 72204

**California Board of
Registered Nursing**
400 R St., Suite 4030
Sacramento, CA 95814

**California Board of Vocational
Nurse and Psychiatric
Technician Examiners**
1414 K St., Suite 103
Sacramento, CA 95814

Colorado Board of Nursing
1560 Broadway, Suite 670
Denver, CO 80202

**Connecticut Board of
Examiners for Nursing**
150 Washington St.
Hartford, CT 06106

Delaware Board of Nursing
Margaret O'Neill Bldg.
P.O. Box 1401
Dover, DE 19903

**District of Columbia
Board of Nursing**
614 H St., NW
Washington, DC 20001

Florida Board of Nursing
111 Coastline Dr., East, Suite 516
Jacksonville, FL 32202

Georgia Board of Nursing
166 Pryor St., SW
Atlanta, GA 30303

**Georgia State Board of
Licensed Practical Nurses**
166 Pryor St., SW
Atlanta, GA 30303

**Guam Board of Nurse
Examiners**
P.O. Box 2816
Agana, GU 96910

Hawaii Board of Nursing
P.O. Box 3469
Honolulu, HI 96801

Idaho Board of Nursing
280 N. 8th St., Suite 210
Boise, ID 83720

**Illinois Department of
Professional Regulation**
320 W. Washington St., 3rd Fl.
Springfield, IL 62786

100 W. Randolph St., Suite 9-300
Chicago, IL 60601

**Indiana State Board of Nursing,
Health Professions Bureau**
402 W. Washington St., Room 041
Indianapolis, IN 46204

Iowa Board of Nursing
State Capitol Complex
1223 E. Court Ave.
Des Moines, IA 50319

Kansas State Board of Nursing
Landon State Office Bldg.
900 S.W. Jackson St., Suite 551-S
Topeka, KS 66612

Kentucky Board of Nursing
312 Wittington Parkway, Suite 300
Louisville, KY 40222

**Louisiana State Board
of Nursing**
912 Pere Marquette Bldg.
150 Baronne St.
New Orleans, LA 70112

**Louisiana State Board
of Practical Nurse Examiners**
3421 N. Causeway Blvd., Suite 203
Metairie, LA 70002

Maine State Board of Nursing
State House Station #158
Augusta, ME 04333

Maryland Board of Nursing
4140 Patterson Ave.
Baltimore, MD 21215

**Massachusetts Board of
Registration in Nursing**
Leverett Saltonstall Bldg.
100 Cambridge St., Rm. 1519
Boston, MA 02202

**Bureau of Occupational and
Professional Regulation, Michi-
gan Department of Commerce**
Ottawa Towers North
611 West Ottawa
Lansing, MI 48933

Minnesota Board of Nursing
2700 University Ave., West #108
St. Paul, MN 55114

Mississippi Board of Nursing
239 N. Lamar St., Suite 401
Jackson, MS 39201

Missouri State Board of Nursing
3605 Missouri Blvd.
Jefferson City, MO 65109

Montana State Board of Nursing, Department of Commerce
Arcade Bldg., Lower Level
111 N. Jackson St.
Helena, MT 59620

Bureau of Examining Boards, Nebraska Department of Health
301 Centennial Mall South
Lincoln, NE 68508

Nevada State Board of Nursing
1281 Terminal Way, Suite 116
Reno, NV 89502

4335 S. Industrial Rd., Suite 430
Las Vegas, NV 89103

New Hampshire Board of Nursing
Health & Welfare Bldg.
6 Hazen Dr.
Concord, NH 03301

New Jersey Board of Nursing
124 Halsey St., 6th Fl.
Newark, NJ 07102

New Mexico Board of Nursing
4206 Louisiana Blvd., NE, Suite A
Albuquerque, NM 87109

New York State Board of Nursing, State Education Department
Cultural Education Center
Rm. 3023
Albany, NY 12230

North Carolina Board of Nursing
3724 National Dr.
Raleigh, NC 27612

North Dakota Board of Nursing
919 S. 7th St., Suite 504
Bismarck, ND 58504

Northern Mariana Islands Commonwealth Board of Nurse Examiners
Public Health Center
P.O. Box 1456
Saipan, MP 96950

Ohio Board of Nursing
77 South High St., 17th Fl.
Columbus, OH 43266

Oklahoma Board of Nursing
2915 N. Classen Blvd., Suite 524
Oklahoma City, OK 73106

Oregon State Board of Nursing
800 NE Oregon St., Suite 465
Box 25
Portland, OR 97232

Pennsylvania State Board of Nursing
Commonwealth Ave. & Forester
Sts., Rm. 611
Harrisburg, PA 17105

Commonwealth of Puerto Rico Board of Nurse Examiners
Call Box 10200
Santurce, PR 00908

Rhode Island Board of Nurse Registration & Nursing Education
Cannon Health Bldg.
Three Capitol Hill, Rm. 104
Providence, RI 02908

South Carolina State Board
of Nursing
220 Executive Center Dr., Suite 220
Columbia, SC 29210

South Dakota Board of Nursing
3307 S. Lincoln Ave.
Sioux Falls, SD 57105

Tennessee State Board
of Nursing
283 Plus Park Blvd.
Nashville, TN 37247

Texas Board of Nurse
Examiners
9101 Burnet Rd.
Austin, TX 78758

Texas Board of Vocational
Nurse Examiners
9101 Burnet Rd., Suite 105
Austin, TX 78758

Utah State Board of Nursing,
Division of Occupational
and Professional Licensing
Heber M. Wells Bldg., 4th Fl.
160 East 300 South
Salt Lake City, UT 84111

Vermont State Board
of Nursing
Redstone Bldg.
26 Terrace St.
Montpelier, VT 05602

Virginia Board of Nursing
6606 W. Broad St., 4th Fl.
Richmond, VA 23230

Virgin Islands Board
of Nurse Licensure
P.O. Box 4247
Veterans Drive Station
St. Thomas, U.S. VI 00803

Washington State Nursing Care
Quality Assurance Commission,
Department of Health
P.O. Box 47864
Olympia, WA 98504

West Virginia Board
of Examiners for Registered
Professional Nurses
101 Dee Dr.
Charleston, WV 25311

West Virginia State Board of
Examiners for Practical Nurses
101 Dee Dr.
Charleston, WV 25311

Wisconsin Department
of Regulation & Licensing
1400 E. Washington Ave.
Madison, WI 53708

Wyoming State Board
of Nursing
Barrett Bldg., 2nd Fl.
2301 Central Ave.
Cheyenne, WY 82002

Appendix B

◆ Directory of Selected Nursing and Health-Related Organizations

International

International Council of Nurses
3, place Jean-Marteau
1201 Geneva, Switzerland

International Council of Nurses, American Nurses Association
1 Park Ave.
New York, NY 10016

Pan American Health Organization
Pan American Sanitary Bureau, WHO Regional Office for the Americas
525 23rd St. NW
Washington, DC 20037

People to People Health Foundation (Project HOPE)
Millwood, VA 22646

World Health Organization
Avenue Appia
1211 Geneva 27, Switzerland

National

Alpha Tau Delta National Fraternity for Professional Nurses
5207 Mesada St.
Alta Loma, CA 91737

American Academy of Nurse Practitioners
Capital Station, LBJ Bldg.
PO Box 12846
Austin TX 78711

American Academy of Nursing
600 Maryland Ave., SW
Suite 100 West
Washington, DC 20024

American Assembly of Men in Nursing
P.O. Box 31753
Independence, OH 44131

600 S. Paulina, 474-H
Chicago, IL 60612

American Association of Colleges of Nursing
One Dupont Circle, Suite 530
Washington, DC 20036

American Association
of Critical-Care Nurses
101 Columbia
Aliso Viejo, CA 92656

American Association for
the History of Nursing, Inc.
P.O. Box 90803
Washington, DC 20090

American Association
of Neuroscience Nurses
224 N. Des Plaines, Suite 601
Chicago, IL 60661

American Association
of Nurse Anesthetists
222 South Prospect Ave.
Park Ridge, IL 60068

American Association
of Nurse Attorneys
720 Light St.
Baltimore, MD 21230

American Association of Occupational Health Nurses, Inc.
50 Lenox Pointe
Atlanta, GA 30324

American Cancer Society
90 Park Ave.
New York, NY 10016

American College
of Nurse-Midwives
818 Connecticut Ave. NW, Suite 900
Washington, DC 20006

American Heart Association
7320 Greenville Ave.
Dallas, TX 75231

American Hospital Association
840 N. Lake Shore Dr.
Chicago, IL 60611

American Journal
of Nursing Company
555 W. 57th St.
New York, NY 10019

American Nephrology
Nurses' Association
East Holly Ave., Box 56
Pitman, NJ 08071

American Nurses Association
600 Maryland Ave. SW
Suite 100 West
Washington, DC 20024

American Nurses
Credentialing Center
600 Maryland Ave. SW
Suite 100 West
Washington, DC 20090

American Nurses Foundation
600 Maryland Ave. SW
Suite 100 West
Washington, DC 20024

American Organization
of Nurse Executives
840 N. Lake Shore Dr.
Chicago, IL 60611

American Psychiatric
Nurses' Association
6900 Grove Rd.
Thorofare, NJ 08086

American Public Health
Association
1015 15th St., NW
Washington, DC 20005

American Red Cross,
National Hdq.
17th & D Sts. NW
Washington, DC 20006

American Society of Plastic
& Reconstructive Surgical
Nurses, Inc.
N. Woodbury Rd., Box 56
Pitman, NJ 08071

American Society of Post
Anesthesia Nurses
11512 Allecingie Pkwy.
Richmond, VA 23235

Association of Operating
Room Nurses
2170 S. Parker Rd., Suite 300
Denver, CO 80231

Association for
Professionals in Infectious
Control & Epidemiology
1016 16th St., NW
Washington, DC 20036

Association of
Rehabilitation Nurses
5700 Old Orchard Rd., 1st Fl.
Skokie, IL 60077

Commission on Graduates of
Foreign Nursing Schools
3600 Market St., Suite 400
Philadelphia, PA 19104

Drug and Alcohol Nursing
Association, Inc.
660 Lonely Cottage Dr.
Upper Black Eddy, PA 18972

Emergency Nurses Association
216 Higgins Rd.
Park Ridge, IL 60068

Frontier Nursing Service
Wendover, KY 41775

National Association of
Hispanic Nurses
1501 16th St., NW
Washington, DC 20036

National Association of
Neonatal Nurses
1304 Southpoint Blvd., Suite 280
Petaluma, CA 94954

National Association of
Orthopaedic Nurses, Inc.
East Holly Ave., Box 56
Pitman, NJ 08071

National Association of
Pediatric Nurse Associates
and Practitioners
1101 Kings Hwy. North, Suite 206
Cherry Hill, NJ 08034

National Association for
Practical Nurse Education
and Service, Inc.
1400 Spring St., Suite 310
Silver Spring, MD 20910

National Association
of School Nurses, Inc.
P.O. Box 1300
Scarborough, ME 04074

National Black Nurses
Association, Inc.
1012 10th St. NW
Washington, DC 20001

National Council of State
Boards of Nursing
676 N. St. Clair, Suite 550
Chicago, IL 60611

National Federation of
Licensed Practical Nurses, Inc.
3948 Browning Pl., Suite 205
P.O. Box 18088
Raleigh, NC 27619

National Federation of
Specialty Nursing Organizations
East Holly Ave., Box 56
Pitman, NJ 08071

National Flight Nurses
Association
6900 Grove Rd.
Thorofare, NJ 08086

National Gerontological
Nurses Association
7250 Parkway Dr., Suite 510
Hanover, MD 21076

National League for Nursing
350 Hudson St.
New York, NY 10014

National Nurses in Business
Organization
1000 Burnett Ave., Suite 450
Concord, CA 94520

National Organization for
Associate Degree Nursing
1730 N. Lynn St., Suite 502
Arlington, VA 22209

National Student Nurses'
Association
555 W. 57th St., Suite 1327
New York, NY 10019

North American Nursing
Diagnosis Association
1211 Locust St.
Philadelphia, PA 19107

Nurses Christian Fellowship
6400 Schroeder Rd.
P.O. Box 7895
Madison, WI 53707

Nurses House, Inc.
350 Hudson St.
New York, NY 10014

Nurses Organization of the
Veterans Affairs
1726 M St. NW, Suite 1101
Washington, DC 20036

Oncology Nursing Society
501 Holiday Dr., 1st Fl.
Skokie, IL 60077

Public Health Nursing/Ameri-
can Public Health Association
1015 Fifteenth St. NW
Washington, DC 20005

Sigma Theta Tau, International
Honor Society of Nursing, Inc.
550 West North St.
Indianapolis, IN 46202

Society of Gastroenterology
Nurses and Associates, Inc.
1070 Sibley Tower
Rochester, NY 14604

Transcultural Nursing Society
College of Nursing & Health,
Madonna University
36600 Schoolcraft Rd.
Livonia, MI 48150

Visiting Nurse Association
of America
3801 E. Florida Ave., Suite 900
Denver, CO 80210

Government

Air Force Nurse Corps, HQ USAF/SGN
Bolling Air Force Base
Washington, DC 20332

Alcohol, Drug Abuse, and Mental Health Administration
5600 Fishers Lane
Rockville, MD 20857

Army Nurse Corps, Office of the Surgeon General, D. of Army
5111 Leesburg Pike
Falls Church, VA 22041

Centers for Disease Control
1600 Clifton Rd., NE
Atlanta, GA 30333

Department of Health and Human Services, Regional Offices

	STATES	ADDRESS
Region I	Connecticut, Maine, Massachusetts, New Hampshire, Rhode Island, Vermont	John F. Kennedy Federal Bldg. Government Center Boston, Massachusetts 02203
Region II	New York, New Jersey, Puerto Rico, Virgin Islands	Jacob K. Javits Federal Bldg. 26 Federal Plaza New York, New York 10278
Region III	Delaware, Maryland, Pennsylvania, Virginia, West Virginia, and the District of Columbia	3535 Market Street P.O. Box 13716 Philadelphia, Pennsylvania 19101
Region IV	Alabama, Florida, Georgia, Kentucky, Mississippi, North Carolina, South Carolina, Tennessee	101 Marietta Tower Atlanta, Georgia 30323
Region V	Illinois, Indiana, Michigan, Minnesota, Ohio, Wisconsin	105 West Adams Street Chicago, Illinois 60603
Region VI	Arkansas, Louisiana, New Mexico, Oklahoma, Texas	1200 Main Tower Dallas, Texas 75202
Region VII	Iowa, Kansas, Missouri, Nebraska	601 East 12th Street Kansas City, Missouri 64106

➤

Department of Health and Human Services, Regional Offices *(continued)*

	STATES	ADDRESS
Region VIII	Colorado, Montana, North Dakota, South Dakota, Utah, Wyoming	1961 Stout Street Denver, Colorado 80294
Region IX	Arizona, California, Hawaii, Nevada, Guam, Trust Territory of Pacific Islands, American Samoa	Federal Office Bldg. 50 United Nations Plaza San Francisco, California 94102
Region X	Alaska, Idaho, Oregon, Washington	Blanchard Plaza Bldg. 2201 Sixth Avenue Seattle, Washington 98121

Federal Bureau of Prisons Director of Nursing Service
320 1st St., NW
Washington, DC 20534

Health Resources and Services Administration, Bureau of Health Professions, Division of Nursing
5600 Fishers Lane
Rockville, MD 20857

Indian Health Service, Division of Clinical Environment Services
5600 Fishers Lane
Rockville, MD 20857

National Institute of Nursing
9000 Rockville Pike
Bethesda, MD 20892

National Institutes of Health
9000 Rockville Pike
Bethesda, MD 20892

National Occupational Safety and Health Administration
200 Constitution Ave.
Washington, DC 20210

Navy Nurse Corps, Director Navy Nurse Corps, Office of the Chief of Naval Operation (OP-093N)
23rd & E Sts.
Washington, DC 20372

Peace Corps, Office of External Affairs
1990 K St., NW
Washington, DC 20526

Public Health Service
200 Independence Ave., SW
Washington, DC 20201

Photography Credits

Chapter 1	© FPG International
Chapter 2	Kathy Kieliszewski
Chapter 3	Kathy Kieliszewski
Chapter 4	David Bacon
Chapter 5	Alain McLaughlin
Chapter 6	Elena Dorfman
Chapter 7	Elena Dorfman
Chapter 8	David F. Singletary
Chapter 9	Esther Kutnick, California Nurses Association
Chaper 10	© Chuck O'Rear/Westlight
Chapter 11	© Chuck O'Rear/Westlight
Chapter 12	Alain McLaughlin
Chapter 13	Esther Kutnick, California Nurses Association

Index

Note: A *b* following a page number indicates boxed material, an *e* indicates an exercise, an *f* indicates illustrative material, and a *t* indicates a table.

AAN. *see* American Academy of Nursing
Abuse, substance. *see* Substance abuse
Acceptance, of change, stages in, 266
Accountability in management
 budgets, 325–326
 performance evaluations, 330–331
 quality assurance, 328–330
 risk management, 326–328
 see also Management process
Accreditation, 76, 152
 by JCAHCO, 83–84
 by nursing boards, 83–84
 NLN and, 39, 86, 105–106
 of practical nursing programs, 33–34
 process of, 82–84
 see also Credentialing; Education; Nursing boards
Acculturation, defined, 128
ACNM. *see* American College of Nurse Midwives
Adaptation, general adaptation syndrome, 341–342*f*
Adaptive organizational structures, 307, 308–309
Administrative law, 231*t*
ADN (associate degree nursing) programs, 40–42
Advanced nursing practice, 45, 76–77, 81, 149
Advanced registered nurse (ARN), 81
Advanced registered nurse practitioner (ARNP), 81
Affirmative action law, 312*t*
Age Discrimination in Employment Act, 376, 390
Agents of change, nurses as, 265, 271–275
AHA. *see* American Hospital Association
Alcohol abuse. *see* Substance abuse
Altruism, defined, 25
Alumni organizations, 91–92

AMA. *see* American Medical Association
American Academy of Nursing, 51, 97–98, 111
American Arbitration Association, 385
American Association of Colleges of Nursing, 105, 111
American Association of Occupational Health Nurses, 111, 416
American College of Nurse Midwives, 76, 81, 150
American Hospital Association, 251
 patient's bill of rights, 252*b*–253*b*
American Journal of Nursing, 51, 91, 97, 211, 436
American Medical Association, 18, 35, 160, 210, 279
American Nurse, 97
American Nurses Association
 activities of, 96–98, 107
 career planning and, 416, 436
 certification programs of, 23, 50, 77–79, 96, 150
 collective bargaining and, 97, 380
 credentialing and, 75–76, 81–82
 disciplinary action and, 75–76
 entry into practice and, 46, 48–49, 57
 ethics code of, 211–212
 functions of, 38, 72, 95–96
 history of, 34, 91–92, 93, 158–159
 model nurse practice acts of, 67, 69, 70*b*–71*b*
 organizational structure of, 93, 94*f*, 95
 political activities of, 96, 105, 173, 181, 279, 282
 purposes of, 95–96
 quality assurance standards and, 328
 recognition activities of, 97–98

standards for practice and, 38, 151
American Nurses Credentialing Center, 77–78, 81, 82, 95, 96
American Nurses Foundation, 38, 95, 97
ANA. *see* American Nurses Association
Analytical ethics, 195
ANCC. *see* American Nurses Credentialing Center
ANF. *see* American Nurses Foundation
Anger, 343–344, 351, 352*b*, 357
Anxiety, defined, 343
Apprenticeships, 11–12, 14, 52
Arbitration, 387–389
ARN (advanced registered nurse), 81
ARNP (advanced registered nurse practitioner), 81
Articulation, of nursing programs, 35
Assertive communication, 320, 356–358
Associate degree nursing (ADN) programs, 40–42
Associative power, defined, 278
Audiovisual materials, for career planning, 436
Audits, quality assurance and, 329
Authoritarian leadership style, 275–276, 280
Autonomy, in nursing 25, 204–206, 251, 409

Baccalaureate programs, 43–44
Bachelor's degree (BSN) programs, 41, 42–45, 57
Ballard, Lucinda, 33
Barton, Clara, 16
Belief systems, 194–195, 303
Beneficence, 202–204
Benefits. *see* Salaries and benefits
Benner, P., 134–135, 136
Bentham, Jeremy, 196
Bickerdyke, Mary Ann, 19

Bill of Rights, US Constitution, 227, 228b–229b
Bioethics, 189, 196
 see also Ethical principles; Ethics
Biologic clocks, 360, 361f, 362
Blackwell, Elizabeth, 19
Blame, as a stressor, 351–352, 354b
Block grants, 162
Boards of nursing. see Nursing boards
Breckinridge, Mary, 21
Brown, Esther L., 38, 46
BSN degree programs, 41, 42–45, 57
Buddy systems, for new staff, 313–314
Budgets 304–305, 325–326
Bureaucratic organizational structures, 307–308f
Burnout, 277, 358–359

California Statewide Nursing Program, 44
Canada, nursing education in, 36, 38, 91, 124
Canadian Nurses Association, 38, 91–92, 107
Capital Update, 282
Capstone programs, 44
Career ladders, 35
Career management strategies
 application forms, 424
 continuing education, 432
 control phase of, 433–436
 cover letters, 424, 425e
 curricula vitae, 419–423e
 follow-up letters, 429, 430e
 interviewing. see Job interviews
 marketing phase of, 419
 negotiating salaries/benefits, 429, 431
 networking, 429, 431–432
 performance evaluations, 433–434
 personal health and safety, 432–433
 production phase of, 432–433
 recordkeeping, 424, 426
 relationships/networking, 429, 431–432

resignations, 434–436, 437e
resumés, 419–420, 421e–422e
setting standards, 433
sources of information, 436, 438
terminations, 434–436, 437e
written communications, 419–424
 see also Career planning
Career perspective, versus job perspective, 397
Career planning
 assessing education/credentials/experience, 402e
 personal characteristics, 399e
 personal interests, 400e–401e
 personal values, 398e
 physical self, 397e
 proficiency levels, 401e
 summary assessment, 403e
 audiovisual materials for, 436
 career plans
 changing, 416
 evaluation of, 417–419
 framework for writing, 418e
 implementation of, 417
 statement of intent, 414e
 timelines for, 417, 418e
 compensation/working conditions and, 411–413
 computer programs to help in, 436
 goal setting for, 413–416
 health problems/nursing specialties and, 403–404
 human responses to health problems and, 404–405
 identifying
 health problems of interest, 404e
 preferred client characteristics, 408e
 preferred compensation/working conditions, 412e

preferred nursing diagnoses, 405e
 preferred nursing functions/services, 406e
 preferred nursing roles, 407e
 preferred nursing specialties, 404e
 preferred work settings, 410e–411e
 preferences assessment summary, 413e
 intent and, general statements of, 414e
 job versus career, 397
 nursing functions/services/prevention levels and, 405–406
 nursing profession options and, 403–413
 practice settings, characteristics of, 408–411
 process of, 416–418
 sources of information for, 436, 438
 statements of intent and, 414e
 values and goals in, 397–403
 working conditions/compensation and, 411–413
 work settings, characteristics of, 408–411
Caring
 Benner's qualities of power with, 134–135
 culture-care theory of, 131–132b
 definitions of, 131–134
 ethic of, developing, 200
 in nursing practice, 134–135
 views on/differences in, 131–134
 Watson's carative factors, 133
 see also Culture; Ethics; Nursing; Nursing practice
Case law, 227, 231t
Case nursing, as a delivery system, 315
Case studies
 of ethical dilemmas, 215–219
 of goal setting, 413–415
 of malpractice, 248–251
Categorical programs, 162
CE. see Continuing education
CEN (certified emergency nurse), 77

Centralized organizational
structures, 307–308f
Certificates, defined, 65
Certification, 96, 152
ANA requirements for,
77–79, 93
of clinical specialists, 79
of foreign-educated nurses,
74–75
generalist, 78
governmental, 79, 81
nongovernmental, 77–80
of nurse assistants, 33–35
of nurse midwives, 81
of nurse practitioners,
78b–79b, 81
in nursing administration,
79
of registered nurses, 81
of specialty nursing, 23,
79–80, 150
see also Accreditation; Education; Licensure; Nurses
Certified emergency nurse
(CEN), 77
Certified nurse midwife
(CNM), 81
Certified nursing assistant
(CNA), 33
Certified registered nurse
(CRN), 81
Change
acceptance of, stages in, 266
agents of, defined, 265,
271–275
authoritarian approach to,
275–276
coercive model of, 275–276
defined, 265–267
democratic approach to,
273–275
diffusion of innovation
model of, 268
driving forces for/against,
271–273
emotional phases of, 267
first-order level of, 269–270
force-field analysis of, 271f,
273f
Havelock-Lippitt model of,
273–275
innovative approach to,
269–270
Lewin model of, 270–273
models of, planned, 268–276
natural models of, 270–275
normative models of,
270–275

paradoxical model of,
269–270
planned, 267, 268–276
rational model of,
268–269
refreezing stage in,
270–273
resistance to, 266,
271–273
second-order level of,
269–270
target systems and, 265,
268, 270–275
types of, 267
unfreezing stage in,
270–273
see also Political action;
Power
Charismatic power, defined,
278, 279
Chronological resumés, 421e
CINAHL. see Cumulative
Index to Nursing and
Allied Health Literature
Civil law, 231t, 234–235,
237–251
assault and battery, 238
defamation of character,
244–245
durable power of
attorney, 239,
242b–243b
false imprisonment,
240–242
good Samaritan laws, 248
informed consent,
238–239
invasion of privacy,
243–244
libel, 244–245
living wills and, 239,
240b–241b
malpractice and, 245
medical records and,
243–244
negligence, 245–247
nursing practice and,
237–251
privacy and, 243–244
privileged
communication, 244
res ipsa loquitur, 245,
247
respondeat superior, 245,
246
right to die, 239–240
slander, 244–245
torts, 237–238

trial process of,
234b–235b
see also Law; Legal aspects
of nursing
Civil Rights Act, 23, 376,
390, 428
Civil trial process,
234b–235b
Client characteristics, assess-
ing preferred, 407, 408e
Client (patient) education,
314
Client satisfaction rating
scales, 329–330
Clinical competence. see
Competence
Clinical nurse specialists, 23,
76, 79
Clinical specialist
certification, 79
Closed systems, 295
CNA (Canadian Nurses
Association), 38,
91–92, 107
CNA (certified nursing assis-
tant), 33
CNM (certified nurse
midwife), 81
Code of Ethics as Applied to
Nursing, 211, 213b
Code for Nurses with Inter-
pretive Statements,
211–212b
Codes of ethics, 25, 210
American Nurses Associa-
tion's, 211–212b
Florence Nightingale
Pledge, 210b
Hippocratic Oath, 210
International Council of
Nurses's, 211, 213b
see also Ethical principles;
Ethics
Coercive model, of planned
change, 268, 275–276
Coercive power, defined,
278–279
Cognitive appraisal, of stress-
ful experiences, 343,
347
Cognitive rehearsal, as a
coping strategy, 349
Collective bargaining
agents for, 380
arbitration process,
387–389
authorization to represent
cards, 382, 383f

(continued)

Collective bargaining *(continued)*
  bargaining units, 380, 382–383
  grievances, 387–390
  history of, 376, 377*t*, 378
  lockouts, 385–386
  mediation process in, 384–385
  National Labor Relations Board and, 376, 380–381, 382–383
  negotiation process in, 384–386
  organizing a bargaining unit, 382–383
  reinstatement privilege, 386
  state nurses associations and, 376, 380
  strikes, 385–386
  terminology of, 378*b*–379*b*
  when negotiations break down, 384–386
  see also Contracts; Union organizations
Collective contracts, 371–372
Collective power, defined, 277, 278, 279
Collegial management organizational structures, 308
Collegial relationships, 429, 431–432
Common law, 227, 231*t*
Communication skills, 320, 356–358
  see also Management process
Community activities, 103, 149–150, 285, 314
Competence, 48
  of associate degree graduates, 42
  clinical, 25
  cultural. *see* Cultural competence
  of diploma graduates, 40
  diversion programs and, 75–76
  educational, 40, 42
  expectations of, 47–49
  of practical nurses, 48–49
  of registered nurses, 48–49
  technological, 302

  see also Licensure; Nursing practice
Computer programs, to assist nurses, 302, 436
Conceptual model, defined, 54–55
Concurrent audits, 329
Conflicts
  preexisting conditions for, 324
  resolution of, 324–325, 326*b*
Consent, informed, 238–239
Constitutional law, 230*t*
Constitution, US, 227, 228*b*–229*b*
Continuing education, 49–50, 77, 106, 314, 432
Contracts
  breach of, 372
  employment, 372–375
  essential features of, 369–370
  termination of, 372
  terminology in, 369–370*b*
  types of, 370–372
  violations of, 387, 389–390
  see also Collective bargaining; Union organizations
Controlling functions
  in career planning, 433–436
  in management, 296–297, 325–332
Coping
  emotion–focused, 346–347
  functions of, 346–349
  problem–focused, 346–348
  see also Coping strategies
Coping personality, 345
Coping strategies, 343, 345–346
  for anger, 351, 352*b*
  assertive communication, 356–358
  balancing demands/resources, 349–350
  changing situational factors, 350–351
  for frustration, 351, 353*b*
  for guilt/blame/shame, 351–352, 354*b*

  relaxation, 355, 356*b*–357*b*
  social support networks, 355–356
  see also Coping
Costs of health care. *see* Health care costs
Courts, federal and state, 232–233
Cover letters, 424, 425*e*
Creative thinking, 120
Credentialing
  accreditation, 82–84
  certification, 77–84
  examinations, 68–69
  licensure, 66–77
  nurse practice acts, 69–77
  registration, 65–66
  types of, 65–66
  uniform system of, 81–82
  see also Accreditation; Certification; Examinations; Licensure
Credentials, 65–66, 402*e*
Criminal law, 231*t*, 236–237
  trial process in, 232*b*–233*b*
  see also Law; Legal aspects of nursing
Critical thinkers. *see* Critical thinking
Critical thinking
  characteristics of, 121, 122*t*, 123
  creative thinking and, 120
  defined, 119–120
  FIRE acronym, to describe, 120
  habits of mind for effective thinking, 122*t*
  in nursing practice, 123–126
  personal dispositions and, 123*b*
  questions that stimulate, 125*b*–126*b*
  skills of, 123–124*t*
CRN (certified registered nurse), 81
Cross-training, of caregivers, 316
Crude death rate, defined, 179
Cultural competence, 127–130*b*
Culture
  attitudes about, 129–130
  caring and, 131–132*b*
  competence in, 127–130*b*
  defined, 127–128
  early, 3–11
  influence of, 128

prejudice and, 129–130
relativism and, 129–130
values and, 190
see also Caring; Ethical principles
Culture-care theory, 131–132*b*
Cumulative Index to Nursing and Allied Health Literature, 51–52, 436
Curricula vitae, 419–423*e*
CV. *see* Curricula vitae

Dark Ages, of nursing, 13–14
Death and dying
durable power of attorney, 239, 242*b*–243*b*
living wills, 239, 240*b*–241*b*
right to die, 239–240
see also Ethical principles; Ethics
Death rates, defined, 175, 179–180
Decentralized management, 298–299
Decision making
case studies of, 215–219
defined, 300–301
ethical dilemmas and, 214–215
Defamation of character, 244–245
Degree nursing programs, 35, 40–45
Delaying tactics, in coping, 349
Delivery of health care
nurses as change agents in, 268–276
nursing organizations and, 285
systems of nursing care, 315–316
uses of power in, 276–281
see also Health care systems; Nursing practice
Democratic leadership style, 273–275, 280
Democratic management, 298–299
Democratic Party, 282
Deontological ethics, 196, 214
Descriptive ethics, 195
Diagnosis-related groups, 167–168
Diffusion of innovation, 268
Dilemmas, ethical, 214–219
Diploma nursing programs, 35, 39–40, 66
Directing in management

communication skills for, 320–321
conflict resolution, 324–325, 326*b*
institution-focused activities of, 319
interpersonal skills required for, 320–325
morale building, 325, 327*b*
motivation and, 322–323*b*
shift reports, guidelines for, 319*b*
staff-focused activities, 319
teaching as aspect of, 321
technical activities of, 318–319
see also Management; Management process
Disciplinary action, 75–76
Discontent, employee, preventing, 390–391*b*
Discrimination, 312*t*, 376, 377*t*, 390, 432
Disease, beliefs about, 3–4, 6–7, 16
Diversion programs, for substance abuse, 75–76, 331
Dix, Dorothea, 19
Dock, Lavinia, 51
Doctor of nursing degree (ND), 45
DRGs. *see* Diagnosis-related groups
Drucker, Peter, 299
Drug abuse. *see* Substance abuse
Durable power of attorney, 239, 242*b*–243*b*
Durant, Henri J., 16
Durkheim, Emil, 194–195
Dying. *see* Death and dying

Education
accreditation of schools. *see* Accreditation
alternative programs, 44
apprenticeships, 11–12, 14
articulation, 35
assessing credentials/experience and, 402*e*
associate degree programs, 40–42
bachelor's programs, 41, 42–45

Capstone programs, 44
client (patient), 314
competencies in, 40, 42
continuing, 49–50
degree programs, 35, 40–45
diploma programs, 35, 39–40, 66
doctoral programs, 45
early training programs, 11–12, 14
external degree programs, 41, 44
health, 314
of home health aides, 33
honor societies, 109–110
hospital-based programs, 35
inservice, 314
internships, 52–53
master's programs, 45
minimum, entry level, 43–44, 46, 49, 57
of nursing assistants, 33
nursing theory and, 54–57
patient (client), 314
postgraduate, 49–50
practical nursing, 33–35
preceptorships, 52–53
research, process of, 53
Second Step programs, 44
standards for, 21–22
studies on, 37–39
trained versus practical nurses, 34
Two plus Two programs, 44
see also Accreditation; Credentialing; Examinations; Nursing schools
Emotional exhaustion, strategies to reduce, 358–359
Emotion-focused coping strategies, 346–347
Emotions
anger, 351, 352*b*
defined, 347
frustration, 351, 353*b*
guilt/blame/shame, 351–352, 354*b*
phases of, during change, 267
Employee health services, 166

Employers
  collective bargaining and,
    380–381
  ways to prevent discon-
    tent, 390–391*b*
  see also Union organiza-
    tions
Employment contracts. *see*
    Contracts
Empowerment, 134–135,
    277, 279, 350
Enculturation, defined,
    127–128
Endorsement license, 75
Entry into nursing practice.
    see Nursing practice
Environmental stressors, 343
Equal opportunity law, 312*t*,
    428
Erikson, Erik, 197
Ethical principles
  autonomy, 204–206, 251
  beneficence, 202–204
  honesty, 206–207
  justice, 208–209
  laws versus, 200
  nonmaleficence, 202–204
  respect for human dignity,
    201–202, 251
Ethics
  analytical, 195
  belief systems and,
    194–195
  bioethics, defined, 189,
    196
  care ethic, 200
  case studies, 215–219
  codes of, 210–213
  committees, 211–212
  decision-making and,
    214–215
  defined, 189, 196
  deontological theories of,
    196, 214
  descriptive, 195
  dilemmas in, 214–219
  Erikson's theory on, 197
  Freud's theory on, 197
  Gilligan's theory on, 200
  Kohlberg's theory on,
    198*b*–199*b*, 200
  metaethics, 195
  morals and, 196–197
  normative, 195–196
  in nursing research,
    53–54
  Piaget's theory on,
    197–200

prescriptive, 195–196
principles of. *see* Ethical
    principles
religions and, 194–195
technological advances
    and, 23
teleological theories of,
    195–196, 214
theories of, 195–200
values and, 189–194
virtue and, 196–197
see also Caring; Moral
    development
Ethnicity, defined, 127
Ethnocentrism, defined, 128
Evaluation
  in career planning,
    417–419
  in management, 296–297,
    325–332
Evaluative thinking, 120,
    122*t*, 125
Examinations, licensure and,
    67–69*t*
  see also Education; Licen-
    sure; NCLEX-PN;
    NCLEX-RN
Exhaustion, emotional,
    341–342*f*, 358–359
Expectations, managing
    unrealistic, 354–355
Expert knowledge, as infor-
    mational power, 278
Expert witness, nurses as,
    234–236
Expressed contracts, 371
External degree programs,
    41, 44
Extrinsic values, 190

FAAN (Fellow of the
    American Academy of
    Nursing), 98
Factual thinking, 120, 122*t*,
    125
False imprisonment,
    240–242
Federal courts, 232
Federal Mediation and
    Conciliation Service,
    376, 385, 388, 389
Feelings, defined, 347
Fellow of the American
    Academy of Nursing
    (FAAN), 98
Felony convictions, and
    licensure, 73
Feminism, 22–23

Fertility rate, defined, 179
Financing of health care. *see*
    Health care financing
FIRE (Factual, Insightful, Ratio-
    nal, Evaluative), 120
First-order change, 269–270
Fiscal year, defined, 304
Fisher, Alice, 17
Fletcher, Joseph, 196, 200
Flexner Report, 18, 158
Fliedner, Frederike, 14–15
Fliedner, Theodor, 14–15
Florence Nightingale Interna-
    tional Foundation, 107
Florence Nightingale Pledge,
    210*b*
FMCS. *see* Federal Mediation
    and Conciliation Service
Food stamps program, 169–170
Force-field analysis, of change,
    271*f*, 273*f*
Forces, for/against change,
    identifying, 270–275
Foreign nursing schools, gradu-
    ates of, 74–75
Formal contracts, 370
Free-form organizational struc-
    tures, 308
Frustration, how to manage,
    351, 353*b*
Fry, Elizabeth Guerney, 14
Functional nursing, as a deliv-
    ery system, 315
Functional resumés, 422*e*

GAS. *see* General adaptation
    syndrome
Gautama Buddha, 5–6
Gender roles, 265, 286–288
  see also Men; Women
General adaptation syndrome,
    to stress, 341–342*f*
General systems theory. *see* Sys-
    tems theory
Gilligan, Carol, 134, 200, 201
Ginzberg Report, 38
Goals, 303
  assessing personal/career,
    397–419
  setting of, 413–415
Goodrich, Anne W., 38, 119,
    127, 135
Good Samaritan laws, 248
Grandfather clause, licensing
    and, 47–48
Grapevines, as communication
    channels, 320
Gretter, Lystra, 210

Grievances, 387–390
Group decision-making management, 298–299
Guilt, as a stressor, managing, 351–352, 354b

Habits of mind for effective thinking, list of, 122t
Hamilton, Alice, 166
Hampton, Isabel, 51
Hardiness scale, 346
Hatch Act, 286
Havelock-Lippitt model, of planned change, 273–275
Hawthorne effect, 298
Health care costs, 145–146, 171–174
planning and, 152, 153–158, 161
see also Health care financing; Health care planning
Health care delivery. see Delivery of health care
Health care facilities, 144–146, 148
types of, 145b
see also Hospitals
Health care financing
block grants, 162
categorical programs, 162
diagnosis-related groups, 167–168
employee health services, 166
funding sources, 163b
health insurance, 164–166
HMOs, 165, 169
managed-fee-for-service, 164–165
philanthropic contributions, 165–166
private funds, 163b, 164–166
prospective payment systems, 167–168
publicly funded programs, 166–171
workers' compensation, 166
see also Health care costs; Medicaid; Medicare
Health care planning, 153–158, 161
federal agencies for, 156b–157b
Health care policy
data collection for, 175, 176t–178t
health status, major indicators of, 175, 179–180

research, defined, 174–175, 180
Health care reform
comprehensive plans, 171–174, 180
managed competition, 173
Nursing's Agenda for Health Care Reform, 173
universal coverage, 172–173
Health care systems
administration of, 152–158
centralized, 148, 150, 155, 158
composition of, 144
comprehensive, defined, 143, 171–174, 180
controls in, 151–152
cooperative, 152
cultural values and, 146
economic influences on, 143–158
entrepreneurial/permissive, 143, 146, 150–151
facilities of. see Health care facilities
federal administration of, 155–158
financing. see Health care financing
functions of, 149–151
influences on, 143–158
organization of, 152–158
personnel of, 148–149
planning. see Health care planning
political influences on, 143–158
primary care in, 145b, 149–150
regulations of, 151–152
resources of, 144–149
scope of practice in, 151
secondary care in, 145b, 150–151
services of, 149–151
socialist, 143, 152
specialty care in, 150–151
standards in, 151
tertiary care in, 145b, 150
United States. see US health care system
welfare-oriented, defined, 143
Health data, sources of, 175, 176t–178t

Health education, 314
Health insurance, 164–166, 172–173, 180
Health maintenance organizations, 165, 169
Health-related organizations
directory of selected, 445–450
federal agencies, 112, 154–158
nursing. see Nursing organizations
state agency program areas, 154b
Health status, 195, 339
indicators of, 146–147t, 175, 179–180
see also Illness
Henderson, V., 132–133
Herbert, Sir Sidney, 15
HHA (home health aide) certificates, 33
Hierarchical organizational structures, 307–308f
HMOs. see Health maintenance organizations
Home health agencies, 168
Home health aide (HHA) certificates, 33
Honesty, 206–207
Honorary organizations
American Academy of Nursing, 97–98, 111
Sigma Theta Tau, 93, 109–110, 111
Horizontal conflict, 324
Hospitals, 144–146, 148
American Hospital Association and, 251–253
collective bargaining and, 376, 382–386
Diagnosis-related groups and, 167–168
ethics committees of, 211–212
job descriptions at, in 1887, 20b
Human rights, in nursing research, 53–54

ICN. see International Council of Nurses
Illness, beliefs about, 3–4, 6–8, 16, 144
cultural influences on, 127–136
Image: Journal of Nursing Scholarship, 110

Implied contracts, 371
Imprint, 103
Impulses, defined, 347
Incident reports, 327–328, 329b
Independent nurse practitioner (INP), 81
Individual contracts, 371–372
Infant mortality, 146–147t, 179
Informational power, defined, 278
Informed consent, 238–239
Injunctions, court, 372
Injury control programs, 170
Innovation, change and, 269–270
INP (independent nurse practitioner), 81
Inservice education, 314
Insightful thinking, 120, 122t, 125
Institutional licensure, 65
Instrumental values, 190
Intensive care units, 23
Interdepartmental conflict, 324
Interests, personal, assessing, 400e–401e
Intergroup conflict, 324
International Classification of Nursing Practice project, 108–109
International Code of Nursing Ethics, 211, 213b
International Council of Nurses, 92–93, 152
  activities of, 108–109
  ethics code of, 211, 213b
  history of, 107
  organizational structure, 107–108
  publications of, 108
International Honor Society of Nursing, 93, 109–111
International Nursing Index, 97, 436
International Nursing Library, 110
International Nursing Review, 108
Internships, 52–53, 313
Interpersonal conflict, 324
Interpersonal power, 280
Interpersonal skills, in management, 320–325

Interviewing
  guidelines, staff nurse selection committees, 311, 312t
  job. see Job interviews
Intrapersonal conflict, 324
Intrinsic values, 190
Invasion of privacy, 243–244

JCAHCO. see Joint Commission on Accreditation of Healthcare Organizations
Job descriptions
  as function of staffing process, 309
  of hospital staff nurses, in 1887, 20b
  sample, 310b
Job interviews
  evaluating performance at, 428–429
  follow-up to, 429, 430e
  personal assessment exercises for, 397e–403e
  preparation for, 426–427
  suggestions for successful, 427–428
  see also Career management strategies; Discrimination; Staffing
Job performance. see Performance evaluations
Job perspective, versus career perspective, 397
Job satisfaction, 298, 390–391b
Joint Commission on Accreditation of Healthcare Organizations, 83–84, 302, 328
Judicial system. see Legal aspects of nursing
Justice, 208–209

Kant, Immanuel, 196, 200, 204–205
Kimber, Diana, 51
Kohlberg, Lawrence, 198b–199b, 200

Labor unions. see Union organizations
Ladders, career, 35
Law
  administrative, 231t
  affirmative action, 312t

case, 227, 231t
civil, 231t, 234–235, 237–251
common, 227, 231t
constitutional, 230t
criminal, 231t, 232–233, 236–237
defending yourself, 255–258
equal opportunity, 312t
federal courts and, 232
how a bill becomes a law, 282b–283b
legislation and, 282b–283b
narcotics, 237
nurse practice acts. see Nurse practice acts
overview, 227–236
proposed, obtaining copy of, 282–283
scope of practice. see Scope of practice
sources of, 230t–231t
state courts and, 233
statutory, 230t
summons, steps, if served with, 255–258
trials, process of, 232b–235b, 236
types of, 230t–231t
versus ethical principles, 200
see also Legal aspects of nursing
Lawsuits. see Legal aspects of nursing
Leaders, compared to managers, 300, 301t
Leadership
  compared to management, 300, 301t
  defined, 300, 301t
  styles of, 273–277, 280
Learning/teaching, principles of, 321b
Legal aspects of nursing
  basis of legal system, 227
  civil law, 237–251
  contracts. see Contracts
  criminal law, 236–237
  defending yourself, 255–258
  how a bill becomes a law, 282b–283b
  laws. see Law
  liability insurance, 149, 255, 256b–257b
  licensure. see Licensure
  malpractice claims, preventing, 254–255
  negligence, 245–247

overview of, 227–236
patient's bill of rights, 251,
    252b–253b
trial process, 234–236
US Constitution and, 227,
    228b–229b
see also Collective bargaining;
    Law; Nurse practice acts;
    Scope of practice
Legislation
    health-related, 105
    how a bill becomes a law,
        282b–283b
Legitimate power, defined, 278
Leininger, Madeleine, 127, 136
    culture care theory, tenets
        of, 131–132b
Leverage point, in planned
    change, 274–275
Lewin model, of planned
    change, 270–273
Liability insurance, 149, 255,
    256b–257b
Liability suits. see Malpractice
Libel, 244–245
Licensed practical nurse (LPN),
    34–35, 71
Licensed vocational nurse
    (LVN), 34–35, 71
Licenses, defined, 65
Licensure, 26, 152, 158, 159,
    236–237
    application process, 73
    by endorsement, 74
    continuing education and, 77
    disciplinary action and,
        75–76
    endorsement, interstate, 48
    examinations for, 67–69
    exemptions from, 73–74
    foreign graduates and, 74–75
    grandfather clauses and,
        47–48
    health care systems and, 152
    history of, 16, 66–68
    institutional, 65
    interim permits to practice,
        74
    interstate endorsement, 48
    mandatory, 67
    permissive, 66–67
    for practical nurses, 34
    reciprocity agreements for,
        74
    for registered nurses, 66–67
    registration acts and, 66–67
    relicensure, 49–50, 432
    requirements, 72–73

temporary permits, 74
see also Accreditation; Cer-
    tification; Credential-
    ing; Nurse practice acts
Life-change events, 339,
    340t, 341, 345
Limit-setting, as a coping
    strategy, 349
Literature, nursing, 51–52
Living wills, 239, 240b–241b
Lockouts, unions and,
    385–386
LPN (licensed practical
    nurse), 34–35, 71
LVN (licensed vocational
    nurse), 34–35, 71

Maas, Clara, 21
MacPherson, K., 133
Mahoney, Mary Eliza, 36
Male nurses, 7–8, 10, 36
Malpractice, 4, 26
    case studies, 248–251
    incident reports and,
        327–328, 329b
    liability insurance and,
        149, 255, 256b–257b
    negligence and, 245–247
    preventing, steps of,
        254–255
    see also Legal aspects of
        nursing
Maltese Cross, 12
Managed care plans,
    164–165, 180
Managed competition, 173
Management
    by objectives, 298–299
    compared to leadership,
        300, 301t
    concepts of, 295–302
    decentralized, 298–299
    decision making in,
        300–302
    definitions of, 296–297
    democratic, 298–299
    group decision making,
        298–299
    levels of, 297
    operations of. see Manage-
        ment process
    participative, 298–299
    problem solving in,
        300–302
    process. see Management
        process
    shared governance,
        298–299

systems theory of, 295–296
technological competence
    and, 302
theories X, Y, Z of, 298
Management by exception,
    305
Management process
    accountability function of,
        325–332
    activating function of,
        296–297, 318–325
    budgets and, 304–305,
        325–326
    bureaucratic structure
        and, 307–308
    communication skills,
        320–321
    conflict resolution,
        324–325, 326b
    controlling function of,
        296–297, 325–332
    coordinating function of,
        296–297, 309–318
    defined, 296–297
    delivery systems, for
        client care, 315–316
    directing function of,
        296–297, 318–325
    evaluation function of,
        296–297, 325–332
    flowchart of, 296f
    goals and objectives and,
        303
    institutional philoso-
        phy/purpose, 303
    interpersonal skills
        required in, 320–325
    interviewing job candi-
        dates and, 311–313
    motivation and, 322–323b
    organizational structures
        and, 307–309
    organizing function of,
        296–297, 307–309
    orientation programs,
        313–314
    performance evaluations,
        330–331
    philosophy statements
        and, 303
    planning function of,
        296–297, 302–307
    policies, procedures and,
        303–304
    quality assurance,
        328–330
    risk management,
        326–328, 329b

(continued)

Management process (con-
tinued)
socialization, of new staff,
313–314
staff development, 314
staffing function of,
296–297, 309–318
time management, effec-
tive, 306–307
total quality management
(TQM), 330
ways to save time, 307
work shifts and, 316–318
Managers, compared to leaders, 301t
Mance, Jeanne, 17
Marketing yourself, careers
and, 419
Martin Chuzzlewit, 14
Maslow's hierarchy, 298,
322, 323b
Matrix organizational structures, 309
Mayeroff, M., 133
MBO. see Management
MCN: American Journal of
Maternal-Child Nurs-
ing, 97
Media relations, 280–281
Medicaid, 155, 161, 166,
168–169, 174, 180
Medical records, privacy of,
243–244
Medicare, 155, 161, 166,
167–168, 174, 328, 329
Medicine, 6–10, 17–19, 54,
158
Men, 18–19, 200
leadership styles of, 277
as nurses, 7–8, 10, 36
power and, 286–288
see also Women
Mental health care, 17,
159–160, 251
diversion programs for,
75–76, 331
Mentorships, 314
Metaethics, defined, 195
Midwifery
American College of
Nurse Midwives, 76,
81, 150
Frontier Nursing Service,
21
history of, 4, 7, 8, 18–19
nurse practice acts and, 76
Military nursing, 9, 21, 22,
34

Mill, John Stuart, 196, 200,
204–205
Model Nurse Practice Act of
1990, ANA, 70b–71b
Models
conceptual, defined,
54–55
of nursing practice,
55t–57t, 70b–71b
of planned change,
264–276
of stress/stressors,
339–343
Moloney, M.M., 24
Montag, Mildred L., 40, 46
Moral development, 134
ethics and, 196–200
Kohlberg's stages of,
198b–199b, 200
men versus women, 200
Piaget's stages of, 197–200
see also Ethical principles;
Ethics
Morale-building activities,
325, 327b
Morbidity rates, 175,
179–180
Mortality rates, 146–147t,
175, 179–180
Motivation, 268, 322–323b
Moulder, Betty, 21

Narcotics abuse. see
Substance abuse
National Council Licensure
Examination for
Practical Nurses. see
NCLEX-PN
National Council Licensure
Examination for
Registered Nurses. see
NCLEX-RN
National Council of State
Boards of Nursing, 47,
49, 67–68, 69–70, 72,
441–444
National health insurance,
160, 163, 166,
172–173, 180
National Labor Relations
Board, 376, 380–381,
382–383
National League for Nursing,
124, 251
as accrediting agency, 34,
39, 82–83, 105–106
activities of, 38, 92,
105–106

"Blue Book" of, 106
CE activities of, 106
functions of, 104–105
history of, 34, 103–107,
158–159
licensure and, 67–68, 72, 75
placement center of, 436
purpose of, 104–105
National League of Nursing
Education, 21–22, 34, 37,
103
National Student Nurses Association
activities of, 92, 102–103
community activities of, 103
membership of, 98–99
organizational structure of,
98–99f
political activities of, 102
purposes of, 100–103
responsibilities of,
100b–101b
Natural models, of planned
change, 268, 270–275
NCLEX-PN, 35, 48, 49, 73, 84
NCLEX-RN, 40, 45, 48, 68, 73,
75, 84
study guide for, 86
subject content of, 68–69t
test plan percentages for, 69t
NCSBN. see National Council of
State Boards of Nursing
ND (doctor of nursing degree),
45
Negligence, professional,
245–247
Negotiation
in collective bargaining,
384–386
of salaries and benefits, 429,
431
Neonatal mortality rate,
defined, 179
Networking, 355–356, 429,
431–432
Nightingale, Florence, 15,
35–36, 107
Florence Nightingale Pledge,
210b
Nightingale School of Nurs-
ing, 12, 16, 36, 66, 158
Nightingale Fund, 15, 16
NLN. see National League for
Nursing
NLRB. see National Labor Rela-
tions Board
Nonmaleficence, 202–204
Normative ethics, 195–196

Normative models, of planned change, 268, 270–275
North American Nursing Diagnosis Association, 404
Notes on Hospitals, 16
Notes on Nursing: What It Is and What It Is Not, 16
NP. *see* Nurse Practitioner
NPA. *see* Nurse practice acts
NSNA. *see* National Student Nurses Association
NSNA News, 103
Nurse assistants, 33–35
Nurse managers. *see* Management process
Nurse midwives. *see* Midwifery
Nurse practice acts
  advanced practice and, 76–77, 81, 149
  ANA Model Nurse Practice Act of 1990, 70*b*–71*b*
  defined, 26, 65, 69
  exception clauses in, 73–74
  models for, 67, 69–71
  titling and, 71
  violations of, 236–237
  see also Legal aspects of nursing; Licensure; Scope of practice
Nurse practitioner, 23, 76, 78*b*–79*b*
  independent, 81
Nurse registration acts, 66–67
Nurses
  certified nursing assistants, 33
  as change agents, 265, 285–286
  clinical nurse specialists, 23, 76, 79
  collective bargaining and, 382–386
  district, 14, 17
  as expert witnesses, 234–236
  home health aides, 33
  job descriptions of, in 1887, 20*b*
  legal roles of, 234–236
  liability insurance and, 149, 255, 256*b*–257*b*
  licensed practical, 33–35, 71
  licensed vocational, 35
  as managers. *see* Management process
  media relations and, 280–281
  as natural leaders, 285

nurse practitioners, 23, 76, 78*b*–79*b*, 81
  political action and, 281–288
  power and, 276–281, 287–288
  practical, 33–35, 46, 48–49
  professional, defined, 46
  public health, 21, 34, 37
  registered. *see* Registered nurse
  roles of, 52, 234–236, 406, 407*e*
  self-employed, 149
  shortages of, 39, 40
  supply of, 148–149
  technical, defined, 46, 70*b*–71*b*
  trained, versus practical, 33
  as witnesses, 234
  see also Nursing; Nursing practice
Nurse theorists, defined, 55
Nursing, 436
Nursing
  altruistic nature of, 24–25
  ANA definition of, 54
  authority and, 26
  autonomy and, 25, 204–206, 251, 409
  burnout and, 277, 358–359
  codes of ethics, 25, 210–213
  commitment and, 25
  "dark ages" of, 13–14
  definitions of, 3, 70*b*–71*b*
  delivery systems of, 315–316
  education. *see* Education
  emotional exhaustion and, 358–359
  ethics. *see* Ethics
  Florence Nightingale Pledge, 210*b*
  focus of, 33
  functions of, 55*t*–57*t*, 405, 406*e*
  future challenges to, 23–24
  history of, 3–24
  job descriptions, in 1887, 20*b*
  knowledge-based, 24
  malpractice. *see* Malpractice

organizations. *see* Nursing organizations
  prestige of, 25–26
  process, models of compared, 55*t*–57*t*
  as a profession, 24–26, 70*b*–71*b*, 265
  purpose of, 54
  roles, 52, 234–236, 406, 407*e*
  services, 25, 405, 406*e*
  shift work, how to survive, 359–362
  specialties. *see* Nursing specialties
  technical, defined, 46, 70*b*–71*b*
  technological influences on, 22
  theories of, 24, 54–57
  uniforms, 12, 37
  see also Codes of ethics; Nurse practice acts; Nurses; Scope of practice
Nursing administration, certification in, 79
Nursing assistants, education for, 33–35
Nursing audits, quality assurance and, 329
Nursing boards, 72, 81–84
  see also National Council of State Boards of Nursing
Nursing DataSource, 106
Nursing diagnoses, 404
  categories of, assessing interests in, 405*e*
Nursing literature, 51–52
Nursing organizations
  alumni, 91–92
  ANA. *see* American Nurses Association
  directory of selected (Appendix B), 445–450
  general-interest, 92–93
  government agencies, 112, 154–158
  health-related, 112–113
  honorary, 93, 97–98, 109–111
  ICN. *see* International Council of Nurses
  International Honor Society of Nursing, 93, 109–111
  NLN. *see* National League for Nursing

(continued)

Nursing organizations *(continued)*
　NSNA. *see* National Student Nurses Association
　political activities of, 285
　special-interest, 80*b*, 110–112
　student, 92–93, 98–103
　see also specific organizations
Nursing Outlook, 51
Nursing practice
　advanced, 45, 76–77, 81, 149
　ANA and, 48–49, 95
　civil law and, 237–251
　competencies of, registered versus practical, 48–49
　controversies in, 47–49
　criminal law and, 236–237
　culture and, 127–130
　definition of, 70*b*–71*b*
　entry into professional, 43–44, 46–49, 57
　ethics of. *see* Ethics
　grandfather clauses in, 47–48
　minimum education for, 43–44, 46, 49, 57
　models of, compared, 55*t*–57*t*
　standards for, 151
　titling and, 47
　work-settings for. *see* Practice settings
　see also Credentialing; Licensure; Nurse practice acts
Nursing process, nurses as change agents and, 265
Nursing research, 53–54, 97
Nursing Research, 97
Nursing schools
　accreditation of. *see* Accreditation
　early, 12, 35–39, 158
　evaluation criteria for, NLN, 83
　first, in United States, 36
　foreign graduates of, 74–75
　licensure and, 66–67
　Nightingale, 12, 16, 36, 66, 158
　see also Education
Nursing specialties, 81 82

list of, assessing interests in, 404*e*
Nursing theory, 24, 54–57
Nutting, M. Adelaide, 37, 42, 51

Objectives, in the management process, 303
Occupational health, 8, 82, 111, 432–433
　nursing, 21, 166
Online Journal of Knowledge Synthesis for Nursing, 110
Open systems, 295–296
Operations, of management. *see* Management process
Oral contracts, 370, 371
Organizations
　health-related. *see* Health-related organizations
　nursing. *see* Nursing organizations
　structures of, types, 307–309
Organizing, in management process, 307–309
Orientation programs, for new staff, 313–314, 411

PACE. *see* Patient Care Expert System
PACs. *see* Political action committees
Paperwork, how to reduce, 306
Paradox, defined, 269
Paradoxical model, of planned change, 268, 269–270
Participative management, 298–299
Passive-aggressive communication, 320, 357
Passive communication, 320
Patient Care Expert System, 302
Patient classification systems, 317
Patient (client) education, 314
Patient-focused care, as a delivery system, 316
Patient's bill of rights, 251, 252*b*–253*b*
Patient Self-Determination Act, 239
Peer review, 167–168, 329

Peers, using power with, 280
Performance evaluations, 330–331, 433–434
Perinatal mortality rate, defined, 179
Personal assessment exercises, 397*e*–403*e*
Personal dispositions of critical thinkers, 123*b*
Personality
　assessment exercises, 399*e*, 400*e*–401*e*
　stress and, 344–345
Personal power, defined, 277, 279
Personal values, 190, 397–419
Personnel management. *see* Management process
Physicians, 4, 7–8, 16, 18–19, 148–149
Physiology, of stress, 341–342*f*
Piaget, Jean, 197–200
Planning
　for change, 267–276
　health. *see* Health care planning
　as a management function, 296, 297, 302–307
Policies and procedures, 303–304
Policy research. *see* Health care policy
Political action
　becoming informed, 281–283
　contacting elected officials, 284
　focus of, 285–286
　Hatch Act and, 286
　how to take, 281–286
　men versus women, 286–288
　power and, 277–278
　proposed laws, obtaining copy of, 282–283
　restrictions to, in the workplace, 286
　strategies for nurses, 286, 287*b*
　voting, 283
　see also Change; Power
Political action committees, 96, 102, 111, 285
Political power, 277–278
Politics. *see* Political action
Positional power, defined, 278
Postneonatal mortality rate, defined, 179
Poverty, 161

Power
characteristics of, 276–277
empowerment, 277
legitimate, 278
men versus women,
286–288
personal, 277, 279
political, 277–278
professional, 278, 280
qualities of, and caring,
134–135
resistance to change and,
268
sources of, 278–279
types of, 277–278
uses of, 279–281
women versus men,
286–288
see also Change; Political
action
Power of attorney, durable,
239, 242*b*–243*b*
PPOs. see Preferred provider
organizations
Practical nursing, 46, 70, 71
certified nursing assistants,
33
competencies of, 48–49
education for, 33–35
foreign-educated nurses as,
75
licensure and, 33–35, 67
scope of practice, 35
see also NCLEX–PN
Practice settings
assessing preferred,
410*e*–411*e*
autonomy, degree of,
204–206, 251, 409
kind of care provided in, 409
organizational profiles, 409
type of industry, 408
see also Health care facilities
Preceptorships, 52–53, 313
Preferred provider organizations, 165, 169
Prescriptive ethics, 195–196
Prestige, of nurses, 25–26
Prevention levels, of nursing,
406*e*
Primary care health services,
149–150
facilities, types of, 145*b*
see also Health care systems
Primary care nursing, as a
delivery system, 316
Primary prevention, 406
Privacy, invasion of, 243–244

Privileged communication,
244
Problem-focused coping
strategies, 346–348
Problem solving, 300,
301–302
versus problem-focused
coping, 348
Professionalism, 40, 190
collective bargaining and,
376
criteria of, 24–26
defined, 24, 46, 278
negligence and, 245–247
Professional nursing practice.
see Nursing practice
Professionhood, 91, 113
Professions
characteristics of, 24–26
collectivism in, 376
liability insurance and,
149, 255, 256*b*–257*b*
organizations of, 279,
280, 285
Proficiency level, assessing,
401*e*
Project management organizational structures, 309
Prospective payment
systems, 167–168
Psychiatric hospitals, change
in, 273*f*
Public health nurses, 21, 34,
37

QA. *see* Quality assurance
Quality assurance, 328–330
Questions that stimulate
effective thinking,
125*b*–126*b*

Race, defined, 127
Rational model, of planned
change, 268–269
Rational thinking, 120, 122*t*,
125
Recovery rooms, 23
Recruitment, 102–103, 309
Referent power, defined, 279
Reflections, 110
Refreezing stage, in planned
change, 270–273
Registered nurse, 71
ARNs, 81
certified, 81
collective bargaining and,
378
competence of, 48–49

defined, 46, 65–67
education of, 35–46
examination for, 68–69*t*
licensed, 65
specialized, 81
SRNs, 81
see also NCLEX–RN
Registration, of nurses,
65–67
Registries, defined, 66
Regulations. *see* Nurse practice acts
Relaxation, to reduce stress,
355, 356*b*–357*b*
Relicensure, 49–50, 432
see also Continuing education; Licensure
Religious values, 190
Republican Party, 282
Research, nursing, 53–54, 97
Resignation, from employ-
ment, 434–436, 437*e*
Res ipsa loquitur, 245,
246–247
Resistance, to change, 266,
268
Respondeat superior, 245,
246
Response model, of stress,
341–342*f*
Restraining forces, in
planned change,
271*f*–273*f*
Resumés, 419–423
assessing education/cre-
dentials/experience for,
402*e*
chronological, 421*e*
functional, 422*e*
Retrospective audits, 329
Reward power, defined, 278
Richards, Linda, 36
Right to die, 239–240
Risk management, 326–328,
329*b*
RN. *see* Registered nurse
RN Magazine, 436
Roles
gender, 265
of nurses, 52, 234–236,
406, 407*e*
of women, 3, 4–10,
13–14, 18–19, 21

Salaries and benefits,
304–305, 411–413
assessment exercise for,
412*e*

(continued)

Salaries and benefits *(continued)*
  guidelines, ANA, 376
  negotiating, 429, 431
  see also Career
    management strategies;
    Career planning; Contracts
Sanger, Margaret, 21
Scheduling, in the staffing
  process, 318
Schools of Nursing. *see* Nursing schools
Scope of practice
  ANA special task force on,
    48
  of certified nursing assistants, 33
  controversies in, 47–49
  defined, 48, 71
  of home health aides, 33
  legal issues of, 67, 151,
    152, 236–237
  mandatory licensure laws
    and, 67
  of practical nurses, 35
  violations of, legal,
    236–237
  see also Nurse practice acts;
    Nursing practice
Secondary care facilities,
  types of, 145*b*
Secondary prevention, 406
Second-order change,
  269–270
Second Step programs, 44
Selection committees, 311
Self-awareness, 279,
  344–345, 346
  assessment exercises for,
    397*e*–403*e*
Self-employed nurses, 149
Self-esteem, strategies to
  build, 354
Self-motivation, steps to
  develop, 322
Selye, Hans, 339, 341
Shame, as a stressor,
  351–352, 354*b*
Shared governance management, 298–299
Shared power, defined, 277
Shaw, Clara Weeks, 51
Shift reports, guidelines for,
  319*b*
Shift work, surviving,
  359–362
Sigma Theta Tau, 93, 109–111

Slander, 244–245
Sleep
  alertness and, 361*f*
  biologic clocks, resetting,
    360–362
  cycle, 360–362
  performance and, 359–360
  shift work and, 359–362
Socialization 40, 313–314,
  411
Social Readjustment Rating
  Scale, 339, 340*t*, 341
Social reform, 14, 15, 17, 21
Social Security program, 21,
  160, 167, 329
  see also Medicaid; Medicare
Social support, as a coping
  strategy, 355–356
Societal values, 190
Special-interest nursing
  organizations, 110–112
Specialized registered nurse
  (SRN), 81
Specialty certification, 23, 79
  list of organizations offering, 80*b*
Spirituality, to reduce stress,
  355
SRN (specialized registered
  nurse), 81
SRRS. *see* Social Readjustment Rating Scale
Staff development, 314
Staffing
  affirmative action Law,
    312*t*
  application process, 311
  case nursing, 315
  interviewing guidelines
    for, 311
  delivery systems for,
    315–316
  equal opportunity Law,
    312*t*
  formulas for, 316–318
  functional nursing, 315
  job analysis, 309
  job descriptions, 309, 310*b*
  patient classification systems and, 317
  patterns, 316–318
  recruitment, 309
  scheduling, 318
  screening applicants, 310
  selecting candidates, 311,
    313
  task-level analysis and,
    317

team nursing, 315–316
  time-and-motion studies, 317
  work shifts, 316–318
  see also Management process
Standards of Nursing Practice,
  328
State courts, 233
State health agencies, program
  areas of, 154*b*
State nurses associations, 376,
  380, 383*f*
State nursing boards. *see* Nursing boards
Statutory law, 230*t*
Stereotyping, defined, 128, 129
Stewart, Ada, 21, 166
Stewart, Isabel M., 37
Stimulus model, of stress,
  339–341
Stress
  causes of, 344
  definitions of, 339
  dynamics of, 345–346
  general adaptation syndrome and, 341–342*f*
  interpretation of, 345–346
  life events and, 339, 340*t*,
    341, 345
  management. *see* Stress
    management
  manifestations of, 343–344
  models of, 339–343
  physiologic response to,
    341–342*f*, 343–344
  psychologic response to,
    343–344
  response model of, 341–342
  self-awareness of, 344–345
  Social Readjustment Rating
    Scale for, 339, 340*t*, 341
  stimulus model of, 339–341
  transactional model of, 343
  see also Stress management;
    Stressors
The Stress of Life, 339
Stress management
  coping strategies for, 349–358
  effective coping, 349
  emotion-focused coping, 347
  problem-focused coping,
    347–348
  self-awareness and, 346
  see also Stress; Stressors
Stressors
  defined, 339, 343–344
  general adaptation
    syndrome to, 341–342*f*
  hardiness and, 346

work-sleep cycle changes as, 359–362
see also Stress; Stress management
Strikes (union), 385–386
Student nurse associations, 92–93, 98–103, 109–111
Substance abuse, 23, 237
diversion programs for, 75–76, 331
licensure and, 75–76
Support networks, as a coping strategy, 355–356
Systems theory, 295–296*f*

Target systems, of planned change, 265, 268, 270–275
Task force organizational structures, 309
Task-level analysis, for staffing needs, 317
Taylor, Susie, 19
Teaching/learning, principles of, 321*b*
Team nursing, as a care delivery system, 315–316
Team power, defined, 277
Technical nursing practice, defined, 46, 70*b*–71*b*
Technology, 22–23, 302
Teleological ethics, 195–196, 214
Terminal values, 190
Termination, of employment, 434–436, 437*e*
Tertiary care health services, 150, 406
facilities, types of, 145*b*
Tests. *see* Examinations
Theories of nursing, 54–57
Theory X, Y, Z, 298
Thinking. *see* Critical thinking
Thiroux, J.P., 201
Time-and-motion studies, 317
Time management, 306–307
Titling, requirements for, 47, 71
Torts, 237–238
Total quality management, 330
TQM. *see* Total quality management
Trained nurses, defined, 33
Transactional model, of stress, 343
Transcultural nursing, 127–136
Trials, legal. *see* Legal aspects of nursing
Tubman, Harriet, 19

Twenty Thousand Nurses Tell Their Story, 38
Two plus Two programs, 44
Type A, B, C personality, 344–345

Unfreezing stage, in planned change, 270–273
Uniform credentialing system, 81–82
Uniforms, nursing, 12, 37
Union organizations, 409
Authorization to Represent card 383*f*
bargaining agents for nurses, 380
history of, 376–378
joining, attitudes toward, 369, 390
National Labor Relations Board, 376, 380–381, 382–383
terminology of, 378*b*–379*b*
see also Collective bargaining; Contracts
Unions. *see* Union organizations
Unusual events, action plan for, 329*b*
US Constitution, 227, 228*b*–229*b*
US health administration and planning agencies, 156*b*–157*b*
US health care system administration of, 152–158
cultural influences on, 158–163
as entrepreneurial/permissive, 143, 146, 150–151
federal involvement in, 160–161
financing of, 163*b*–171
free-market economy and, 143, 146
Hill-Burton Act and, 161
history of, 158–163
HMOs, 165, 169
Medicaid. *see* Medicaid
Medicare. *see* Medicare
mental health care, 159, 160
national health insurance and, 160, 163
personnel, 148–149
planning and, 152, 153–158, 161

PPOs, 165
public health, history of, 159–160
special programs in, 169–171
see also Health care system
US House of Representatives, 282–284
US Senate, 282–284
Utilization review, 329

Values, 303
acquisition of, 190–191
clarification, 191–194, 192*b*, 397–419
conflicts in, 194
functions of, 189–190
valuing process, 193*b*
see also Ethics
Vertical conflict, 324
Virtue, 196–197
Voting, 283

Wages. *see* Salaries and benefits
Wagner Act, 376
Wald, Lillian, 21
Watson, J., 133, 136
Weir, George, 38
Winslow-Goldmark Report, 37, 46
Women, 23, 265
leadership styles of, 277
moral development in, 200
politics and, 286–288
power and, 277, 286–288
roles of, historical, 3, 4–10, 13–14, 18–19, 21
see also Men
Woolsey, Jan Stuart, 19
Workers' compensation insurance, 166
Working conditions, 410–413
assessing preferences in, 410*e*–411*e*, 412*e*
Work-life plan. *see* Career planning
Work settings. *see* Practice settings
Work-sleep cycle, stress and, 359–362
World Health Organization, 22, 150, 436
Written contracts, 370, 371

POINT LOMA NAZARENE COLLEGE
RYAN LIBRARY